**Also by Dick Cheney with Liz Cheney**

*In My Time*

# HEART

## AN AMERICAN MEDICAL ODYSSEY

## DICK CHENEY AND
## JONATHAN REINER, MD

### WITH LIZ CHENEY

SCRIBNER

New York   London   Toronto   Sydney   New Delhi

Scribner
A Division of Simon & Schuster, Inc.
1230 Avenue of the Americas
New York, NY 10020

First Scribner hardcover edition October 2013

SCRIBNER and design are registered trademarks of The Gale Group, Inc., used under license by
Simon & Schuster, Inc., the publisher of this work.

For information about special discounts for bulk purchases,
please contact Simon & Schuster Special Sales at
1-866-506-1949 or business@simonandschuster.com.

The Simon & Schuster Speakers Bureau can bring authors to your live event.
For more information or to book an event contact the Simon & Schuster Speakers Bureau
at 1-866-248-3049 or visit our website at www.simonspeakers.com.

Manufactured in the United States of America

1   3   5   7   9   10   8   6   4   2

Library of Congress Control Number: 2013030129

ISBN 978-1-4767-2539-0
ISBN 978-1-4767-2541-3 (ebook)

*To my family, my medical team,*
*and the donor of my heart*

—DICK CHENEY

*To Charisse, Molly, and Jamie,*
*who fill my heart with joy*

—JONATHAN REINER, MD

# Contents

# Prologue

## VICE PRESIDENT CHENEY

June 2010

*If this is dying,* I remember thinking, *it's not all that bad.* It had been thirty-two years since my first heart attack. I'd had four additional heart attacks since then and faced numerous other health challenges. Now, in the summer of 2010, seventeen months after I left the White House, I was in end-stage heart failure.

On a trip to Jackson Hole, Wyoming, in May, it had become clear my weakened heart could not tolerate the high altitude. I returned to Washington on an emergency flight, and as the plane took off, I realized I might never see my beloved Wyoming again. Since then, my wife, Lynne, and I had been at our house in McLean, Virginia. When I got up in the morning, all I wanted to do was sit down in my big easy chair, watch television, and sleep.

What was happening to me was hardly a surprise. I had lived with coronary artery disease for many years, and I had long assumed it would be the cause of my death. Sooner or later, time and medical technology would run out on me. Now my heart was no longer providing an adequate supply of blood to my other vital organs. My kidneys were starting to fail. I believed I was approaching the end of my days, but that didn't frighten me. I was pain free and at peace, and I had led a remarkable life.

I thought about final arrangements. I wanted to be cremated and have my ashes returned to Wyoming. It was a difficult subject to broach with my family. They weren't eager to discuss it. For them, talking about it made an already difficult situation even worse. But I needed them to know. And I needed to say good-bye.

As my condition deteriorated that summer, my cardiologist, Dr. Jonathan Reiner, had raised the possibility of having a left ventricular assist device (LVAD) implanted in my chest, and I agreed to be briefed on it at Inova Fairfax Hospital in Northern Virginia, which has one of the most active LVAD programs in the country. The LVAD transplant team showed me the device, which connects to the left ventricle, the main pumping chamber of the heart. The LVAD passes blood through a small pump operating at nine thousand revolutions per minute and returns it to the aorta, the largest artery in the human body, ensuring an adequate blood supply to the vital organs. The device is powered by a driveline that passes through the wall of the chest to an external set of batteries or an electrical outlet.

The idea of being kept alive by a battery-driven piece of equipment operating at high speed inside my chest was a bit daunting at first, but it soon became apparent that this option offered real hope and the possibility of extending my life long enough to be eligible for a new heart. Previously we had never really considered a heart transplant as an option for me because I clearly wouldn't live long enough to work my way up the transplant list to become eligible for a heart. The average wait was about twelve months. The medical team explained that although the LVAD was originally designed as a bridge to a transplant, some patients were deciding to live with the device.

I was impressed with the individuals on the LVAD/transplant team: they clearly knew their business. It was also apparent that they respected and welcomed Jon Reiner, who although he practices at George Washington University Hospital, would be included as an integral part of the team. That carried great weight with me given all that Jon and I had been through together over the past fifteen years.

The preceding weeks had been challenging. I not only had many of the symptoms of a failing heart, I was also, due to the anticoagulants I was taking, suffering severe nosebleeds, including one so massive it required emergency surgery and a number of blood transfusions. On more than one occasion that spring, we had found ourselves speeding down the George Washington Parkway in Northern Virginia toward my doctors and the emergency room at George Washington University Hospital in the District of Columbia. In addition, my heart failure was causing severe sleep apnea. As soon as I nodded off to sleep, I would find myself awake again, gasping for air.

On July 4, I'd experienced internal bleeding in my thigh and was rushed to George Washington University Hospital as fireworks lit up the night sky. At the hospital, they gave me narcotic painkillers, which, as we were on the way home and stuck in holiday traffic, caused me to be sick to my stomach. The list of things I could not do grew. I'd stopped climbing the stairs. I could no longer walk to the end of the driveway to pick up the morning newspapers. I barely had the strength to walk the length of the hallway between our bedroom and my office. My world shrank until I was barely able to leave my bed. By the time I was admitted to Inova Fairfax Hospital on July 6, 2010, it was clear that there really was no choice: without the LVAD surgery I would not survive.

My last memory of that evening is of Jon Reiner and the other doctors and my family gathered around my bed in the intensive care unit. The doctors explained that although they had originally scheduled the surgery for July 8, my situation was worsening and they recommended taking me immediately to the operating room. After I listened to the doctors, I asked Lynne and our daughters, Liz and Mary, what they thought. One by one, they each agreed that we should not delay. "Okay," I said, "let's do it."

## DR. REINER

July 6, 2010

The numbers in the morning were bad; now, after 8:00 p.m., they were even worse. Dr. Shashank Desai and I agreed to meet in the cardiac surgery intensive care unit (ICU) to check on our patient one last time before we left for the night. Shashank runs the advanced heart failure program at Inova Fairfax Hospital just outside Washington, DC, where we had admitted Dick Cheney, the former vice president of the United States, earlier in the day. When I entered the second-floor cardiac surgery ICU, I found Shashank standing just outside the vice president's corner suite. Through a glass partition, I could see Cheney staring at a television across the room. He had an oxygen cannula under his nose and a glowing red pulse oxymetry sensor taped to his thumb. Telemetry leads ran from under his hospital gown, coalesced into a loose bundle, and spilled over the raised bedrail on their way to the adjacent rack of electronics. A blood pressure cuff around his bicep automatically inflated and deflated every few minutes, displaying its relentless march of numbers, waveforms, and alarms on a wall-mounted touch-screen monitor. A nurse exited the room and handed us a flow sheet with the patient's latest labs. "These can't be right," I said softly, although I knew they probably were.

The prior months had not been good for Cheney. In December an arrhythmia would have killed him had his implanted defibrillator not delivered a resuscitating twenty-five joule shock. Six weeks later, an exsanguinating arterial nosebleed, intensified by anticoagulants, required emergency late-night surgery. At the end of February, Cheney had chest pain while staying on the Eastern Shore of Maryland and was taken by helicopter to George Washington University Hospital for treatment of a heart attack. In May, he had acute shortness of breath within hours of arriving in Wyoming that necessitated an immediate turnaround and admission to GW's intensive care unit. Now, for the last week and a half, Cheney had required a continuous home infusion of milrinone, intravenous "rocket fuel" administered via a small, portable pump.

Milrinone typically is reserved for use in end-stage congestive heart failure, when the heart's declining ability is no longer capable of sustaining vital organ function. Cheney's initial response to the drug was impressive: his breathing and energy improved almost immediately. The benefit was short-lived, however, and at the end of June, his condition took an abrupt turn for the worse. The vice president's weight rose by several pounds, indicating retention of fluid, and his energy sharply waned, largely limiting him to a reclining chair or bed. On July 4 he again bled spontaneously, this time into his leg. The next day, labs obtained by a visiting nurse at Cheney's home in Northern Virginia revealed a precipitous drop in his kidney function, triggering our decision to admit him to the hospital.

The kidneys, which are essential not just for fluid management but also for the regulation of blood pressure, electrolytes, and acid-base balance, account for only about 0.5 percent of a human's total weight but receive about 25 percent of the total cardiac output (the volume of blood ejected by the heart each minute). So in patients with congestive heart failure, the kidneys act like a canary in a coal mine. When cardiac performance drops, the kidneys are often the first to take the hit.

In the morning, we escalated the milrinone infusion in an effort to squeeze just a little more function from Cheney's depleted heart. Now, ominously, after several hours on the higher dose, his cardiac output had dropped, not risen. A normal cardiac output is about 5.5 liters per minute; Cheney's was barely 2.

"Where's Nelson?" I asked.

"He's in North Carolina trying to get back," Shashank replied.

Dr. Nelson Burton, a talented, senior surgeon at Fairfax, had extensive experience implanting ventricular assist devices (VADs) in patients with advanced heart failure. Although all VAD surgeons perform the more familiar cardiac surgical procedures like coronary artery bypass and valve replacement, relatively few cardiac surgeons have experience implanting VADs. Burton had been on the Outer Banks of North Carolina with his family celebrating his son's homecoming after a tour of duty with the Marines in Afghanistan. Surgery for the vice president to implant a VAD had originally been scheduled for the following week, and Nelson was planning to return in a day or two. That was going to be too late.

Mrs. Cheney and Liz were with the vice president. I couldn't hear what they were talking about, but I knew they weren't prepared to hear what I was about to say. Liz saw us outside the room and came out to talk.

"Where's Mary?" I asked.

Liz told me that her sister had a cold and was afraid to expose her father to it.

"Tell her to come," I said.

Liz understood immediately and, without asking for an explanation, turned to call Mary.

I had taken care of Dick Cheney for about fifteen years. I was young, just a few years out from training, when I assumed his care after his prior cardiologist, Allan Ross, a mentor to me, retired. In many ways, my career and life had become inextricably entwined with this patient. Although deep down I always knew one day we would arrive at this moment, the realization hit me very hard. Dick Cheney was dying.

## CHAPTER 1

# A Prime Candidate

## VICE PRESIDENT CHENEY

I loved my mom's dad, Granddad Dickey, very much. He and my grandmother lived a life that seemed full of adventure. At the start of World War II, they had left their home in Syracuse, Nebraska, when they got work on the Union Pacific Railroad. They lived in a railcar and cooked for the section gangs that repaired and maintained the tracks. For my brother, Bob, and me, visiting grandparents who lived and worked on a train was a dream come true. My granddad taught us two of the most important things a man can learn in life: how to cook and how to fish. He combined the two skills in a "recipe" he had for catching catfish. He'd take the guts he'd cleaned out of a chicken he'd fixed for dinner, put them in a glass jar, and let them "ripen" for a day or two. He swore the ripening made them especially appealing as bait for catfish. Judging from his success as a fisherman, he was on to something.

Granddad loved to laugh. He also loved good bourbon, a game of cards, and a smoke. He had nicotine stains on his fingers from the unfiltered Camels he smoked until his first heart attack in the late 1940s. His doctors tried to get him to quit smoking then, and he compromised with them: he cut down to four cigarettes a day, but he switched from Camels to the much longer, and also unfiltered, Pall Malls.

After my grandmother died in 1951, Granddad Dickey moved between the homes of his three kids every several months. One afternoon when he was staying with us, my parents were working in our yard, and I heard him call out to me from his bedroom: "Dickey, go get your mother." I ran to the yard. Mom came inside, and moments later she was on the phone that sat on a desk in our hallway calling the ambulance. My dad sent me outside to wave down the ambulance driver and make sure he found our house.

The paramedics rushed through our front door with their stretcher and medical equipment. Soon they were wheeling my grandfather down the hallway, toward the living room. I stood on the front porch, holding open the screen door as they carried him out to the ambulance. It was the last time I ever saw him. He had suffered a massive heart attack and died later in the afternoon. He was sixty-six. I was fourteen.


My mom and dad both smoked when I was growing up. My dad mostly stuck to pipes and mom smoked cigarettes. I smoked my first cigarette when I was twelve. Our Boy Scout troop met every week in the basement of the Baptist church near our home in Lincoln, Nebraska. There was an older, cooler kid named Jim Murphy who was the head scout in our troop. Jim also had a job at a local drugstore, which gave him access to the packs of cigarettes he brought to Scout meetings. On our way home from the meetings, a group of us would stop by the park near the church and smoke a cigarette or two.

By the time I got to high school, my buddies and I smoked cigars every once in a while. In the winter, we went ice fishing at Alcova Lake near Casper. While we waited for the fish to bite, we split a six-pack of beer and a five-pack of cigars.

I went on to college where I smoked some. I wasn't a heavy smoker then, mostly because I couldn't afford it. I was saving every penny I could to make phone calls to Lynne, who was at college in Colorado.

By 1964, Lynne was in graduate school, and I was just about to wrap up my bachelor's degree. (I had been on a somewhat slower path than she was, but that's another story.) That year the US surgeon general issued his first report on the dangers of smoking. I remember sitting in Lynne's apartment at the University of Colorado campus in Boulder and hearing a story on the radio about the report. It registered enough that I remember it all these years later, but not enough to make me quit smoking back then.

My habit really picked up once I got to Washington and was working for Don Rumsfeld, who was a counselor to President Nixon. In those days, just about everyone smoked in meetings, at meals, at home. It was pervasive. When Rumsfeld and I started working for President Ford, both Don and the president smoked pipes, and I had a supply of free cigarettes. Tobacco companies kept the White House stocked with presidential cigarettes that came in gold-trimmed white boxes stamped with the presidential seal. You could also get matches from Air Force One, Marine One (the presidential helicopter), and even Camp David. There was a certain cachet to pulling out a box of presidential cigarettes and using a match from a pack labeled "Air Force One" to light up.

Despite the growing evidence that smoking was bad for your health, we all did it. Even in a meeting in the Oval Office, it wasn't unusual for most of the participants to be smoking. In one photo, taken by President Ford's official photographer, David Kennerly, I am reaching across the president's desk—while the president is sitting there—to put out my cigarette in his ashtray. We didn't even think twice about it. Smoking seemed to keep you from gaining weight, and all the advertising made it appear cool and sophisticated.

By the time I was in my early thirties, I'd developed a heavy smoking habit, my diet was terrible, and I didn't get nearly enough sleep or exercise. I basically ate whatever anyone put in front of me. Many nights, dinner consisted of high-calorie, high-fat hors d'oeuvres at Washington receptions. Other nights, I'd arrive home late and whip up some eggs and bacon for dinner. Sunday mornings meant a trip to the local Krispy Kreme for a dozen doughnuts. I told myself the doughnuts were a treat for the kids, but Liz and Mary didn't eat nearly as many as I did.

I rarely got regular exercise. I was more of a weekend warrior, not always with good results. One weekend, I was playing a game of touch football and tore the cartilage in my right knee, leading to two months in a cast and ultimately surgery to remove all the cartilage. My sporadic activity increased my risk of injury without giving me much, if any, cardiac benefit.

At that stage of my life, I believed there was a direct relationship between how well I did my job and how many hours I was at the office. I hadn't yet learned to pace myself or recognize the difference between quantity of hours and quality of work. Nor did I feel that I was under stress. The fact that I was in a high-pressure job tackling challenging problems enhanced its attractiveness. I literally couldn't wait to get up and go to work each morning. At thirty-four, I was White House chief of staff. I began and ended most days in the Oval Office with the president of the United States, the most powerful and influential man in the world. And not just any president but Gerald Ford, a man for whom I had and have tremendous admiration, a man who healed the nation after Watergate and the first-ever resignation of a sitting president. The war in Vietnam was coming to an end. We were negotiating major arms control agreements with the Soviet Union. We had signed the Helsinki Accords, putting human rights on the table for the first time in negotiations between the United States and the Soviets, and by late 1975 we were gearing up for a historic presidential campaign. Most of the people I knew in Washington would have killed for this job. And I absolutely loved it. I knew we were living through historic times, and I wasn't just an observer; I was a participant.

Like most other people in their thirties, I didn't give a lot of thought to my mortality, and I operated as though I'd live forever. Bad habits and their long-term consequences frankly didn't concern me much.

Although we came very close, we didn't win the 1976 election. One of the hardest things I've ever had to do in politics was read President Ford's concession to Jimmy Carter the morning after the election. While the campaign hadn't seemed to take much of a toll on my health, by Election Day the president was suffering a bout of laryngitis. The next morning, just after 11:00, sun streaming through the windows of the Oval Office, his family gathered around him, he told me to have the White House operator get Governor Carter on the line. After some brief words of congratulations, President Ford turned things over to me, and I read the concession telegram that was on its way to Plains, Georgia:

*Dear Jimmy:*

*It is apparent now that you have won out in our long, intense struggle for the presidency, and I want to congratulate you on your victory. As one who has been honored to serve the people of this great land—both in Congress and in the presidency—I believe that we must now put the divisions of the campaign behind us and unite the country once again in a common pursuit of peace and prosperity.*

*Certainly there will continue to be disagreements over the best means of reaching our goals, but I assure you that you will have my complete and wholehearted support as you take the oath of office this January. I also pledge to you that I and all the members of my administration will do all we can to ensure that you begin your term as smoothly and effectively as possible.*

*May God bless you as you undertake your new responsibilities.*

*Sincerely,*

*Jerry Ford*

The call lasted three minutes.

Shortly after Election Day, job offers began coming my way. Lynne and I decided we would take a much-needed vacation and spend some time carefully considering what we'd do next. I decided this would also be a good time to see a doctor for a routine physical exam. I wasn't having any problems and thought of myself as very healthy. The doctor told me that given my smoking, cholesterol levels, bad diet, and family history on my mom's side, I was a prime candidate for a heart attack.

I didn't believe him.


Losing a presidential campaign is painful, as anyone who has ever been through it will tell you. I had huge admiration for Jerry Ford and still believe he should have won that race. But the loss convinced me that I didn't want to be in that position again with my future dependent on someone else. I loved politics, and I loved public policy even more. *If I am going to continue to do this,* I thought, *I want it to be my name on the ballot.* I knew if I were going to run, I had to get out of Washington and go home to Wyoming. When school ended that June, Lynne and I packed up the girls and our basset hound and headed out in a U-Haul for our hometown of Casper.

On June 11, 1977, at the annual convention of the Wyoming Stock Growers Association, Wyoming's senior senator, Cliff Hansen, announced he would be retiring the following year. "When my wife, Martha, and I go home at the end of the 1978 session," Hansen said, "we are coming back for good." A rancher and member of one of the first families to settle in Jackson Hole, Cliff had also served as Wyoming's governor and was loved throughout the state. His decision to retire meant that a lot of folks would be thinking about a run for the Senate. I was one of them. Later that summer, after we'd gotten settled in back in Casper, I drove down to Cheyenne to visit one of my mentors, former Wyoming governor Stan Hathaway. Hathaway had given me my first political job as an intern in the state legislature when I was a student at the University of Wyoming. He knew Wyoming politics and issues better than just about anyone else.

I sat across from Stan in his law office and told him I was considering running for Cliff Hansen's seat. "Well," Hathaway said, "you could do that, but Al Simpson is going to kick your butt." At that point, Al had served for twelve years in the Wyoming State House of Representatives. He was a natural: he loved people and they loved him. He remains one of my closest friends to this day. And I remain glad I took Hathaway's advice and didn't run against Al in that first campaign. In 1977 I didn't yet know Al well, but Stan's warning meant a lot. I headed home to Casper resigned to the possibility that I wouldn't be running for office after all in 1978. All that changed on September 17, 1977, at a football game in Laramie between the University of Wyoming and the University of Texas at El Paso. During half time, Congressman Teno Roncalio, a Democrat who held Wyoming's only House seat, went up to the press box in the stands and announced he would not be seeking another term. Three months later, on December 14, 1977, I announced I would be a candidate for Congress. I was thirty-six, and there was no doubt in my mind that I was perfectly capable of running for and serving as Wyoming's congressman. As far as I was concerned, I had no health problems whatsoever aside from a bum knee.

The idea of a statewide campaign in Wyoming was daunting, but I didn't think of it as jeopardizing my health. Any obstacles to success in my mind were purely political, and I was confident I could overcome them.

At the beginning of the campaign, I traveled the state alone, talking to as many Wyoming citizens as I could, looking folks in the eye, asking for their support, and building an organization. Wyoming covers nearly a hundred thousand square miles and has only one congressman, making it one of the largest congressional districts in the country geographically. In a primary, I could expect there would be less than one voter per square mile. Running for office for the first time meant long hours and many miles of travel.

In November 1977 I attended my first political event—a spaghetti dinner at the high school gym in Lusk, Wyoming, hosted by the state auditor Jim Griffith—and spoke for the first time as a candidate for Congress. Lots of candidates were in attendance, and each of us was given ninety seconds to make our case. I had worked hard to prepare my remarks. I had rehearsed in front of Lynne and had my notes in large print on a stack of note cards for the event. Unfortunately, when I got to the gym, I discovered there was no podium, so no place to put my cards. There was just a bare microphone. I had to do the best I could from memory, and I was very nervous. The master of ceremonies for the event had a huge gong—*The Gong Show* was a big hit on TV in those days—and the challenge for all candidates was to say what we had to say before our time ran out and we were gonged off stage. I slid in under the wire. The whole thing was a bit disconcerting, but it taught me a valuable lesson: never to assume I could predict the conditions under which I'd have to speak.

Eventually it would become the closest race I ever ran in Wyoming, but things didn't really heat up until June 1978. When the filing deadline came that month, three of us were in the race. Fortunately for me, a potential fourth candidate, Tom Stroock, decided at the last minute not to run. Tom was an oilman in Casper and would later become US ambassador to Guatemala. He would have been a strong opponent, and he and I would have split the vote in Casper. In the primary, I faced two men, both formidable opponents. Ed Witzenburger was a decorated World War II Air Force pilot and the incumbent state treasurer, who had been elected four years earlier. Jack Gage was the Republican son of a former Democratic governor with solid name recognition throughout the state.

All five statewide elected officials were also up for reelection in 1978, and from the start I had to assume that if I made it through the primary, I could well be in for a tough general election fight. Although Wyoming is traditionally a Republican state where Republicans outnumber Democrats by two to one, over the years the state's voters had elected Democrats every once in a while. Gale McGee served for eighteen years in the US Senate, Teno Roncalio represented Wyoming for ten years in the US House of Representatives, and Ed Herschler served three terms as governor. By mid-June, the race was taking shape, and I was in Cheyenne campaigning. The day before Father's Day, we went to two events: a square dance contest and the Cheyenne Kiwanis Club clambake, which was nonpolitical but an important event for those running for office.

We stayed that night with Joe and Mary Meyer. Joe and I had known each other since we'd started playing football together at Natrona County High School when we were fourteen years old, and he had been in our wedding. Joe, who would go on to serve as Wyoming's treasurer, attorney general, and secretary of state, was the deputy director of the state legislative services office in 1978. This was a nonpartisan appointed position, so he couldn't participate in the campaign. But he and Mary were happy to help out, providing us with a place to sleep whenever we were in Cheyenne. Around 2:00 a.m. on Father's Day, I awoke with a tingling sensation in the two small fingers of my left hand. I had no chest pain or any other symptoms, but I thought immediately of my cousin, Gene Dickey, who had recently had a serious heart attack. I knew instinctively that I should have this odd feeling in my arm checked out. I woke Lynne up and told her I needed to go to the hospital. Then I went downstairs and woke up Joe. As Joe drove Lynne and me to the hospital, I remember telling them that this was probably nothing to worry about. I just wanted to be cautious.

When we arrived at the emergency room, I walked in on my own, sat down on an examining table, and passed out. When I regained consciousness, there was a good deal of excitement in the emergency room, and I suddenly realized it was focused on me. I was having a heart attack.

## DR. REINER

Over an eighty-year life, a human heart beats, uninterrupted, 2.5 billion times, an astonishing example of physical durability seldom, and maybe never, replicated by even the most sophisticated human engineering. An automobile motor, for comparison, will make less than 500 million revolutions if you're lucky enough to keep it running for 100,000 miles.

The heart is powered by nutrient- and oxygen-rich blood delivered through slender arteries, fuel lines for the human engine, that arise from the aorta, adhere to the surface of the heart, and then dive deep into the muscle. These vessels are not simple passive pipes; they are complex, living conduits capable of dilating, or contracting, when provoked, and they are lined with a single layer of cells that, when healthy, discourage the formation of blood clots. When these arteries are diseased, however, blood flow to the heart is imperiled, a condition that can yield catastrophic consequences, a harsh lesson I learned early in my career.

In July 1986, on my third day of internship, only my third day on the job as a doctor, I am paged stat to the exercise lab. North Shore University Hospital on Long Island is a sprawling place, and I have to run through a maze of corridors and stop to ask directions before I find the suite where cardiac stress tests are performed. When I finally arrive, I see one of my patients—I'll call him Bob—lying on the floor, his legs propped on the stopped but still-inclined treadmill ramp. The patient, in his fifties, had been admitted a week before with a myocardial infarction (MI), that is, a heart attack. The cardiology fellow who had been supervising the test is kneeling next to the man, frantically trying to insert a large-bore IV into the patient's arm. The fellow said that everything was fine until the patient's knees suddenly buckled. Bob is still conscious but he doesn't look good, and his blood pressure is barely detectable.

Bob's recovery from the heart attack had been relatively uncomplicated, notable only for a bout of pericarditis, a painful inflammation of the fibrous sac that encases the heart. Pericarditis is not usually dangerous, but its appearance in this setting was a bit ominous because it suggested that Bob's MI was not, as we'd previously suspected, small, involving only a limited inner rim of tissue, but instead involved the death of the full thickness of one of the walls of the heart, resulting in a significant loss of muscle. The stress test had been ordered as part of the standard procedure to determine if it would be safe to discharge him later in the day. Bob's wife is already en route to the hospital intending to take him home.

Suddenly Bob stops breathing. We pull Bob off the treadmill, start cardiopulmonary resuscitation (CPR), and call for the "code team." Over the hospital-wide loudspeaker, the page operator intones "9-9-9 stress lab," the euphemism at North Shore for the more widely known "code blue." In less than a minute, a breathless parade of residents, nurses, cardiologists, fellows, and assorted other onlookers rushes through the doorway. A nurse opens the code cart, a rolling, fire-engine-red Sears Craftsman cabinet with a defibrillator on top and rows of drawers below, housing an array of drugs, drips, catheters, and emergency paraphernalia—an end-of-life toolbox. An anesthesiologist intubates the patient, placing a transparent plastic tube into the airway below Bob's vocal cords, enabling us to breathe for the patient with the aid of an Ambu bag, a hand-squeezed, plastic, barrel-shaped bellows connected to 100 percent oxygen. I do chest compressions for a while, a laying on of hands equal parts resuscitative and ritual, until my effectiveness wanes and I am relieved by fresher arms.

It's a choreographed chaos accompanied by a sound track of monitor beeps, pump alarms, and desperate voices all simultaneously struggling to be heard. Time is not our ally, and every minute that passes without restoration of a pulse makes it less and less likely that this is going to turn out well. Bob's exercise clothes have been cut away to facilitate the placement of central lines and defibrillator paddles. Now remnants of shredded clothing lie scattered on the floor. Unadorned we come into this world and, in a hospital, unadorned we go out.

After multiple rounds of drugs and shocks and after what seems like a very long time, but probably not much more than about half an hour, chest compressions stop. The room gets very quiet and someone palpates the patient's carotid. There is no pulse. The team is polled for suggestions. There are none. Very little is said as someone records the time of death, and people file out of the room leaving behind soiled gloves and gauze and IV bags still tethered to the now lifeless man and an electrocardiogram (EKG) monitor with a horizontal green line stretching into eternity.

Bob's wife arrives at the hospital unaware of this terrible terminal event. She is informed only that her husband has had a complication, and hospital staff take her to a room to wait. No one has told her that he is dead, a final responsibility left for me. The chief resident, David Cooper, who accompanies me on the short walk to the conference room, offers some quick advice on how to speak to the family and tells me to get permission for an autopsy. Postmortem examinations have been performed for millennia, and even today, when a patient dies unexpectedly, sometimes only an autopsy can determine the cause of death.

We introduce ourselves when we enter the room and sit down to talk. It is obvious that she is dreading what we are about to say, probably because of the way she was sequestered after she arrived at the hospital. Maybe she knows in the way that husbands and wives and mothers and fathers just seem to know when something bad has happened. I tell Bob's wife that he collapsed while walking on the treadmill and, despite the efforts of many people, we were unable to resuscitate him. I don't use euphemisms like *passed* or *gone* and instead say simply that I am so sorry to have to tell her that her husband has died. It's an awful moment. I search without success for words of comfort. She asks us if he suffered at the end, and I tell her that I'm sure he did not.

Nurses clean Bob and dress him in a hospital gown before bringing him to a room where his wife spends some time with him before he is taken to the morgue. Cooper and I wait outside the door. When Bob's wife finally comes out, I tell her that although we know he had a heart attack earlier in the week, we don't know why he died today. I explain that an autopsy will answer some of these questions, and after some thought she gives her consent.

Bob's autopsy removes all doubt as to why he died: a week out from his heart attack, his weakened myocardium ruptured, filling the pericardial space with blood, essentially strangling his heart. Although heart disease has been with humans for millennia and traces can be found in the remains of four-thousand-year-old Egyptian mummies, detailed knowledge of this affliction is relatively new.

• • •

## A Prime Candidate

In 1500, Leonardo da Vinci returned to Florence where he served as an engineer for Cesare Borgia, painted the *Mona Lisa*, and rekindled his prodigious interest in anatomy. In the winter of 1507, Leonardo visited a one-hundred-year-old man in Florence's Hospital of Santa Maria Nuova a few hours before the man's death. After performing an autopsy on the centenarian da Vinci wrote:

> And I made an anatomy in order to see the cause of a death so sweet, which I found to proceed from debility through lack of blood and deficiency of the artery which nourishes the heart and the other lower members. I found this artery very dessicated, shrunken and withered. . . . The tunics of the vessels behave in man as in oranges, in which the peel thickens and the pulp diminishes the older they become.

Da Vinci is undoubtedly describing atherosclerosis.

The term *atherosclerosis* is derived from the Greek words *athere* (gruel) and *skleros* (hard). Examine an artery afflicted with this disease, and you appreciate the aptness of its name. While a normal artery has an elastic quality, an atherosclerotic vessel is often stiff ("hardening of the arteries"), a consequence of cholesterol, calcium, and various cellular elements that have been deposited in the blood vessel wall. Over many years, the accumulating material can impede blood flow and become prone to blockage by blood clots. Until fairly recently, the disorder was thought to result mainly from the accumulation of lipids (fats). It is now known that the disease, which develops over decades, is caused by a complex interaction among lipids, inflammatory cells, and components of the immune and clotting systems.

Although noted for hundreds of years, atherosclerotic heart disease is largely a malady of the twentieth and twenty-first centuries, killing more people than any other disease in the United States every year since 1900 with the sole exception of 1918, when the Spanish influenza pandemic infected 28 percent of Americans and killed a staggering 675,000 people. Atherosclerotic disease developed in the United States during an era of increasing life expectancy brought about by a precipitous decline in death due to infectious causes and a concomitant improvement in nutrition and wealth.

In 1971, Abdel Omran, an epidemiologist, published an influential paper, "The Epidemiologic Transition: A Theory of the Epidemiology of Population Change," in which he described how a population's death rate changes as a country industrializes. This landmark work described three progressive stages in the evolution of population longevity. In the United States, the first stage, what Omran called the "Age of Pestilence and Famine," a period of high mortality and low life expectancy, when the top ten causes of death were all infectious diseases, persisted until about the year 1900. Prior to that time, the average life expectancy in the United States was only forty-eight years.

The second stage, the "Age of Receding Pandemics," a time when mortality began to decline, occurred in the first half of the twentieth century. During this period, there were steep reductions in deaths in this country from diseases such as dysentery, typhoid fever, and tuberculosis. Food-borne diseases declined following key improvements in food quality fostered by safeguards like the Pure Food and Drug Act of 1906. The discovery of penicillin by Alexander Fleming in 1928 led to the antibiotic era. Polio mortality dropped sharply after the introduction of the Salk vaccine in 1955. These steep declines in deaths from infectious diseases contributed to a significant increase in the nation's average life expectancy, which reached sixty-eight years by midcentury, ushering in the third stage (the modern era), in which chronic diseases and cancer predominate, and no other disease kills more Americans than heart disease.

The rise of coronary heart disease occurred in part because Americans were living long enough to develop this illness, which most commonly presents in the fifth through seventh decades of life and also because life itself was changing in this country. As we became more affluent and more urbanized, the nation shifted away from a traditional low-fat, agrarian diet and toward a diet high in saturated fats, found mostly in beef, pork, and lamb, as well as associated by-products such as lard, cheese, and cream.

On the eve of World War II, the US Army solicited the assistance of a University of Minnesota physiologist to help design a mobile diet for paratroopers. The components of the meal, initially acquired from a Minneapolis grocery store, were hard biscuits, dried sausage, chocolate, and hard candy; they were intended to provide soldiers with thirty-two hundred calories per day in a compact and easy-to-carry package. The final product, which also included Spam, Wrigley's spearmint gum, and a four-pack of Chesterfield cigarettes, was assembled in a rectangular cardboard container resembling a Cracker Jack box and was called a "K-ration" in honor of its developer, Ancel Keys.

Following the war, Keys returned to the University of Minnesota interested in deciphering the puzzling increase in US deaths from heart attacks. Despite harsh conditions during World War II, the incidence of heart attacks had dropped significantly in many parts of Europe, but they were on the rise in the United States, where people had been relatively well fed. Beginning in the late 1940s and continuing over the next fifteen years, in what was likely the first-ever prospective cardiac epidemiology study, Keys followed several hundred businessmen from Minneapolis and St. Paul and demonstrated that the higher their cholesterol levels were, the greater their risk was of developing coronary heart disease.

In the 1950s there remained much uncertainty concerning the interaction between diet and cardiovascular risk, which was reflected in the conclusion of a somewhat ambivalent 1957 American Heart Association report:

The evidence at hand suggest a general association with high rates of consumption of fat, but it is difficult to disentangle this from caloric balance, exercise, changes in body weight, and other meta-bolic and dietary factors that may be involved. Thus the present evidence does not convey any specific implications for drastic dietary change, specifically in the quantity or type of fat in the diet of the general population, on the premise that such changes will definitely lessen the incidence of coronary artery disease.

Ancel Keys continued to investigate the interaction between diet and cardiovascular disease and conceived an enormous, international epidemiological project, called the Seven Countries Study, which began in 1958 and has continued for more than fifty years. The study followed nearly thirteen thousand men from the United States, the Netherlands, Finland, Italy, Croatia, Serbia, Greece, and Japan and collected detailed diet and risk factor data such as cholesterol levels and blood pressure. Keys found that meat consumption was high (more than 7 ounces a day) in the United States, Italy, and parts of Yugoslavia and almost nonexistent in Japan. In contrast, fish consumption predominated in Japan but was very low in the United States. The higher the content of dietary saturated fat and the more prevalent meat was in the diet, the higher was the average serum cholesterol level, and the higher was the death rate from heart disease.

In 1961, the American Heart Association appeared a little more convinced about the role of fat in the genesis of heart disease:

> The reduction or control of fat consumption under medical supervision with reasonable substitution of polyunsaturated for saturated fats is recommended as a possible means of preventing atherosclerosis and decreasing the risk of heart attacks and strokes. . . . More complete information must be obtained before final conclusions can be reached.

Later that same year, Ancel Keys was profiled in a cover story in *Time* magazine, titled "The Fat of the Land," in which he promoted his version of a lower-fat diet:

# A Prime Candidate

Eat less fat meat, fewer eggs and dairy products. Spend more time on fish, chicken, liver, Canadian bacon, Italian food, Chinese food, supplemented by fresh fruits, vegetables and casseroles.

As the nation's diet changed, so did its addiction to cigarettes. According to the American Lung Association, at the turn of the last century, Americans smoked 2.5 billion cigarettes per year. Over the next several decades the US population tripled, but cigarette consumption increased by a factor of 250, peaking at 640 billion cigarettes sold in 1981.

Despite a greater than 50 percent decline in the prevalence of smoking over the past fifty years, 46 million people in the United States currently smoke, and the drop in tobacco use has not occurred with equal vigor in all socioeconomic groups. For instance, although the overall prevalence of tobacco use in adults is about 21 percent, it is about 28 percent for those with less than a high school education, those living below the federal poverty line, and those with no health insurance.

Several years ago a sixty-five-year-old obstinate smoker in my practice with severe coronary artery disease inquired whether my sister had been able to stop smoking. This patient, who resumed smoking after multiple operations, including both heart and leg bypass surgeries, knew that my older sister, Melanie, also struggled with smoking, a habit she hesitated to abandon for fear of gaining weight.

"Yes," I told her. "As a matter of fact she did quit."

My patient's eyes brightened, and a smile came across her face when she asked me how Melanie did it.

"She got lung cancer," I replied, mustering all the verbal tenderness of a punch in the nose.

Melanie didn't fit into any of the disadvantaged groups. She was well educated and had an MBA in marketing, she wasn't poor, and she did have health insurance, but she started smoking when she was a teenager and she couldn't stop. Currently, about one in five US high school students smoke, and each day about four thousand kids under the age of eighteen try cigarettes for the first time. About a third of those who become regular smokers ultimately will die as a consequence. When Dick Cheney attended Natrona County High School in Casper in the 1950s, more than half of American high school students smoked.

Once begun, smoking is an extraordinarily difficult habit to break. The American Cancer Society estimates that only 4 to 7 percent of people will succeed in quitting on any given attempt, a statistic that increases to only about 25 with the aid of medications like nicotine patches, bupropion (Wellbutrin), or varenicline (Chantix). For many patients, however, a heart attack is a potent behavioral modifier, and at five years following the event, about half the patients who smoked prior to their heart attack remain abstinent from tobacco.

We now know that cigarette smoking is unsafe at any dose. There are more than seven thousand chemical substances in tobacco or tobacco smoke, including hydrogen cyanide, cobalt, benzene, and arsenic. The complex chemistry of cigarette smoke likely contains many more carcinogens and hazardous constituents and results in increases in blood pressure, coronary plaque deposition, arterial wall injury, and the propensity for blood to clot, a perilous mix increasing the likelihood and decreasing the age at which coronary disease will develop. On average, active smokers experience their first heart attack five to ten years earlier than people who have never smoked.


On a hot July day in 2007, my smart and successful sister, a woman who loved fashion, family, and all things wonderful, died at age fifty-two. Her cancer was in no rush, first taking Melanie's left lung and a piece of her esophagus, then her ability to eat or talk, and then her ability to breathe without a ventilator. My sister had the longest ICU stay of any patient I have ever come across in my twenty-seven years as a physician. Melanie was brave and beautiful and doggedly refused to leave her husband, Marty, the love of her life, until the relentless disease finally consumed her with its singular, terrible malice. I remind patients who continue to smoke that there are consequences even worse than another heart attack. There are some that are even worse than death.

The identification of individual behavioral and physiological character-istics associated with an increased likelihood of developing atheroscle-rotic heart disease (risk factors) was achieved in large measure through the efforts of a long-term study run jointly by the National Heart Lung and Blood Institute and Boston University. The study, which began in 1948, enrolled 5,209 men and women from the town of Framingham, Massachusetts, and followed these subjects every two years with physi-cal examinations, blood work, and detailed interviews with the goal of identifying common factors associated with the development of heart disease. Over the past sixty-five years, the still ongoing Framingham Heart Study has identified hypertension, diabetes, tobacco use, high cholesterol, obesity, physical inactivity, and male gender as risk factors for heart disease.

Framingham investigators have developed a variety of tools, now accessible with online calculators, that use readily available clinical data such as age, weight, blood pressure, and cholesterol to predict an indi-vidual's risk of developing heart disease. At the time of Dick Cheney's heart attack in 1978, he was thirty-seven years of age, had a blood pressure of 125/70 mmHg (normal) and serum cholesterol of 271 mg/dl (high), was an active smoker, and was 5 feet 9 inches tall weighing 196 pounds. Using these variables, the Framingham model estimates that Mr. Cheney had an 8.2 percent ten-year risk of developing heart disease (similar to that of a fifty-year-old man) compared to a normal risk of 3.4 percent and "optimal" risk for a man his age of 2.6 per-cent. Subtract the history of cigarette smoking from the model, and Mr. Cheney's ten-year cardiac risk drops in half to 4.1 percent.

Although disease of the coronary arteries typically announces its presence in middle age, a heart attack is usually the culmination of a process that begins decades earlier, typically when we are still children. It's in childhood that we develop our eating habits and exercise patterns and, importantly, when we have our first cigarette. In the 1970s, doctors at Walter Reed Army Medical Center examined the hearts of soldiers killed in Vietnam and noted that although the young men were on average only twenty-two years old, evidence of atherosclerosis was identified in almost half.

The seeds of heart disease are planted early.

CHAPTER 2

# Echoes of Ike

## VICE PRESIDENT CHENEY

Although I'd suspected something was wrong when I woke up in the middle of the night with a strange sensation in my arm and hand, hearing the words was a blow: "You're having a heart attack, Mr. Cheney." Hours earlier, I was a thirty-seven-year-old in what I thought was great health, going all out, working around the clock, to try to win Wyoming's congressional seat. I felt young and invincible. Now I was lying in the ER at Cheyenne Memorial Hospital, having passed out shortly after I arrived. I came to as physicians and nurses scrambled around me. I had a million questions. How could this have happened to me? Was my life at risk? How would this change my life? How would it change my race for Congress? Would I have to drop out of the race?

Nobody had many answers in those first few hours. I was admitted to the hospital and began what would be an eleven-day stay. Although there were no cardiologists in Cheyenne in 1978, I was fortunate that my case was assigned to an internist named Dr. Rick Davis. I have never forgotten the advice he gave me in the first days after my first heart attack: "Hard work never killed anybody, Dick." He told me that spending time doing work you don't want to be doing is far more stressful and potentially harmful. I took his words to heart as I thought about how this heart attack might have to change my life.

The humor and thoughtfulness of my friends certainly helped lighten my mood during the long hospital stay. James Naughton, a well-known reporter for the *New York Times*, had covered the 1976 presidential race. He loved a good prank and was constantly playing practical jokes on his colleagues. Several of them came to me just after the election with an idea for a prank we could pull on Naughton. We convinced him to travel to the Catoctin Mountains in Maryland for what he thought would be an exclusive interview at Camp David with President Ford. We in fact set it up for a time when the president wasn't in residence at the camp. Then we all enjoyed a good laugh when we heard the Marines at the Camp David gates had turned away a crazy reporter who had tried to gain entry to the presidential retreat. A few days after my heart attack, Lynne came into the hospital room laughing and handed me the one-line telegram from Jim. It said, "I didn't do it. Naughton."

Another dear friend, Foster Chanock, a brilliant young man who had worked for me in the White House when I was chief of staff, spent a good deal of time calling all of our mutual friends telling them not to even think about sending flowers. Send campaign contributions, he told them.

It may surprise some, but I wasn't viewed as the most conservative candidate in the race. Most thought Ed Witzenburger, who had been the Air Force liaison to the Senate when Barry Goldwater was on the Senate Armed Services Committee, was more conservative than I was. Before my heart attack, I'd heard that Goldwater was planning a trip to Wyoming and thinking of endorsing Ed. The last thing I needed was a nationally known conservative endorsing one of my opponents. Before I had my heart attack, I'd placed a call to Dean Burch, one of Goldwater's closest aides. I knew Dean from my time in the White House when he'd been a counselor to both Presidents Nixon and Ford. I told him I knew Goldwater was coming to Wyoming and asked if the former senator might avoid endorsing anyone in this hotly contested primary. Dean didn't make any commitment to me, but he heard me out.

Three days after my heart attack, Barry Goldwater came to Wyoming. He stopped in Cheyenne, and he didn't endorse anyone. I am sure my call to Dean may have helped, but I imagine the fact that I was lying in a hospital bed having suffered a heart attack seventy-two hours before his arrival was also a pretty big factor in his decision not to endorse my opponent that day.

When I was released from the hospital on June 29, I knew that I wanted to continue the campaign. Dr. Davis told my hometown paper, the *Casper Star Tribune*, "The prognosis is excellent for Dick's full and complete recovery. After a period of rest and recuperation at home he can expect to be able to resume a full and active schedule." I spent most of my rest and recuperation in the shade of a large spruce tree in the backyard of our house in Casper. A good friend had just finished working with President Nixon on his memoirs and got me an advance copy, which I read while I thought about what to do next. Looking back thirty-five years later through the medical records from that period, I found something I hadn't remembered. Both Dr. Davis and my hometown cardiologist, Dr. Wes Hiser, had noted their concerns about my continuing the campaign. Dr. Davis wrote:

> He and his family have been terribly concerned about the congressional campaign, and whether he should quit or not. It was my own personal feeling that it would probably be wisest to drop this at the present time, but I certainly didn't press this on them at all. He understands that he has at least a two months convalescence without any active campaigning and it is currently his choice to keep the options open and continue with the campaign.

I can understand why the doctors felt that way. I am confident neither of them had ever before treated a cardiac patient who was simultaneously a candidate for Congress. What is significant, though, is that neither of them wanted to focus solely on their personal responses. They listened to me and thought about the negative impact it might have if they placed limits on my aspirations. Thirty-five years later, I still consider Dr. Davis's reminder that "hard work never killed anyone" some of the finest medical advice I have ever received. I believe it sustained me through my four subsequent heart attacks and the numerous other cardiac challenges I faced as I pursued my career in public service. For that, I will always be grateful.

# HEART

• • •

As I rested in Casper over the next few weeks, for the first of what would be many times in my life, I had to contemplate heart disease as a political issue. Even after I got the go-ahead from the doctors to continue the campaign, I considered what the voters would think. Would they be concerned that I might not be physically up to the job? Would my opponents try to use my heart attack against me? How would I explain to the voters exactly what had happened—and why, in spite of the heart attack, I wanted to go forward and pursue my political aspirations to represent them in the US Congress?

I convened a number of people I trusted to discuss the way forward. Bob Teeter was my pollster. We had met on the Ford campaign, and he would remain a close confidant until his untimely death in 2004. Bob Gardner, another Ford campaign veteran, was my advertising director. The best man at our wedding and my campaign chairman, Dave Nicholas, also joined us. And of course Lynne was my most trusted adviser. We got together and explored the idea of conducting a statewide poll to ascertain what impact the heart attack had on public attitudes toward me. We realized pretty quickly, though, that we didn't know what questions to ask. No one had ever tried to measure the impact of a candidate's heart attack in the middle of a campaign. We decided to try to put together an ad to address voters, thinking the direct approach would be best. There had been plenty of coverage of my heart attack in the Wyoming media, so the ad took the issue head-on. We gathered a group of friends and supporters, and we all sat on the lawn in our backyard. With the cameras rolling, we discussed famous political leaders who'd suffered heart attacks. We talked about Lyndon Johnson and Dwight Eisenhower and how they'd continued in the highest office in the land after their coronaries. When we showed the finished product to a small group of friends, it bombed. People said it was way too depressing and jarring. We scrapped it.

While we thought of other ideas and approaches, Lynne spent a good deal of time filling in for me on the campaign trail. She spoke at

30

Republican events all across Wyoming. She was so good that many of my supporters suggested, only half-jokingly, that we might be better off if she were the candidate.

We finally settled on the idea of writing a letter that we'd send to every registered Republican voter in Wyoming explaining the facts of my heart attack and why I had decided to continue my campaign for Congress. I addressed why I had decided to run in the first place, laying out the issues that had initially inspired my candidacy. Then I continued:

> A man's political beliefs are only a part of what motivates him, and in June an event in my life gave me reason to evaluate why I am running for Congress from a different perspective. While I was campaigning in Cheyenne, I suffered a mild heart attack.

I explained that I'd been given a green light by the doctors to go ahead with my run, that there was no health reason I couldn't run for and serve in Congress. Then I wrote:

> An event like a heart attack, however mild it might be, causes a man to reflect upon himself and what is important to him. I must admit that when I found out what had happened, it occurred to me that there are certainly easier ways for a man to spend his life than in running for Congress and being a public official, ways of life which are easier on his family, on his privacy, and on his pocketbook.
>
> But as I talked to my family, it became clear to me that while public life is sometimes difficult, it is also, for the Cheneys at any rate, immensely satisfying. All of us, Lynne, our two daughters, and myself, like being involved in an effort which goes beyond our own personal interest. Trying to achieve goals which benefit many people gives all of us a good feeling, an uplifting sense of purpose.

On July 11, 1978, I invited a few members of the Wyoming press to our home in Casper and announced that I would be continuing the race. I explained that I would continue to rest for the next few weeks and then would be back out on the campaign trail.

I traded in the Ford Mustang I had been using to drive myself to campaign events for a large motor home. My dad joined us as our driver, and my mom came along as our cook. Both of them, along with Lynne, made sure I got plenty of rest in the back of the RV between campaign events and I had healthy food to eat. A note from Dr. Hiser to Dr. Davis on July 26, 1978, indicates how closely they were watching my progress:

> Dick Cheney returned to this office on 25 July 78. He looks extremely well and feels as well. Because he is doing well I have permitted him to have two short appearances in his campaign this coming weekend. Overall I think he is doing nicely and I will keep you informed.

Dr. Hiser had some specific instructions for me:

> We will permit him to have two short appearances this weekend in Douglas and Torrington. He is to ride there in an air-conditioned travel van. He is to rest while going there, he is to maintain his exercise program, and he is to assure that he will get 8 hours sleep each night.

With my wife and parents along for the ride, I am confident we followed Dr. Hiser's orders to the letter.

The heart attack, as daunting as it was, probably helped my campaign. The letter gave me an opportunity to communicate with the voters of the state without asking for anything other than their understanding. And it allowed me to talk to them as a husband and a father, not as a politician. A congressional candidate suffering a heart attack midcampaign was big news, and the event probably increased my name recognition across the state. When primary day rolled around, I won the three-way race with 42 percent of the vote.

## DR. REINER

On September 23, 1955, President Dwight David Eisenhower developed what he thought was indigestion while playing golf at a country club outside Denver. The president had already completed eighteen holes and was in the middle of his second round when the discomfort convinced him to leave the course and return to the home of his mother-in-law in Denver, Colorado, where President and Mrs. Eisenhower were staying. The president, who was sixty-five, had no prior history of heart disease, but he had been an avid smoker, at one point consuming four packs of cigarettes per day. Eisenhower painted for a few hours, ate a light dinner, and went to bed around 9:30 p.m., but at about 2:45 a.m., he awoke with pain in his lower chest. When milk of magnesia failed to provide relief, the president's physician was summoned to the Doud residence. Major General Howard Snyder, an army surgeon, arrived at 3:11 a.m. and noted that the president's blood pressure was 160/120 and his pulse was 90 beats per minute, both elevated, typical for a patient in pain. Although there are conflicting accounts of what occurred next, a handwritten note, which Major General Snyder maintained he wrote at the president's bedside, states:

> As soon as I arrived, listened to the president's heart and took blood pressure, I realized it was a heart injury.

This would have been an impressive diagnostic achievement for a physician not trained in cardiology and not having ready access to an EKG. Nonetheless, Snyder asserted that the president was immediately treated with amyl nitrate, an inhaled vasodilator; papaverine, also a vasodilator, this one administered in an injection; morphine for pain; and heparin, an anticoagulant injected intramuscularly. Because the patient was sweaty, cold, and restless, Snyder asked Mrs. Eisenhower to get into bed with the president in the hope that this would calm and warm him (a curious strategy not currently recommended for a patient with a suspected heart attack). Snyder later administered a second dose of morphine, which eased the president's pain and lowered his blood pressure to a closer-to-normal 140/80. The morphine allowed the president to fall asleep around 5:00 a.m., but when he awoke at 11:00 a.m., his chest pain was still present. At 12:30 p.m. (ten hours after the president's chest pain began and about twenty-four hours after his initial discomfort), Dr. Snyder requested an EKG machine; forty-five minutes later he documented an anterolateral myocardial infarction (a heart attack involving the front wall of the heart). The president was then walked downstairs and transported by car to the hospital.

In his exhaustive book *Eisenhower's Heart Attack*, from which this chronology is obtained, Clarence Lasby casts doubt about whether Snyder's note was indeed a contemporaneous depiction of the events that night and instead suggests that Snyder wrote the memorandum much later to cover up for misdiagnosing the president's symptoms and for erroneously treating him many hours for a presumed gastroenteritis.

After arrival at Fitzsimons Army Hospital, President Eisenhower was placed in an oxygen tent, not permitted to see his cabinet for two and a half weeks, ordered to remain at bed rest for a month, and kept out of Washington for seven weeks. Two hundred thousand people lined the streets to view the motorcade when he returned to the nation's capital. After only a weekend in the White House, Eisenhower left Washington to continue his recovery at his farm in Gettysburg, Pennsylvania, and didn't return to work at the White House until after the New Year.

Regardless of whose version of events one accepts, Eisenhower's case illuminates the standard of care for a heart attack at midcentury. For the first eight decades of the twentieth century, the standard therapy for a heart attack mostly involved bed rest and pain control, usually with morphine, palliative treatments intended to keep the patient quiet and comfortable in the hope that no further catastrophe would befall the damaged heart. In the 1950s, oxygen was introduced as a standard therapy and papaverine and nitroglycerin, blood vessel dilators, were often given to prevent coronary spasm. Sometimes warfarin (an oral anticoagulant) or heparin (an injectable anticoagulant) was prescribed to prevent another heart attack or pulmonary embolism (a real hazard because of the prolonged bed rest); however, no strategy was employed to reopen the culprit vessel and limit the damage to the muscle. Patients spent on average four to six weeks in the hospital, and 30 percent died during the hospitalization, a toll reflecting the dismal progress achieved in the management of this disease through much of the twentieth century.

The term *infarction*, derived from the Latin *infarcire*, "to stuff," refers to the death of tissue resulting from interruption of nutrient-rich blood. In 1880, Karl Weigert, a German pathologist, first made the association between an occluded coronary artery and a myocardial infarction, but most physicians of the time, including the legendary Sir William Osler, considered a heart attack a nonsurvivable event. In his classic 1892 textbook, *The Principles and Practice of Medicine*, Osler incorrectly noted, "Complete obliteration of one coronary artery, if produced suddenly, is usually fatal." Twenty years later, at the 1912 meeting of the Association of American Physicians, Dr. James Herrick, a master clinician who two years earlier was the first to describe sickle cell anemia, proposed the revolutionary idea that a patient could survive an MI:

> Obstruction of a coronary artery or any of its large branches has
> long been regarded as a serious accident. . . . But there are reasons
> for believing that even large branches of the coronary arteries may
> be occluded—at times acutely occluded—without resulting death,
> at least without death in the immediate future.

Not only did Herrick understand that a myocardial infarction need not be fatal but he also suggested that it was caused by a thrombus (blood clot) and was among the first to suggest strategies that might ameliorate the damage:

The hope for the damaged myocardium lies in the direction of securing a supply of blood through friendly neighboring vessels so as to restore so far as possible its functional integrity.

Although the concept that a heart attack results from obstructed coronary blood flow was accepted as fact by the early 1900s, Herrick's notion that a newly forming blood clot was the cause of that obstruction was the subject of continuing debate for most of the century. As recently as 1974, only four years before Dick Cheney's first heart attack, Dr. William Roberts, head of cardiac pathology at the National Heart, Lung and Blood Institute at the National Institutes of Health, wrote an editorial in *Circulation*, the journal of the American Heart Association, in which he rhetorically asked, "Which comes first, coronary thrombosis or myocardial necrosis?" (Which comes first, a blocked coronary artery or the heart attack?) His answer, like that of many physicians before him, that coronary thrombosis was the consequence rather than the precipitating cause of acute myocardial infarction, would soon be proven incorrect.

Without a clear consensus in the cardiology community that the usual culprit during a heart attack was a thrombus, a dynamic and potentially reversible problem, treatment was mostly limited to prodigious amounts of rest. In his brief remarks to the five thousand well-wishers who greeted him at the airport upon his return to Washington after his heart attack, President Eisenhower acknowledged the caution of his doctors and the torpid pace of his recovery:

I am happy the doctors have given me at least a parole if not a pardon. I expect to be back at my accustomed duties, although they say I must ease my way into them and not bulldoze my way into them.

The treatment administered for Dick Cheney's myocardial infarction was remarkably similar to that received by Eisenhower twenty-three years earlier, both focusing mostly on rest. After an uneventful eleven days in the hospital, Cheney was advised by Dr. Davis to remain "homebound with in-house activity" for an extended period of time.

Dick Cheney's care did differ in one important aspect from that delivered to President Eisenhower: Mr. Cheney was monitored in a coronary care unit, an innovation introduced just a few years after Eisenhower's hospitalization and the first advance in the treatment of heart attacks that actually lowered mortality.

In the 1920s, as electrical power was being disseminated throughout homes and businesses in the United States, it was becoming common for utility linemen to die after accidental electrical shocks. It had been known since the mid–nineteenth century that electricity could cause a chaotic and fatal arrhythmia called ventricular fibrillation, but the prompt restoration of a normal heart rhythm remained an elusive problem. Ventricular fibrillation, also a dreaded complication of acute myocardial infarction, causes cardiac output to cease and blood pressure to drop to zero, halting the delivery of oxygen to the tissues, a condition called anoxia. While some organs can tolerate anoxia for an extended period of time, the brain cannot, and after just a few minutes, irreversible brain damage occurs.

In 1933, William Kouwenhoven, an electrical engineer, and colleagues at Johns Hopkins University reported experiments, funded by the Edison Electric Institute, in which for the first time they were able to reverse ventricular fibrillation and restore a normal rhythm by applying a "countershock" of electricity to the thorax of a fibrillating dog. The first successful defibrillation of a human patient occurred in 1947, but only after the chest of the fourteen-year-old boy was opened and electrical current was applied directly to the surface of the quivering heart. The boy made a full recovery.

In the years that followed, more patients were resuscitated from in-hospital cardiac arrest in this manner but only after enduring an emergency thoracotomy in which an incision was made along the left side of the chest, the ribs spread to expose the heart, and defibrillator paddles placed directly against the muscle. Although a step forward, this technique was hampered by two major drawbacks. First, it required an around-the-clock in-house team of skilled surgeons to "crack" the patient's chest, and second, and just as important, it was time-consuming, a major disadvantage when the time window for resuscitation is a very few minutes. There was thus a need for technology that could promptly detect life-threatening arrhythmias, enable defibrillation of the heart without having to open the chest, and, perhaps of paramount importance, keep the patient alive until defibrillation could be accomplished. Within several years, all three pieces would come together.

In 1956, one year after President Eisenhower's heart attack, Dr. Paul Zoll, a Harvard cardiologist, successfully resuscitated a sixty-seven-year-old man using a new external defibrillator, for the first time obviating the need to open a patient's chest.

One year later, Zoll developed a method to display a patient's cardiac electrical activity on an oscilloscope equipped with an alarm capable of detecting a cardiac arrest. This revolutionary technology permitted real-time surveillance of cardiac patients for life-threatening arrhythmias.

The final piece of the resuscitation puzzle came in 1960 when researchers at Johns Hopkins University described a method of "closed-chest massage" capable of pumping blood in and out of the heart without opening the chest. William Kouwenhoven (who twenty-seven years earlier pioneered defibrillation), James Jude, and Guy Knickerbocker, in a landmark paper published in 1960 in the *Journal of the American Medical Association,* reported their simple method to squeeze the heart between the sternum and spine by compressing forcefully with the heel of a hand. Kouwenhoven and colleagues wrote:

Cardiac resuscitation after cardiac arrest or ventricular fibrillation has been limited by the need for open thoracotomy and direct cardiac massage. As a result of exhaustive animal experimentation a method of external transthoracic cardiac massage has been developed. . . . Anyone, anywhere can now initiate cardiac resuscitative procedures. All that is needed are two hands.

The stage was set for a new way to monitor and resuscitate cardiac patients, and at the meeting of the British Thoracic Society at Harrogate in North Yorkshire, England, on July 15, 1961, Dr. Desmond Julian presented a paper in which he described the rationale for the first coronary care unit:

> Many cases of cardiac arrest associated with acute myocardial ischaemia could be treated successfully if all medical, nursing, and auxiliary staff were trained in closed-chest cardiac massage and if the cardiac rhythm of patients with acute myocardial infarction were monitored by an electrocardiogram linked to an alarm system.

Years later, Julian noted that it was essentially the success of closed chest cardiac resuscitation that triggered the creation of the coronary care unit (CCU). Julian opened the first CCU in Sydney, Australia, in November 1962 and was soon followed by colleagues in Kansas City, Toronto, New York, and Miami.

Concentrated monitoring in a coronary care unit enabled physicians to rapidly recognize and reverse a variety of complications after a heart attack. Crucially, nurses were given the responsibility for the detection of ventricular fibrillation and its treatment with defibrillation. The nursing staff could quickly attend to ventricular fibrillation, often before the arrival of a physician. Continuous EKG monitoring could detect heart blockage or other slow heart rhythms, allowing treatment with a pacemaker prior to a cardiac arrest. Patients with low blood pressure or other symptoms of shock could receive medication such as norepinephrine from a staff specially trained to administer and adjust these drugs.

The net result of this new model of acute cardiac care was a substantial drop in in-hospital deaths. During the 1950s, when President

Eisenhower experienced his myocardial infarction, 30 percent of patients died during their hospitalization. In the era of the coronary care unit, the in-hospital death rate declined to 15 percent.

Eleven days after Dick Cheney was admitted to the CCU in Cheyenne Regional Hospital with an acute inferior wall myocardial infarction, he went home. The sole medication prescribed to him on discharge was Anturane (sulfinpyrazone), a drug typically used to lower uric acid levels in patients with gout, but used in his case to prevent a recurrent heart attack because of its aspirin-like inhibitory effect on platelets, the blood cells that are essential to clot formation.

Today, a patient discharged following a heart attack will be treated with a host of medications, including antiplatelet drugs like aspirin and clopidogrel (Plavix), statin medications like atorvastatin (Lipitor) or rosuvastatin (Crestor) to reduce cholesterol, beta blockers to slow the heart rate, and ACE inhibitors to prevent congestive heart failure.

Following an exercise stress test three weeks after the heart attack, during which Cheney had no chest pain or concerning EKG changes, Dr. Hiser prescribed an exercise program consisting of thirty minutes per day of walking at a target heart rate of 120 beats per minute. Even with the reassuring stress test, Hiser remained cautious and somewhat ambivalent about Cheney's return to the campaign. In a July 10, 1978, letter to Dr. Davis, he wrote:

> His plans for the campaign are now familiar to you . . . he will resume the campaign, but not actively until late July or early August. Jumping fully into the campaign will be delayed until mid-August. Even at that time he has been admonished to not excessively fatigue himself and to maintain his exercise program and to get a full eight hours sleep every night. . . . The campaign is so important to him that I am reluctant to tell him that he should drop out of it.

At the end of July, Cheney was allowed to resume limited campaigning but only after Dr. Hiser issued strict conditions, underscoring the fragility of a post-MI patient. In September 1978, with the campaign for Congress in full swing, Dr. Hiser ordered blood tests that documented an elevated total cholesterol of 271 mg percent (the normal range 110 to 253) and a triglyceride (a type of lipid) of 334 mg percent (normal range 29 to 201). In view of these abnormal results he reminded Cheney of the importance of adhering to the restricted diet and advocated weight reduction and continued exercise. Dick Cheney didn't need to be reminded about tobacco; he smoked his last cigarette the day he had his first myocardial infarction.

CHAPTER 3

# Into the Heart

## VICE PRESIDENT CHENEY

On election night, November 7, 1978, we watched the returns with friends and campaign aides at our home in Casper. We set up extra TVs in the dining room and study so we could watch all three networks and the local Casper station, KTWO. I had won the three-way primary that August with 42 percent of the vote, the smallest total I would ever receive during my congressional career. I suspected that the primary fight would be tougher, and the outcome closer, than the general election, but no successful politician takes anything for granted. Watching the returns come in and seeing that I'd been elected to the US House of Representatives with 59 percent of the vote that November night was a life-changing experience. I felt privileged to be selected by the people of Wyoming to represent them in Congress. Thirty-five years later, after holding other positions of high office, no title ever made me prouder than being known as the Gentleman from Wyoming.

The morning after the election, I called Congressman John Rhodes of Arizona, the Republican leader in the House of Representatives. Rhodes had succeeded Jerry Ford as the minority leader in the House in December 1973 when Nixon selected Ford to be his vice president, and I got to know Rhodes when I served as White House chief of staff. As the minority leader in the House, Rhodes would have a major voice in committee assignments for the newly elected Republican members of the Ninety-Sixth Congress. I asked him to consider me for a seat on the Committee on Interior and Insular Affairs. As a public lands state where the federal government owns 50 percent of the surface and 65 percent of the mineral rights, Wyoming is affected greatly by decisions that come within the jurisdiction of the Interior Committee.

Rhodes said he thought there wouldn't be any problem with fulfilling my request. Then he added that he wanted me to take a seat on the Committee on Standards of Official Conduct, better known as the Ethics Committee. The committee's jurisdiction includes conducting investigations of alleged wrongdoing by members accused of violating House rules. If members are found guilty, the committee is charged with recommending appropriate sanctions to the full House up to and including expulsion.

The power invested in the Ethics Committee to sit in judgment and sanction members has led to a set of rules that are unique. The committee always has an equal number of members of both parties (six Republicans and six Democrats in 1978). Although the chair was of the party that controlled the majority in the House, no significant action could be recommended to the House without at least seven votes. The leaders are careful to appoint only members they believe will understand the significance of the responsibility and will conduct themselves in a manner that puts the interest of the House of Representatives ahead of personal or partisan interests. Freshmen are rarely selected to serve on the committee. Rhodes's decision to appoint me indicated he had confidence in my experience and judgment to handle the assignment. I readily accepted.

A week after the election, Lynne and I took the girls to Hawaii. We spent some time on the big island of Hawaii at the home of our friend Jack Ellbogen. We also spent a few days in Honolulu with Congressman Bill Steiger and his wife, Janet. Bill, who'd been my first boss in Washington, was a rising star in the Republican Party. We enjoyed a wonderful few days of rest and relaxation before we all went to Washington to take up our places in the Ninety-Sixth Congress.

A few weeks later, I was in Washington for the orientation sessions for new members. Many of our meetings were held at the Dulles Marriott Hotel, but we also gathered for introductory meetings at the Capitol. On December 4, 1978, I stepped out of the organization meeting of the Republican conference for a photo shoot with *U.S. News & World Report*. As I emerged onto the steps of the Cannon House Office Building, I noticed the flag over the Capitol was being lowered to half-staff. I asked one of the Capitol police officers standing nearby why they were lowering the flag, and he explained it was because a member of Congress had just died. "Who?" I asked. "Bill Steiger of Wisconsin," came the answer. I was stunned to learn that Bill had died of a heart attack in his sleep. He had just turned forty, only two years older than I was. When I'd had a heart attack in the middle of my first campaign six months earlier, Bill had urged his donors to write a check to me in Wyoming.

Bill's funeral was held in Oshkosh, Wisconsin, a few days later. Though I hadn't yet been sworn in, I was granted permission to fly with the official delegation of Bill's colleagues from the House. The service was especially poignant because Bill had been so young and because we all knew he'd had such a bright future ahead of him. His death was a tragedy for his family, for those of us who knew him, and for the nation.

Even the death of such a close friend and mentor from a heart attack did not cause me to think much about my own mortality. I considered my heart attack as a one-off event, and I basically thought of myself as healed.

I was leading an active life physically, playing tennis and planning a ski trip for the upcoming holidays. I'd quit smoking, was watching my diet, and trying to exercise regularly. I was doing what a prudent man would, but I also was in denial to some extent. I told myself I had dealt with my heart problem by quitting smoking. I certainly didn't think of myself as sick or even as someone suffering from coronary artery disease.

I maintained a busy and demanding schedule in Washington and back home in Wyoming. I was especially focused in my first term on solidifying my electoral base in the state. I wanted to lay the political groundwork at home so I would have the freedom to get involved in difficult and often controversial issues at the national level.

During the week in Washington, I was busy with committee hearings and meetings, as well as regular sessions of the House. On weekends, I flew home to spend time with my constituents. Because Wyoming has only one congressional district, I was responsible for covering the entire state. As one of my friends remarked when he first traveled across my district, "In Wyoming, it's a long way between voters."

Traveling home was made difficult by the fact that there were no direct flights between Washington, DC, and Wyoming. I usually left late in the day and arrived in Denver after the last connecting flight to Wyoming had departed. I'd spend the night at an airport hotel, and the next morning I'd fly or drive to whatever part of the state I was scheduled to visit. Sometimes we would charter a plane to get to as many communities as possible because much of Wyoming had no commercial air service. During congressional recesses, I visited communities throughout the state, attending and speaking at events or holding office hours. I would announce that I was planning on being in a town on a certain date and time and invite anyone who wanted to see their congressman about an issue or a particular problem to stop by. During my first term, I spent roughly 170 days in or traveling to Wyoming. The schedule was tough and demanding seven days a week, but I loved being Wyoming's congressman.

In that first term, my committee assignments generated a fair amount of activity. The Interior Committee had some jurisdiction over nuclear power. When there was an accident at the Three Mile Island nuclear facility in Pennsylvania, we were involved in visiting the plant, holding hearings, and trying to understand what had happened. The accident eventually had a huge impact on the future of nuclear power in the country. For many years afterward, lingering questions in the public mind about safety discouraged the construction of any new nuclear power plants, which also had consequences for Wyoming, the largest uranium-producing state in the nation.

The Ethics Committee had one of the most active agendas in its history in the Ninety-Sixth Congress. I gave my first speech on the floor of the House as a member of the committee. Congressman Charles Diggs of Michigan had been convicted of accepting kickbacks from members of his congressional staff; however, after his conviction, the voters of the Thirteenth District had reelected him. The case forced the Ethics Committee to make a decision about Article I of the Constitution. Article I grants the House the power to expel a member for misconduct if approved by two-thirds of his colleagues. It also specifies that members will be elected by popular vote. Which was to take precedence: the power of Congress to expel a member for misconduct or the right of the voters to pick their representative?

I agreed with the committee that we had to accept the judgment of the voters of the Thirteenth District and supported the committee's recommendation for censure. A number of members disagreed, however, and argued for expulsion. The motion to censure nevertheless prevailed, and we accepted the voters' decision about whom they wanted to represent them. The following year when Diggs's conviction was upheld on appeal, he resigned.

The biggest scandal the committee had to handle while I was a member was ABSCAM. A number of House members, as well as one senator, were caught up in an FBI sting operation. Undercover agents posing as representatives of a wealthy Middle Eastern sheikh offered cash payments to members as bribes. All of the transactions were captured on videotape, so there wasn't a shred of doubt about the guilt of those who had been caught. All of them were either defeated or resigned except Congressman Ozzie Myers of Philadelphia, who refused to resign and was not subject to an intervening election. Myers insisted on taking the matter to a vote of the whole House and became the first congressman since the Civil War to be expelled.

At the end of my first term in December 1980, I was elected by my colleagues to be chairman of the House Republican Policy Committee, the fourth-ranking leadership post. It was unusual for someone to be elected to the leadership after only one term in office, and it was only the second time that Wyoming's congressman was part of the elected leadership. The first time had been from 1919 to 1923, when Congressman Frank Mondell had served as the majority leader. My selection as part of the House Republican leadership had an enormous impact on my career. By 1988 I rose to the number two position as the House Republican whip and was in line to become the GOP leader when Bob Michel retired or Speaker of the House if we won the majority.

As policy chairman, I was a regular participant in meetings to determine our legislative strategy and our positions on key issues that came before the House. During the Reagan years, we met regularly with the president. Being policy chairman led to my appointment as a member of the Intelligence Committee and as the ranking Republican member on the committee to investigate the Iran-contra affair. Working with my Senate colleague, Al Simpson, part of the Republican leadership in the other body, we were often able to push policies important to the people of Wyoming. In later years when I became secretary of defense, the relationships that I developed during my years as part of the House leadership were instrumental in my work on Capitol Hill.

I maintained a significant international travel schedule during the early 1980s as well. A partial list of delegations in which I participated includes visits to the Soviet Union, Egypt, Grenada, Singapore, Japan, England, El Salvador, Israel, and France.

I never felt during these years that my health interfered with my ability to do my job, but I did experience a number of false alarms, instances when I felt something wasn't quite right, when I thought I might be having a heart attack but it turned out I wasn't.

One of the most important lessons I had taken from that first heart attack was "When in doubt, check it out." Some people are hesitant to go to a hospital and embarrassed if they do rush to the ER only to find out they aren't having a heart attack. I have never understood this. I knew that getting to the hospital could mean the difference between life and death if I *were* having an attack, so for me there was never any question of getting it checked out. There were some memorable false alarms, though.

## Into the Heart

One I will never forget occurred during a delegation visit to Tokyo in September 1981. Lynne and I were in Japan with a small group of congressmen and senators under the auspices of the Center for Strategic and International Studies. One evening in our hotel, I felt some chest discomfort and consulted the hotel physician, who recommended I go to the local hospital. The doctor summoned the ambulance, which arrived carrying an emergency team of six paramedics, all of whom wore yellow hard hats and none of whom spoke English. My Japanese was nonexistent. The language barrier didn't prevent me from noticing the paramedics' intense interest in the cowboy boots I was wearing, and with all the pointing and gesturing that went on, I got the idea that they thought my footwear was pretty exotic. The blaring sirens of the ambulance that rushed me to the hospital sounded exactly like the ones in the movie *Godzilla*. I couldn't get the images of a giant monster rampaging through the streets of Tokyo from my mind.

While I was in the emergency room, I was pleasantly surprised when the US ambassador to Japan, former senator Mike Mansfield, walked in. Mike was a longtime senator from my neighboring state of Montana and had been the majority leader of the Senate for many years. I deeply appreciated his gracious act of coming to the hospital to check on me.

Another rush to the hospital occurred while I was hosting a staff retreat at Flat Creek Ranch near Jackson Hole. I began to have some chest discomfort and told Lynne we needed to get to the hospital in Jackson to have it checked out. Lynne got my state representative, Merritt Benson, to drive both of us into town. The road in and out of the ranch was actually a National Forest Service jeep track for about two-thirds of the way, and it was like driving on a dry, rocky riverbed. Though the ranch is only fifteen miles from the town of Jackson, the road conditions can make the trip as long as two hours. It turned out I wasn't having a heart attack, but bouncing along the dirt road as Lynne urged Merritt to go faster was in itself a somewhat stressful experience.

So I was careful about heeding alarm bells, but I didn't spend a whole lot of time thinking about my heart condition. Of course, in hindsight, that first heart attack in 1978 was the initial manifestation of what would become a lifelong battle with coronary artery disease. At the time I didn't think of it in those terms. I thought of my heart attack as something behind me, something I could avoid a repetition of by taking care of myself. The heart attack and the surrounding publicity had in no way impaired my election campaign or my career in Congress. Indeed it was possible to believe it had had a positive effect to the extent it raised my name recognition across Wyoming. And perhaps most important of all, it had made me quit my smoking habit cold turkey. I had not had a cigarette since the night I passed out in the emergency room at Cheyenne Memorial Hospital. If I hadn't been inspired to do that, my life would have undoubtedly ended long ago.

## DR. REINER

An eclectic playlist streams softly in the background as I back through the doorway, warm water dripping from my arms. The staff, wearing masks, scrubs, and several pounds of protective lead, go about their jobs with an efficient, good-humored professionalism. The patient, covered neck to toe by a blue surgical drape, lies cruciform on a narrow gantry, eyes closed in a fentanyl-induced fugue, his right arm strapped to a board, palm up and perpendicular to the table, an oval opening in the drape exposing his wrist painted orange with antiseptic scrub. Two palm-sized patches on his chest are attached to the defibrillator perched on a rolling cart near the wall, its reassuring beeps quickly fading into familiar white noise. I dry my hands with a towel and slip into the sleeves of a sterile gown that unfolds with a quick downward flip. I pull on a pair of gloves, the latex issuing its characteristic *thwack* as I release each cuff. A nurse ties the back of my gown, and I step toward the patient preparing for a routine procedure that not long ago was impossible.

• • •

# Into the Heart

For millennia, the human heart remained mysterious and inviolable, the center of the physical body and the immortal soul, the sacred well-spring of character, intelligence, and valor.

In ancient Egypt, the heart was the only internal organ left in place during mummification, believed indispensable in Duat, the underworld, where it would be weighed against a feather, the symbol of Maat, goddess of truth and justice. Should the scales balance, the deceased would be deemed worthy of admission to the afterlife. If, however, the heart was heavy, Ammit, the devourer of the dead, a fearsome creature with the head of a crocodile, body of a lion, and hindquarter of a hippopotamus, would consume the heart, leaving the soul without rest.

Although the Greeks of the fourth century B.C. knew that the heart had four chambers and understood its anatomical relationship to the large blood vessels arising from it, knowledge they derived principally from the dissection of animals, luminaries like Aristotle and Hippocrates did not understand the organ's role in the circulation of blood. Aristotle believed that the heart was the center of human consciousness, and in many of the languages that evolved over the millennia, the word *heart* represents more than just the cardiac structure. Mandarin uses the same character (xīn) for both "heart" and "mind." The English word *courage* is derived from the Latin *cor* (heart), as are its Italian, French, and Portuguese counterparts, and the word *core* literally means heart.

At the beginning of the third century B.C., human dissection was permitted in Alexandria, and it was there that important advances were made in understanding the structure of the vascular system. The Greek physician Herophilus correctly considered the atria part of the heart (as opposed to part of the vessels leading into the heart) and was the first to describe the differences between the thick-walled arteries and the thin-walled veins, noting correctly that the vessel exiting the right ventricle was an artery, not a vein, and the vessels leading into the left atrium were veins, not arteries. Herophilus is also credited as being the first physician to count the pulse, though he incorrectly believed that the pulsations were caused by the contraction of the arteries.

Galen, a second-century Greek physician who lived in the Roman Empire and whose writings would dominate medicine for fifteen hundred years, believed that the heart was the source of the body's heat and moved pneuma (air, vital spirits) around the body. Although Galen did not believe that the heart was a muscle, he clearly understood its unique attributes:

> Its flesh is hard and not easily injured, being composed of fibres of many different kinds, and because of this, even if it would appear to be like muscles it is clearly different from them. . . . And in its hardness, tone, or tension and general strength and resistance to injury, the fibres of the heart much surpass all other fibres. For no organ functions so continuously, or moves with such force as the heart.

The classic view of circulation, which would perpetuate into the seventeenth century, can be summarized. The veins, it was thought, were the principal blood vessels and arose from the liver; the arteries contained only a small amount of blood mixed with pneuma; the heart provided the body's heat and vital spirits; blood was propelled by inspiration; and the pulse was caused by contraction of the arteries.

Even Leonardo da Vinci, whose detailed dissections and subsequent drawings so elegantly depicted the anatomy of the heart, could not break with the Aristotelian and Galenic view of the purpose of the heart, though he came close to articulating its role in circulation when he wrote, "The heart is the seed which engenders the tree of the veins."

William Harvey, an English physician born in Folkestone, Kent, on April 1, 1578, had a different idea, and in 1628 he published a ninety-page book, *On the Motion of the Heart and Blood in Living Beings (De Motu Cordis)*. In the introduction to an 1889 English translation from the original Latin, Alexander Bowie succinctly summarizes Harvey's theory:

> That there is one blood stream, common to both arteries and veins; that the blood poured into the right auricle, passes into the right

ventricle; that it is from there forced by the contraction of the ventricular walls along the pulmonary artery through the lungs and pulmonary veins to the left auricle; that it then passes into the left ventricle to be distributed through the aorta to every part of the animal body; and that the heart is the great propeller of this perpetual motion, as in a circle; this is the great truth of the motion of the heart and blood, commonly called the circulation, and must forever remain the glorious legacy of William Harvey.

Although Harvey describes for the first time the physiology of the circulatory system, he does not refute the heart's incorporeal role:

The heart of animals is the foundation of their life, the sovereign of everything within them, the sun of their microcosm, that upon which all growth depends, from which all power proceeds.

Until the twentieth century, entry to the heart, be it accidental, intentional, or surgical, was believed to lead to certain death. In 1902, the surgeon Harry Sherman described the heart:

An organ . . . particularly vulnerable—in fact, so vulnerable that any interference, even for surgical purposes, might be followed by immediate fatal results.

In 1929, Werner Forssmann, a German physician, set out to challenge the dogma that declared the heart sacrosanct. Forssmann, twenty-five years old at the time, was interested in finding a safe route into the chambers of the heart. Although studies in cadavers demonstrated the technical feasibility of his idea, Forssmann's hospital chief forbade him from performing the experiment on a patient. Undeterred, Forssmann decided to perform it on himself. In a now legendary and visionary display of both arrogance and bravery, a colleague placed a large-bore needle into the brachial vein of Forssmann's right arm and then advanced a well-lubricated ureteral catheter a short distance. A week later, now without assistance, Forssmann anesthetized his own left arm, punctured a vein, and inserted the catheter its entire sixty centimeters length. In a 1929 paper describing his experiment, Forssmann wrote:

> I checked the catheter position radiologically, after having climbed stairs from the OR to the radiology department. A nurse was holding a mirror in front of the X-ray screen for me to observe the catheter advance in position. The length of the catheter did not allow further advancement than into the right atrium. I paid particular attention to the possible effects on the cardiac conduction system, but could not detect any effect.

Forssmann's maverick work proved that an intrusion into the heart need not be deadly and thus unlocked the door to the heart. For the next quarter-century, other physicians, including Dr. André Cournand and Dr. Dickinson Richards of Columbia University (who would share the Nobel Prize with Forssmann in 1956), refined Forssmann's technique, conducting hemodynamic and dye studies within the cardiac chambers that exponentially expanded knowledge of the structure and physiology of the heart. Imaging of the coronary arteries, however, remained out-of-bounds as physicians believed that a direct injection of dye into a coronary vessel would cause cardiac arrest.

Another paradigm shift occurred in 1958 when Dr. Mason Sones, a Cleveland Clinic cardiologist, made one of medicine's great serendipitous discoveries after his catheter accidentally engaged the origin of a twenty-six-year-old patient's right coronary artery and dye was mistakenly injected. A great commotion ensued in the procedure room, but the patient did not die, and Sones's accident became the world's first coronary angiogram. Finally there was a way to create a detailed road map of the arteries supplying the heart.

• • •

In the early years, cardiac catheterization was an audacious and cumbersome procedure requiring an overnight hospital stay. The X-ray dye was quite toxic, frequently causing nausea and vomiting and, occasionally, cardiac arrest. Patients were instructed to cough violently, a primitive but effective way of maintaining a minimal cardiac output should the heart rate suddenly drop. Manipulation of rigid catheters in diseased arteries was hazardous work, occasionally resulting in vessel injury, perforation, or closure. The mortality rate was a risky 1 percent when cardiac catheterization was originally introduced and dropped steadily thereafter, but the procedure continued to carry hazards. My uncle Henry died during a cardiac catheterization in 1980 while I was a junior in college. I remember my father calling to give me the sad news that his older brother was dead and then trying to describe the procedure that had killed him. I had never before heard of heart catheterization; I remember thinking how terrible it was that an ostensibly healthy man could die while undergoing it.

I stand on the right side of the patient facing a huge, flat panel screen suspended from ceiling-mounted rails by a thick metal post. Not your typical big-screen TV, the glossy $100,000 ultra-high-resolution monitor is capable of simultaneously displaying a dozen medical-grade inputs and is powered by a six-foot-tall rack of video servers in the next room. Interventional cardiologists are often gadget geeks who wouldn't be caught dead with last year's phone, and a cath lab is a multimillion-dollar cathedral to the latest technology.

With the patient asleep and the lights in the room dimmed, I reach up to focus a small surgical spotlight on the upturned right wrist. In most patients, blood is supplied to the hand through the ulnar and radial arteries, redundant vessels that meet in a vascular arch in the palm. Like the interstate highway system, all arteries eventually connect, and the radial artery, easy to identify and compress, lying just under the skin, makes an ideal entry point.

# HEART

In the 1960s and 1970s, coronary arteriography required a surgical cut-down to expose the brachial artery, located in the crook of an elbow. In the late 1980s and 1990s, the preferred route of entry became the femoral artery, a large vessel in the groin accessible by needle, but often located deep under the skin and occasionally prone to severe or fatal bleeding. In the United States, use of the radial artery for access is relatively new, but European cardiologists have used this method for years, recognizing its superior safety and comfort compared with puncturing the leg. American doctors have been slow to adopt the technique because, until recently, very few were taught it during their years of training, there is a learning curve that requires several dozen cases before flattening out, and some physicians are reluctant to learn new tricks. I learned the procedure from my former fellow, and now colleague, Dr. Ramesh Mazhari, who quite patiently taught her former teacher.

Using a very fine needle, I inject a small amount of lidocaine under the skin on the thumb side, about two finger breadths above the horizontal wrist crease. After allowing the anesthetic to take effect, I pinch an IV catheter between my right thumb and forefinger and, with my other hand, get a fix on the location of the pulsating vessel lying a millimeter or two below. Very deliberately, as if demonstrating the procedure in slow motion, I pierce the skin aiming for the target under my left hand, and a few seconds later a crimson flash appears in the IV announcing the needle's arrival in the slim radial artery. I step on a foot pedal to turn on the X-ray tube mounted in the large C-shaped arm encircling the patient and watch on the monitor as the curved tip of a thin wire slides through the radial artery sheath and up the arm toward the shoulder. A one-meter-long catheter is threaded onto the wire, and together they are navigated through the radial and brachial arteries of the arm to the axillary and subclavian arteries of the shoulder and finally down into the aorta to the level of the aortic valve, from where the coronary arteries arise.

Through my latex gloves, I can feel the familiar supple smoothness of the catheter. With a subtle clockwise torque I engage the origin of the coronary, the two-millimeter polyethylene catheter now swinging in synchrony with the moving muscle. I glance quickly at the patient and then at the EKG and blood pressure waveforms while I work the controls to position the digital detector above the patient's head for the first set of images. A programmable power injector delivers six milliliters of iodinated X-ray contrast into the coronary artery; on the monitor, a gray-scale road map of the vessel plays back in a continuous loop, the angular borders of the vessel flexing in concert with the underlying myocardium. I repeat the imaging in multiple projections before switching catheters to assess the other coronaries. Finally, I pass a rounded catheter, shaped like a pig's tail, across the aortic valve and inject dye into the heart, inside the left ventricle, creating a vivid image of the contracting heart. The images acquired during the cardiac catheterization are stored in an array of servers, immediately reviewable on workstations around the hospital, and over the Internet, on my iPad, smart phone, or computer anywhere in the world.

The patient occasionally stirs but will not remember the half-hour procedure, accomplished through a 2-millimeter puncture in his wrist.

Two weeks after the November 1978 election, and five months after his heart attack, Dick Cheney underwent a follow-up stress test at Natrona County Memorial Hospital in Casper. Now back at unrestricted activity, walking every day for exercise, weighing a slimmer 179 pounds, and no longer smoking, the newly elected congressman achieved a peak heart rate of 200 beats per minute without chest pain or EKG abnormalities.

Although he was demonstrating reassuring cardiac fitness at the outset of his congressional career, the stress test could not delineate the amount of Cheney's underlying coronary disease or whether another heart attack was imminent. In a February 1979 letter to Dr. Freeman Cary, the attending physician of the US Capitol, Dr. Hiser had raised the possibility of coronary arteriography (that is, cardiac catheterization) to further define Cheney's coronary anatomy:

Dick Cheney suffered an inferior myocardial infarction in 1978. He has had several treadmills performed since then and has done quite well on them. . . . He had been recommended to have coronary arteriography performed because of his young age and the brilliant career he should have before him. He has not made a final decision as to whether he would desire to have this done.

The day before Thanksgiving in 1979, almost a year and a half after his heart attack, Cheney finally underwent cardiac catheterization to define the extent of his coronary artery disease. Dr. Al Del Negro performed the procedure at Georgetown University Hospital in Washington, DC, employing a now archaic surgical cutdown to expose the brachial artery in the patient's right arm. Using fluoroscopy, a series of catheters were passed to the heart through the incision in the arm, and a hand-powered syringe forcefully injected contrast into the congressman's coronaries. The images were captured on 35 mm movie film, processed in a darkroom at the conclusion of the procedure, and reviewed later with the aid of a projector.

Mr. Cheney was found to have a 50 percent narrowing in the right coronary artery, the vessel supplying the underside of the heart (a moderate lesion) and a 75 percent blockage in the circumflex branch, which supplies the side of the heart, the likely culprit for the heart attack a year and a half earlier. Overall, the test demonstrated not enough disease to warrant coronary artery bypass graft surgery, but much more disease than one would want to see, or expect to find, in a thirty-eight-year-old man.

## CHAPTER 4

# *Cura Personalis*

*No one cares how much you know, until they know how much you care.*

—THEODORE ROOSEVELT

## DR. REINER

It's said that law school doesn't teach students the law; it teaches them how to think like lawyers. Medical school, on the other hand, teaches plenty of science but very little of the art of being a doctor. Humanism, the notion that a physician should focus on the care of the patient rather than the treatment of the disease—what the Jesuits at Georgetown call *cura personalis,* or care for the whole person—is difficult to incorporate into medical training. How does a student learn to combine competence with compassion or optimism with realism? You learn from your patients and your peers, senior physicians, and those only a step or two ahead, mentors with attributes to be emulated and others with traits to avoid. It's an education that continues for a lifetime, and it began for me at the end of medical school when I found myself in the belly of the beast.

I awoke one morning in my junior year of medical school covered in hives. The textbooks call it urticaria, "an allergic skin eruption characterized by multiple, circumscribed, smooth, raised, pinkish, itchy wheals, developing very suddenly, usually lasting a few days, and leaving no visible trace." The lesions are the end result of the release into the skin of histamine, a chemical mediator of inflammation. The list of potential triggers of urticaria is long: foods, medications, insect bites, animal dander, viral infections, autoimmune diseases, pollen, heat, cold, emotional stress, and, very rarely, malignancy.

Blanketed with red welts and distinctly uncomfortable in my own skin, I made my way to Georgetown's ER where the attending physician asked about the usual suspects.

"Did you eat anything new?"

No.

"Have you changed your laundry detergent?"

No.

"Any recent viral illnesses?"

No.

In about half the cases of urticaria, the etiology remains unknown, or idiopathic, which is not the same as saying there is no cause. Everything has a cause; the trick is finding it. After getting some Benadryl and a hefty dose of prednisone, I was sent on my way. A few days later, the hives came back, prompting a visit to an allergist who asked similar questions, drew some blood, and ultimately came to the same conclusion: idiopathic urticaria.

Over the next eighteen months, I used antihistamines to suppress the hives. Medical students are often world-class hypochondriacs, miraculously manifesting fatal diseases they just studied. Still, I felt uneasy about the fact that my immune system was apparently duking it out with a phantom irritant.

In the late winter of my last year of medical school, I developed an intermittent and difficult-to-localize pain in the back of my mouth, at first vague and easy to ignore, coalescing over the next several weeks into a subtle soreness that I treated with periodic ibuprofen.

*Probably a wisdom tooth,* I thought. *The pain will go away.*

In the beginning of April, when the pain had not gone away and eating was becoming increasingly uncomfortable, I went to my bathroom mirror to take a look. After gently pulling my tongue toward the left with one hand and aiming a penlight with the other, I identified the obvious source of my discomfort. Illuminated in the narrow beam of light, midway back, along the right edge of my tongue, was an angry-looking, inch-long, and exquisitely sensitive mass.

*Okay. No reason to panic. Maybe I bit myself.*

I decided to wait a week or two to see if the lesion would disappear, a plan based more on principles of magical thinking than the principles of medicine.

Two weeks later, after gathering a critical mass of courage, I checked again. The growth was even larger, its center now discolored and starting to look necrotic (dead). I forced myself to suppress a rising wave of panic as I vaguely remembered a lecturer describing how a tumor will sometimes outgrow its blood supply.

*Oh, this is definitely not good.*

I made an appointment to have an ear, nose, and throat (ENT) surgeon at Georgetown take a look at my mouth. ENT surgeons, also known as otolaryngologists, and now more simply described as head and neck surgeons, are the people to see for chronic ear infections, sinusitis, nosebleeds, hoarseness, and also neoplasms (tumors) of the mouth, throat, and neck.

Lest anyone mistake me for a patient, I arrived for my Monday afternoon evaluation wearing my white coat. With it on, I am a healer, possessor of special powers and privileges, the saver and not the sick.

No one else was in the clinic waiting room in Georgetown's Gorman Building when I checked in for my appointment. After filling out the usual paperwork, I was brought to an exam room where I scanned the equipment with both curiosity and dread. In a few minutes, a young woman entered the room.

"Hi, I'm Catherine, one of the residents. What can I do for you?"

"I have something on my tongue that hurts like hell," I said.

"Oh, okay, let's take a look," she responded gently as she grabbed some gloves and adjusted a light.

Reclining in the examination chair, I tilted my head back, opened my mouth as wide I could, and stared at Catherine through the glare of her light. I noticed her squint slightly as she fixed her gaze on the side of my tongue.

"Did you bite yourself, Jon?"

"Not that I remember."

"It almost looks like there could be a little piece of a chicken bone embedded in the muscle," she said.

"I don't think so."

"I'm going to get my attending and have him take a look," Catherine said as she took off her gloves and left the room.

She returned quickly with an attending ENT surgeon, an all-business, middle-aged man who repeated some of Catherine's questions before also peering into my mouth and probing the sides and base of my tongue.

"Could be an inflammatory disease," he said. "Just to be safe, let's do a biopsy."

I didn't ask, "If you think it could be an inflammatory process, why do you want to do a biopsy? Why don't we try some more anti-inflammatory drugs before we snip off a piece of my tongue? What are you really worried about?"

I knew what he was really worried about and instead simply said, "Okay."

I took a deep breath and opened my mouth. The attending wrapped a dry piece of gauze around the tip of my tongue and got a firm grip before handing it off to a student to hold.

*This is going to hurt.*

Suddenly, a white-hot flame exploded in my mouth, like someone had taken a torch to the side of my tongue. I groaned as tears dripped down my cheeks and heard Catherine say, "I'm sorry, Jon."

Ironically the pain was the anesthetic; the biopsy itself I didn't feel. There wasn't much else to talk about. I was told to return Friday when the pathology report would be back.

It was an extraordinarily long week, particularly when I wasn't distracted by work. At dinner with friends or while walking alone in a quiet hospital corridor or in the drowsy still darkness before sleep, the pending biopsy report was never far away.

As I sat in the clinic before my Friday appointment, I spotted Catherine standing behind the reception desk checking something in a thick textbook.

*If she's reading about me I'm screwed.*

I was brought to the same exam room in which I had the biopsy four days earlier. Catherine opened the door and, after briefly inquiring about my week, cut right to the chase.

"Jon, it is cancer. I am very surprised."

It was hard for me to hear much else of what she said. Her attending came in and examined my neck, searching now for enlarged lymph nodes that would signify spread of the disease and maybe portend the end of my life. I caught only bits and pieces of the diagnosis and his proposed surgery, like I was listening to him on a phone with a bad connection: *squamous cell carcinoma, hemiglossectomy, tracheostomy, neck dissection.*

If I understood the attending correctly, he was going to remove half of my tongue, dissect the right side of my neck, and place a tube through my throat with which I would breathe. I reminded him that I was due to start my residency in two months.

"This is cancer," he replied starkly.

Catherine, so much her attending's junior but in some ways so much wiser, instinctively knew that the point to reemphasize was not the diagnosis, which I undoubtedly would remember, but the much more important prognosis. It was a lesson, and a kindness, I have never forgotten: show the patient that the glass is still half full.

"This is curable," Catherine said.


Physicians don't typically experience or imagine the whirlwind of terrible tasks that envelops a patient in the aftermath of a serious diagnosis. I had to tell my girlfriend, Betty, also a Georgetown medical student, that I had cancer. I found her working in the ER at Arlington Hospital, and we cried together in the ambulance bay. From there we went to the Armed Forces Institute of Pathology to get another opinion from a pathologist who specialized in head and neck cancers. He graciously reviewed the slides while we waited and concurred with the diagnosis. Next, it was back to Georgetown to tell the school administration that I needed some time off. I met with the dean who told me that even if I didn't get back before the end of the school year, I could still graduate with my class in May. I thanked him but told him I would be back in a couple of weeks. He also suggested that I consider deferring my internship a year, but I told him I had no intention of doing that. Most difficult of all, I had to fly up to New York for a painful conversation with my parents.

Although I was already tentatively scheduled for the operating room at Georgetown, when the smoke inside my head cleared, I realized I needed to consult another surgeon. Patients grossly underuse second opinions, but there are many good reasons to get one, among them to confirm the diagnosis (we did that at the Armed Forces Institute of Pathology), to validate the proposed treatment, and to ensure that you have the right doctor.

I had already matched for my internal medicine residency in New York at a Cornell program that included Memorial Sloan Kettering, the legendary cancer center in Manhattan, so seeking a second opinion there was the obvious choice. My mother knew of a head and neck surgeon there who specialized in the type of surgery I needed, and on Saturday morning I called Memorial and asked the operator to page Dr. Ronald Spiro, who promptly returned my call. I told Dr. Spiro I was a soon-to-graduate medical student and tried to describe my problem as dispassionately and professionally as I could manage, as if I were a colleague discussing a mutual patient.

"Oh, my God," Spiro replied, genuine concern obvious in his voice. "I can see you Monday morning. I'll alert my secretary you're coming."

"One other thing," he added. "Do you have medical insurance? Memorial doesn't take patients without insurance."

I did, but I'd almost gone without. At the beginning of my fourth year, Georgetown had changed the way medical students acquired insurance, but I had neglected to buy it. When I discovered the error in December, I toyed with the idea of going without it for the last half of the school year. Millions of young adults forgo health insurance either because of the expense or a mistaken sense of immortality. I was twenty-six years old. What could happen? Ultimately I decided that it was worth the few hundred dollars and bought the insurance, a fortuitous decision that probably saved my life.

Occupying an entire city block on the Upper East Side of Manhattan, Memorial Hospital is the oldest cancer hospital in the United States and in the world, an elite institution that attracts the best and the brightest clinicians. After registering and receiving a blue and white patient card embossed with my name, definitely not the type of hospital ID I was hoping for, my parents and I took a seat in the filled waiting room of the head and neck clinic. I tried not to notice the people breathing through tracheostomies or speaking with the harsh robotic sound of an artificial larynx, as if refusing to acknowledge their presence would somehow prevent me from joining their club.

When my name was called, my parents and I were ushered to a small, spare examination room where we waited in silence until the doctor entered. In his mid-fifties, with short salt-and-pepper hair and matching mustache, Dr. Spiro projected confident competence. A warm smile softened his steely seriousness, forged by years of treating people with very bad problems. He asked me about some of the typical risk factors for my type of cancer.

"Do you smoke?"

"Never."

"How much do you drink?"

"A couple of beers on the weekend."

After a thorough head and neck exam including a look at my vocal cords, Dr. Spiro described a less extensive approach for removing a tumor like mine. He would take many of the lymph nodes from the right side of my neck but would be able to spare most of my tongue.

I asked why his surgery would not require the removal of as much tissue or the tracheostomy planned by the surgeons in Washington.

"With all due respect to Georgetown, we do more of this surgery in a month than they do in a year," he said without a hint of bravado. "This is a procedure that I developed."

He swiveled on his stool and faced my parents.

"I want you to know that many patients do very well after an operation like this," he said, "but some don't do well."

"I know that," I replied.

"I know you do, Jon," he said modulating his voice with a paternal benevolence. "I need to tell your parents."


A procession of fluorescent lights and acoustic ceiling tiles waft past the stretcher as I float through the hallways on benzodiazepines, swaddled like an infant in warm blankets. I enter the operating room headfirst, able to see from where I have come but not where I am going.

After I am moved to the table, Dr. Spiro appears directly above me, his masked face silhouetted in the round OR lights above his head.

"Are you ready, Jon?"

*Absolutely.*

From somewhere behind. I hear the anesthesiologist say, "Okay, Jon, this stuff works pretty quick." There is a faint burning in my hand, and then nothing.


A moment later I am lying in a noisy, brightly lit space. An oxygen mask is covering my nose and mouth. I do a quick systems check, reach a hand up to my neck, and find a thin length of clear tubing draining

66

into something resembling a plastic hand grenade that is pinned to my gown and half-filled with bloody liquid. A nurse, noticing I am now awake, asks how I feel. I don't have any pain, but I am very nauseous, a side effect of the general anesthesia. I start to tell her, but my words are unintelligible, as if I'm trying to talk with golf balls in my mouth.

"Comp-a-zine," I say again, pronouncing each syllable of the anti-nausea medication very slowly.

"Compazine? Sure, I'll go get it," she said.

*I can talk.*

I remained in the hospital for another week fed through a nasogastric tube until it was deemed safe for me to eat. Outside the hospital, the world continued to spin. A nuclear reactor in the Soviet Union exploded, there was a lunar eclipse, my classmates continued their final rotations. On post-op day five, I learned that the final pathology report showed no spread of tumor to the lymph nodes, remarkably good news. I was discharged from Memorial a few days later, a little more than two weeks after I first visited the ENT clinic at Georgetown. My hives disappeared.

On a shelf in my closet sits a beautiful inlaid wooden box in which I keep a variety of mementos: expired passports, an old watch, keys to long-forgotten locks. Inside the box are both IDs from my time at Memorial Hospital. The tag labeled "House Physician" has a photo of a bearded young doctor resplendent in his white coat; the other card contains the account number of an incredibly lucky patient.

## CHAPTER 5

# A Tale of Two Drugs

## VICE PRESIDENT CHENEY

On September 10, 1984, I was at work on Capitol Hill when I began to experience discomfort in my chest and throat. It wasn't painful, but I could tell something was not right. I took the elevator down to the Capitol physician's office on the ground floor of the Capitol to have it checked out. The physician thought I should head to Bethesda Naval Hospital to be safe and called an ambulance to take me there. Although an EKG performed that night at the hospital showed none of the changes you would expect to see with a heart attack, cardiac enzyme tests the next day did show elevation consistent with a mild heart attack.

September 11, the day the enzyme tests confirmed I'd had a heart attack, was also the day of the 1984 Republican primary in Wyoming. I was unopposed. President Reagan called me on September 13 to wish me a speedy recovery, and we laughed together as he told me about the dinner he attended the evening before roasting our mutual friend, the retiring senator from Tennessee, Howard Baker.

I was in the hospital for a week and then went home for rest and recuperation. I had a good deal of time during those weeks to think about my heart and my health. It was then that I made one of the most important decisions of my life.

The second heart attack was a true wake-up call. For the previous six years, I had believed my heart attack had been a onetime event that I had taken the necessary steps to fix. I played tennis, took annual pack trips into the Wyoming wilderness, skied in the Rockies, and worked overtime as Wyoming's congressman and as part of the House GOP leadership. In no way was I limited physically by my heart.

In retrospect, my refusal to accept the notion that I had a chronic disease may have been helpful from the standpoint of my being able to aggressively pursue my political career and enjoy the active pursuits I loved. I didn't think of myself as a patient, and I didn't act like one. If I had, I might not have run for Congress, put in the long hours required, or sought a House Republican leadership position. My view of my health also affected the way others perceived me. My colleagues in Congress, for example, a group of highly motivated, ambitious political figures, might have been unlikely to select me as one of their leaders if they had thought of me as "the guy with the bad heart."

The reality, however, was that I was a patient with coronary artery disease. This second heart attack forced me to acknowledge that I had a significant chronic heart problem that would likely worsen over time.

When I'd had false alarms in the years preceding my second heart attack, I was treated by whichever physician was on call at that moment. Most of them had never seen me before. Though I'd had excellent care, the realization that this was going to be a lifelong challenge convinced me I needed to find a single physician to follow my case and know my heart and my disease better than anyone else.

Lynne was working then at *Washingtonian* magazine where one of her colleagues was John Pekkanen, a renowned journalist who specialized in health care. She sought John's advice about the best cardiologists in the DC area, and he recommended several good physicians, including Dr. Allan Ross at George Washington University Hospital. Dr. Ross was focused primarily on research at that point, but he agreed to take me on as a patient. I remained in his care until he retired and passed me on to Dr. Jonathan Reiner, who has handled my care for the past fifteen years.

The decision to develop a long-term relationship with a top-flight physician was one of the most important I ever made. I am convinced that I would not be writing this history if it hadn't been for the outstanding work, knowledge, and commitment I've benefitted from as a result of that choice. When we were discussing the possibility of doing this book together, Dr. Reiner told me he does not know any other patient who suffered a heart attack in the 1970s and is still alive today. My longevity is directly due to the expertise of the doctors who have treated me, and primarily to my cardiologists, Dr. Ross and Dr. Reiner.

Though it coincided with my reelection campaign for my fourth term in the House of Representatives, the 1984 heart attack did not lead me to question my choice to serve in elective office or my commitment to a long-term career in politics. I spent the next several weeks recuperating at home in McLean, Virginia.

On October 2, 1984, I went to the Capitol when the Wyoming Wilderness Act was up for a vote in the House of Representatives. Along with my Senate colleagues Al Simpson and Malcolm Wallop, I had worked very hard on this legislation, which set aside nearly a million acres in wilderness area in my home state. I wanted to be sure it passed, and I wanted to be there to cast my vote for it.

I spent the last two weeks in October campaigning in Wyoming and was reelected to my fourth term with 74 percent of the vote that November. I felt no aftereffects from my second heart attack and had been able to resume a full and active schedule.

In February 1985, I took on additional responsibilities in the House when I was named to the Permanent Select Committee on Intelligence, which has responsibility for congressional oversight of all matters relating to the nation's intelligence agencies, including the CIA, the Defense Intelligence Agency, and the National Security Agency. It is the kind of assignment some members don't relish. The work is mostly highly classified, and you can't explain to your constituents how you are spending your time. Studying the materials and intelligence reports is a significant commitment of many hours and must be done only in the secure committee facilities in the Capitol. But it is an assignment of real significance in terms of the security of the nation, and I found the work fascinating.

In 1986, I was reelected as the House Republican Policy chairman for the Ninety-Ninth Congress. That November, Al Simpson and I had been planning to go elk hunting. The day before we were scheduled to leave, House Republican leader Bob Michel called and asked me to attend a meeting the White House had just called. It seemed I was the only member of the House Republican leadership in town that day.

As it turned out, the meeting, on November 12, 1986, was a briefing delivered by national security adviser John Poindexter in the White House situation room. I sat around a table with the Senate majority leader, Bob Dole, the Senate minority leader, Robert Byrd, House Speaker Jim Wright, and a number of members of President Reagan's cabinet. Poindexter explained to us that in an attempt to secure the release of American hostages being held by Iran's ally, Hezbollah, the United States had been selling arms to what they believed were moderate factions in Iran. Some of the hostages had been freed, but the policy was badly misguided. It violated an existing arms embargo and put the United States in the position essentially of negotiating with terrorists.

A few weeks later, we learned the picture was even more complicated when it was revealed that proceeds from the arms sales were being sent to the Contras, a rebel group in Nicaragua. Congress had prohibited the president from providing any assistance to the Contras when it passed a series of amendments, collectively known as the Boland amendment, in the early and mid-eighties. In the aftermath of the revelation about the diversion of funds, a joint select committee was formed in Congress to investigate what had happened. I was the ranking House Republican on the committee and presided, along with chairman Lee Hamilton, over committee hearings on the arms sales and fund diversion throughout the first half of 1987.

The issues raised by Iran-Contra were significant and concerning. Clearly the administration made mistakes in carrying out a policy of essentially negotiating with terrorists. But there were also legitimate questions to be asked about the proper role of Congress in the conduct of US foreign and national security policy. And the political atmosphere in Washington meant that, in my view, many of the Democrats on the select committee were more interested in scoring partisan points against President Reagan than they were in understanding what truly went wrong and finding ways to prevent it from happening again.

Against the backdrop of my involvement in the significant, highly scrutinized, and time-consuming Iran-Contra committee, I was still dealing with matters of my heart. On January 27, 1987, President Reagan was scheduled to deliver his annual State of the Union address to a joint session of Congress. This would be the One Hundredth Congress and the beginning of the year marking the bicentennial of our Constitution. I was booked to appear on several news programs that night after the speech. I was at work in my office and began to feel some chest discomfort. I took two nitroglycerin pills and called Pete Williams, my press secretary, and Patty Howe, my legislative director, into my office. I asked them to cancel my interviews for the evening and then asked Pete to walk with me over to the Capitol physician's office. We walked the length of the hallway to the elevator. I was feeling worse by the minute and didn't think I could make it over to the Capitol. Pete and I turned around and headed back to my office to call an ambulance.

I took a few steps, and there, in front of the Capitol policeman's desk, fainted. Pete, pretty scared by this point, asked the policeman to call for a doctor. Instead, he called his superior and shouted, "Member down." Pete ran down the hall to our office and had Patty call the House physician. The Cannon House Office Building nurse was on duty. She came out with a pillow and checked my blood pressure. Apparently, as I lay there sprawled out and unconscious on the marble floor with my shirt open, several of my colleagues walked by. As Pete tells it, they didn't quite step over my body, but it was close.

Eventually an ambulance came, and Pete rode with me to the George Washington University Hospital emergency room. Pete was understandably pretty worried and didn't think I was getting medical attention quickly enough. At one point, he started yelling to no one in particular, "This is a United States congressman!" Either in light of that information or, more likely, because they wanted to get Pete to quit yelling, I was taken back for evaluation. After a few hours and tests, the doctors determined I had not had a heart attack but probably had an adverse reaction to the nitroglycerin. They released me to go home.

I was somewhat surprised, given the dramatic nature of the event and the fact that several of my colleagues had strolled past me while I was unconscious on the floor, that the story never made the media. Pete Williams, a dear friend to this day, felt guilty that he'd been standing there when I passed out and hadn't caught me. I couldn't resist giving him a hard time about it when I got back to the office the next day. "Thanks, Williams," I told him. "You dropped me!"

A few months later, in May 1987, after I'd had an abnormal stress test, Dr. Ross performed another catheterization. In 1987, the standard procedure was to access the femoral artery through the groin. The area was shaved and prepped with antiseptic and a local anesthetic was administered. I was given mild sedation but was sufficiently awake to be aware of what was going on around me. On occasion, I remember being asked to cough during the procedure. I was sometimes able to see the screen the doctor used to steer the catheter into the arteries of my heart. When the dye was injected, I felt a warm flush. The only uncomfortable part of the procedure occurred after the catheter was withdrawn and the entry wound closed. The final step, to ensure there was no subsequent bleeding from the entry point, was to apply heavy pressure to the wound for approximately half an hour. This task was usually assigned to the largest member of the surgical team. The procedure has since been significantly improved.

It wasn't until I was reviewing my own medical records in preparation for writing this book that I realized this particular catheterization included some worrying moments. In the words of Dr. Ross:

> Unfortunately, during one injection he developed ventricular fibrillation requiring cardioversion x3 with 300 joules

As happens sometimes, but not often, the dye had prompted my heart to fibrillate in a potentially deadly rhythm. It took three electric shocks to set things right.

This catheterization showed that my right coronary artery had begun to narrow, but there had been no further progression of the plaque in other vessels in the heart. At my follow-up appointment a few weeks later, Dr. Ross advised that I should restrict my most strenuous activities, particularly at high altitudes, in the hope that I would be able to continue to participate in less strenuous recreational pursuits without risking damage to muscle deprived of oxygen. We also agreed that given the results showing narrowing of an artery that had previously been plaque free, I would now have more regular stress tests.

As I was receiving news of a worsening heart condition, my responsibilities on the Hill continued to increase. On June 4, 1987, I moved up in the House leadership when I was elected chairman of the House Republican Conference, the number-three elected position in Republican leadership. Meanwhile I was still engaged in the high-stakes hearings about the Iran-Contra affair. At first glance, it might seem that my professional activities would have added to the stress of the somewhat negative health report. I think it was actually just the opposite. The job of ranking member on the Iran-Contra committee involved me in critically important matters—issues relating to the constitutional roles of the president and Congress, questions about how far the United States should go to secure the release of our hostages, and inquiries about how best we could prevent the Soviets from gaining a foothold in Latin America. I think it was the import of these issues and the sense that I was an important participant in a set of historic events that enabled me not to dwell on the negative developments with respect to my heart. I didn't have time and was not inclined to sit around and feel sorry for myself. I believed Dr. Ross had laid out a reasonable course of action that involved some curtailing of my activity. He had also scheduled me to begin the new cholesterol-lowering drug, lovastatin, as soon as it received approval from the Food and Drug Administration (FDA). The combination of comfort with my physician and his judgments, a sense that we were doing all we could do to deal with the disease, and a knowledge that I had important work to do for the nation allowed me to continue to participate fully in all I was called on to do.

## DR. REINER

You're not sure what is happening, but somehow, in a visceral way you can't articulate, you know that it is not good. At first, the symptoms were subtle. Maybe you awoke not feeling right; you might have had some of these symptoms yesterday, but you're not really sure when it began. You thought it might be indigestion because you're a bit nauseated, and you took some antacid a little while ago, but the discomfort hasn't eased. Now you're feeling something in your shoulder and chest, and your left arm is tingling. Someone tells you that you look pale, and you realize your shirt is drenched even though it is not warm in the room. You're asked if you are having chest pain, and you say no, it's not a pain, it's more like a pressure or maybe a tightness. When you try to describe what you're feeling, you subconsciously place a clenched fist over your chest. You have the sense that if you could manage to burp, you would feel better, but you can't, and to make matters worse, you're a little short of breath.

You don't know it yet, but a blood clot, smaller than a pencil's eraser, is forming inside one of your coronary arteries, and if it is not dealt with quickly, it can kill you.

That's what was happening when Dick Cheney awoke with chest pain in the early-morning hours of June 29, 1988, and was brought to George Washington University Hospital, in DC's Foggy Bottom neighborhood, six blocks from the White House. When he arrived in the emergency room Congressman Cheney's blood pressure was 115/70, and his pulse was 64, both normal. But his EKG showed signs of a new MI in the same region affected by heart attacks in 1978 and 1984. This was his third. Cardiologists Allan Ross and P. Jacob Varghese evaluated

Cheney and recommended urgent cardiac catheterization to determine the site of the likely coronary occlusion.

Dr. Ross had come to GW from Yale about a decade earlier and was an internationally known expert in the management of acute myocardial infarction, having helped to pioneer some of the revolutionary new drugs. Dr. Varghese, a legendary clinician, had come to GW from Johns Hopkins around the same time and was the director of the cardiac care unit.

After puncturing the femoral artery at the top of Cheney's right leg, Ross guided a catheter to the heart, maneuvering it into the aorta and the origin of the coronary arteries where an injection of contrast dye revealed an old occlusion of the circumflex branch (unchanged from 1984) and a new clot blocking the right coronary artery. Ross intended to open the artery with a balloon, but a mechanical malfunction in the cath lab forced him to change his plan. Instead Cheney was administered tissue plasminogen activator (tPA), the new intravenous "clot buster" approved by the FDA seven months earlier.

In the late 1970s, Dr. Marcus DeWood set out to prove once and for all that blood clots caused heart attacks. DeWood and his colleagues at the University of Washington performed coronary angiography in about three hundred heart attack patients admitted to hospitals in Spokane and Seattle. The demonstration that it was both feasible and safe to perform cardiac catheterization during an acute heart attack was itself a groundbreaking achievement. DeWood found that when angiography was performed within a few hours of symptom onset, it showed that almost 90 percent of the patients had a totally blocked coronary artery, and in many of these patients, a culprit blood clot could be extracted from the vessel. Importantly, when other patients in the study were imaged later, up to twenty-four hours after the onset of pain, fewer arteries were closed, suggesting that with time, some clots spontaneously dissolve, raising the possibility that this intrinsic "clot-busting" process might be induced therapeutically.

At about the same time that DeWood's study was under way, several groups were working to prove that not all of the at-risk heart muscle (the myocardium) died immediately after a coronary artery closed. Using a laboratory model involving the temporary occlusion of a dog's coronary, Keith Reimer from Duke University and Robert Jennings from Northwestern demonstrated that myocardium died over hours, limited initially to the innermost layer of the heart (subendocardium) and over time extending through the full thickness of the muscle to the outermost layer (subepicardium). They showed that if blood flow was restored within fifteen minutes, no permanent heart damage occurred. Progressively longer occlusions resulted in progressively larger amounts of muscle death, and restoration of blood flow after about six hours would not salvage any muscle at all. The implication of this work was profound: a heart attack could be interrupted, but time was of the essence.

With the cardiology community finally convinced that a typical heart attack resulted from a blood clot and with a potential therapeutic window of several hours, the approach to the management of heart attacks changed from the old largely defensive, watch-and-wait strategy, to a new offensive attempt to open the occluded vessel and salvage heart muscle. But how to open the artery?

Each of us has more than sixty thousand miles of blood vessels, mostly comprising a microscopic maze of billions of capillaries. The five liters of blood coursing through this complex vascular network must be kept in careful biochemical balance, also known as homeostasis. If blood is too "thin," spontaneous hemorrhage may occur, and if it is too "thick," clots may develop.

In 1933, William Tillett and R. L. Garner, working at the Johns Hopkins Medical School in Baltimore, discovered the novel ability of cultures of streptococcal bacteria to completely liquefy a previously solid blood clot. This bacterial protein, which was later called streptokinase, was found to exert its "fibrinolytic" effects by activating a naturally occurring protein in human blood called plasminogen and converting it to the active enzyme plasmin, which dissolves the fibrin meshwork of a thrombus.

Tillett and his colleagues initially used streptokinase to treat patients with pneumonia or tuberculosis who had developed large gelatinous collections in the pleural space that surrounds the lung. A direct injection of streptokinase into the pleural space between the lung and the chest wall dissolved much of the thick material, enabling drainage from the space and reexpansion of the lung. In 1951, Tillett showed that an experimentally induced clot in an ear vein of a rabbit could be opened when streptokinase was administered systemically, and in the late 1950s, intravenous streptokinase was evaluated in patients with acute myocardial infarction. Despite some data suggesting a potential mortality benefit when the drug was administered relatively early, streptokinase was largely abandoned in the United States because we did not yet know enough about the mechanics of a heart attack.

Twenty years later, with the pathophysiology of heart attacks much clearer, interest in clot-busting drugs returned. In the late 1970s, Evgenii Chazov in the Soviet Union and Peter Rentrop in West Germany separately demonstrated that a direct injection of streptokinase by catheter into an occluded coronary could restore the flow of blood, and in 1984 the FDA approved streptokinase for intracoronary use during myocardial infarction. The downside of this approach was that it was fairly complex, took a significant amount of time to perform, and required the use of a cardiac cath lab, at the time available in only a limited number of hospitals in the United States.

In the years that followed, several very large international clinical research trials, enrolling tens of thousands of patients, proved that streptokinase and tPA, a new drug at that time, produced using recombinant DNA techniques (a process whereby different strands of DNA are combined to produce a "designer" molecule), could open many of the arteries with a relatively simple intravenous administration, and compared with placebo, both drugs significantly improved a patient's likelihood of surviving a heart attack. In November 1987, the FDA granted approval for the intravenous use of streptokinase and tPA in the United States. Manufactured by Genentech (and at $2,200 a dose, ten times the cost of streptokinase), tPA was enthusiastically embraced by the medical community in the United States. Accelerated by a study in the early 1990s that found myocardial infarction death rates lower after treatment with tPA than after treatment with streptokinase, annual tPA sales soared to more than $300 million.

At the same time that tPA and streptokinase were revolutionizing the treatment of heart attacks, intense research was under way to identify drugs that would help to prevent such events. In the 1950s and 1960s, driven by the increasing body of data linking serum cholesterol to heart disease, numerous pharmaceutical companies developed an interest in the complex biology governing how cholesterol is manufactured in the body. In 1956, researchers at one of these companies, Merck, isolated mevalonic acid, a key precursor of cholesterol, and three years later, scientists at the Max Planck Institute in Heidelberg, Germany, discovered the enzyme HMG-CoA reductase, which regulated the key step in mevalonic acid production. Theoretically, inhibition of this enzyme should inhibit the production of cholesterol, and over the next twenty years, researchers around the world hunted for a drug that would do that.

The first HMG-CoA reductase inhibitor was discovered in 1976 in the fermentation broth of the bacterium *Penicillium citrinum* by Japanese researcher Akira Endo. The drug, called compactin, was soon found to be effective at lowering cholesterol levels in rabbits, monkeys, and dogs. Meanwhile, in fall 1978, Merck scientists isolated a substance produced by the fungus *Aspergillus terreus*. The agent, a pure inhibitor of HMG-CoA reductase, was given the name lovastatin, and a US patent was filed in June 1979. In April 1980, Merck began clinical trials of the drug.

In September 1980, the Japanese pharmaceutical company Sankyo abruptly ended development of compactin amid concerns regarding cancers in dogs. Although there had been no such adverse safety signals with lovastatin, Merck quickly terminated development of lovastatin, citing the safety issues with the closely related compactin. Almost two years later, several clinicians petitioned Merck and the FDA for access to lovastatin for patients with severely elevated cholesterol that could not be controlled by treatment with any commercially available drug. Patients with superaggressive coronary disease and off-the-chart cholesterol levels saw their cholesterol drop by 30 percent or more after just a few weeks of lovastatin therapy. Merck promptly reinstituted animal testing in the drug, including long-term toxicology studies in dogs. Even after high doses, no tumors were found in the animals. Human clinical trials of lovastatin resumed in 1984. Merck found that lovastatin was well tolerated, and resulted in great reductions in LDL cholesterol levels. In November 1986, Merck filed a new drug application with the FDA comprised of 160 volumes of lab, animal, and human data. On August 31, 1987, only nine months after the application was filed, the FDA approved lovastatin for use in patients with high cholesterol not controllable by diet. Sold under the trade name Mevacor, the drug was an immediate commercial success, with annual sales eventually reaching $1 billion.

Hospital admissions for acute myocardial infarction began to drop sharply in 1987, the same year that lovastatin was introduced in the United States. Four years later, pravastatin (Pravachol), a derivative of compactin, and simvastatin (Zocor), a synthetic derivative of lovastatin, were approved by the FDA, and collectively the "statins" became some of the most widely prescribed medications in the world. Although the drugs unequivocally and profoundly decreased cholesterol levels, there remained uncertainty about whether improved lab results would translate to improved outcomes such as a reduction in myocardial infarction or death.

Questions concerning the clinical impact of these drugs were put to rest in 1994 when the Scandinavian Simvastatin Survival Study was published. The trial had assigned several thousand patients with high cholesterol to treatment with simvastatin or placebo and followed these patients for five years. The group of patients treated with simvastatin demonstrated a 30 percent or greater reduction in mortality, coronary events, or need for angioplasty or bypass surgery. This study became a landmark, effectively removing any lingering doubt concerning the benefit of cholesterol reduction. The studies that followed, using a variety of statins, including the newer atorvastatin (Lipitor) and rosuvastatin (Crestor), confirmed these results for patients both with and without a prior history of coronary disease, as well as those with a history of diabetes, peripheral vascular disease, and stroke.

Throughout most of the 1980s, Dick Cheney's cholesterol proved resistant to a variety of drugs like cholestyramine and gemfibrozil. In late 1987, Allan Ross started him on newly approved Mevacor, carefully increasing the dose over the next several months and ultimately reaching 80 mg, the maximum daily dose. In October 1988, Cheney's total cholesterol level, which a year earlier was over 300, was down to 133. The low-density lipoprotein (LDL) component (aka "bad cholesterol," because elevated levels are associated with an increased risk of heart disease) had plunged from 163 to 65, a 60 percent reduction.

The clinical impact of this effect in this patient cannot be overstated. In the ten years prior to beginning statin therapy, Dick Cheney was hospitalized six times and experienced three myocardial infarctions, resulting in a loss of about 30 percent of his heart's ability to contract. In the twelve years that followed, even during periods of high stress, including time as secretary of defense during the Gulf War and CEO of a large multinational corporation, Cheney had not a single cardiac event.

CHAPTER 6

# Bypass

## VICE PRESIDENT CHENEY

The year 1988 was shaping up to be an active and important one for the nation and for me personally. Ronald Reagan's second term as president was coming to an end, and there was a major battle in the Republican Party for the nomination to succeed him. I did not get involved in the presidential contest because I was focused on my own campaign to win the second-ranking leadership post among House Republicans.

The incumbent GOP whip, my good friend Trent Lott of Mississippi, was stepping down to run for the Senate. If I could win the race to replace him by a unanimous vote of the GOP Conference, I would be well positioned to succeed Bob Michel as GOP leader or even become the first GOP Speaker in more than thirty years if we captured the majority. As chairman of the House Republican Conference, I was slated to serve as the chair of the Convention Rules Committee. I wanted to take advantage of that assignment to get a rule adopted that would grant floor access at national conventions to all GOP members of Congress. The existing rule allowed only members who had been elected as convention delegates from their home states to have floor access. In addition, I had to get reelected to Congress by the voters of Wyoming for my sixth term in the House.

On the morning of June 29, 1988, believing that I might be having another heart attack, I checked myself into George Washington University Hospital. As before, I didn't experience any major chest pain or other significant symptoms that I can remember, just a general sensation that something was wrong. EKG and enzyme tests confirmed that I was indeed having my third heart attack. Dr. Ross recommended that we try to reopen the offending heart artery by administering a newly approved clot-busting drug designed to clear a blocked artery. It seemed to work initially, but two days later, the pain returned, and I was given a second dose. Of my five heart attacks, this one did the most damage. I have a distinct memory of a crisis, with many hospital personnel hurrying into my room trying to deal with my "crashing blood pressure." During that period, I also recall lying in bed listening to reports that an American cruiser, the USS *Vincennes*, had accidentally shot down an Iranian airliner, with significant loss of life, in the Persian Gulf.

After checking out of the hospital, I issued a press release on July 9 indicating that I planned to attend the Republican National Convention in New Orleans in August. I made it clear that my recent stay in the hospital would not alter my political plans. The heart attack did not force me to make a single major change in my professional schedule, but it did require me to back out of a wilderness pack trip with Jim Baker. We had planned it for July while the Democrats were holding their national convention, but given my health situation, I couldn't justify a weeklong horseback trip into the Yellowstone backcountry. (When I told Jim I couldn't make it, he quickly found a replacement: George H. W. Bush.) I returned to work in the House of Representatives on July 22.

After further tests showed there clearly had been some progression in my coronary artery disease, Dr. Ross raised with me the possibility of undergoing bypass surgery. He didn't present it as necessary to save my life, but thought it was advisable because of my lifestyle. I noticed I was having some difficulty traveling through airports carrying luggage. I found it necessary to stop and rest occasionally. I clearly lacked the stamina I'd once had. Having open heart surgery wasn't something I looked forward to, but if I wanted to continue my career in the Congress and continue my skiing and pack trips in Wyoming and all of the other activities I loved, it was necessary.

# Bypass

My confidence in the outcome grew when I learned that Dr. Ben Aaron, the surgeon who had saved President Reagan's life in March 1981, would perform the operation. On August 9 I announced that I would undergo bypass on August 19, after the GOP convention. "While for me the bypass surgery is optional," the statement said, "I have decided to do it now so that in the future, I can lead the same kind of active life I have in the past."

My August 9 statement also noted that my dad had just undergone coronary bypass surgery in our hometown of Casper. Since my first heart attack ten years before, I had been asked frequently if there was any history of heart disease in my family. I always answered that Mom's dad had died of a heart attack at age sixty-six, but that as far as we knew, there was no history of heart disease on Dad's side of the family. Dad never talked about his health, and as far as I knew, he had rarely if ever seen a doctor since he had been discharged from the Navy at the end of World War II.

In early August 1988, Mom had finally persuaded him that he needed to have a doctor take a look at him, so he made an appointment. During that appointment, the doctor discovered that his condition was so serious that they took him directly into surgery and performed a six-way bypass on him. When they opened him up, they found he also had a large aneurysm in his aorta and evidence that he had experienced two previous heart attacks that he never told anyone about. The doctors didn't believe he would survive the bypass and aneurysm repair if they did both at the same time, so they completed the bypass and sent him home to recover for eight weeks, then brought him back in to repair his aorta. He lived another ten years. Now I knew I had a history of heart disease on both sides of my family.

In Wyoming, I had primary opposition for the GOP nomination for Congress but won comfortably with 87 percent of the vote. That same day, I convened a meeting of the Convention Rules Committee and successfully passed the rules change that would allow all Republican members of Congress to have floor access at national conventions. Since George Bush had already sewn up the GOP nomination for president, the only excitement focused on his choice of Senator Dan Quayle for vice president.

For me, one of the most memorable moments of the convention was the private talk I had with Larry King, then a correspondent for CNN. Larry and I sat on the steps going up to the CNN broadcast booth during one of the regular convention sessions and talked about my scheduled coronary bypass surgery. Larry had recently undergone a similar procedure, and I had a lot of questions. He walked me through his experience and was very helpful.

On Wednesday night of the convention, George Bush was officially nominated for president. The following day, I flew back to Washington and checked into George Washington University Hospital. That evening, George Bush gave his acceptance speech and delivered the memorable line: "Read my lips, no new taxes." What was memorable for me was that I watched his speech flat on my back in a hospital bed while a male nurse shaved the hair off my body to prep me for surgery the next morning.

Since this was my first open heart surgery, I was introduced to a number of technologies and procedures I had never before experienced. I was told at the outset that the anesthesia would have the effect over time of diminishing my memory of the operation. That was probably true, but I still have a recollection of certain aspects of the procedure twenty-five years later. I have a memory of being aware during part of the operation of what was going on around me. When I asked, the doctors explained they really had no idea what goes on inside an unconscious patient's brain.

This was also my first experience with being on a respirator. When I came out from under the anesthetic, I discovered I was breathing with the aid of a machine that had been inserted into my throat, and I couldn't speak. The discomfort I felt was more psychological than it was physical. I felt the same way about the catheter that had been placed in my bladder. The idea of being dependent on these devices bothered me.

On the second day of my recovery, my chest and back felt as if I'd been hit by a truck. Obviously the anesthetic had worn off by then, and I was feeling the effects of having my chest opened wide and my rib cage separated to get at my heart. For two or three days, it was very hard to find a comfortable position in the bed. In my subsequent open heart surgeries I didn't experience that kind of discomfort, no doubt in part because there have been significant improvements in pain management. Other things have changed too. Lynne had purchased a CD player for me that allowed me to listen to music through a pair of earphones. In 1988 it played only one CD at a time.

After I checked out of the hospital on August 26, I spent several weeks getting my strength back. I had time to reflect on the fact that my dad and I both had bypass surgery within a few weeks of each other. He was seventy-three and I was forty-seven.

In October I returned to Wyoming in time to do some campaigning and easily won reelection with 67 percent of the vote. On December 5, my Republican colleagues unanimously elected me House GOP whip.

Four months after my surgery, I was skiing at Vail and Beaver Creek in Colorado, something I could never have done without the bypass.

## DR. REINER

An assignment to Dr. Robert Wallace's service was a lucky break for me as a third-year medical student: I had the opportunity to learn from a famous heart surgeon and decide once and for all if surgery was for me.

Dr. Wallace had come to Georgetown from the Mayo Clinic where he had trained under the legendary John Kirklin, one of the pioneers of cardiac surgery. In 1968, Wallace became the first surgeon in the United States to perform the Rastelli procedure to correct transposition of the great arteries, a devastating congenital heart defect, where the aorta and pulmonary arteries arise from the wrong chambers of the heart. Dr. Wallace was old school, and rounds began in the ICU way before sunrise and moved forward at a rapid pace before concluding in time for the first OR case of the day. There was talk that he didn't approve of students or residents with facial hair, a perhaps apocryphal story recounting a patient's fatal infection and the beard Wallace had allowed the patient to keep at the time of his operation. On rounds the day before, I thought I saw Wallace take note of my well-groomed whiskers, the last vestige of my college years.

"Don't worry about it," one of the residents said.

Not reassured and not taking any chances, I wore a surgical hood for my first case, a kind of OR trapper's hat replete with ear flaps. Now with my mask in place and revealing less of my face than a typical mummy, I tried to make myself invisible as Wallace entered the operating room. After donning his gown and gloves and moving quickly to the table, ignoring a series of "Good morning, Dr. Wallace" salutations, the chief leaned toward me, his head lamp and loupes (magnifying OR lenses) inches from my head, and fumed, "Step away from the table and cover your face! There's no place for a beard if you want to be a surgeon."

An inauspicious beginning.


The British often refer to an operating room as an operating theater. It is part anachronistic description of the old tiered galleries from which young physicians once observed surgical procedures and part apt depiction of a highly choreographed space in which only dramas are staged.

You enter the cardiac OR through a door adjacent to a deep, stainless-steel sink and notice the discarded antiseptic scrub brushes littering the base. When you push through the door, you immediately notice that the room is very bright, and very cold, and filled with a lot of people. At the head of the table, separated from the surgical field by a sterile drape suspended between two poles, is the anesthesiologist who has inserted an endotracheal tube, which protrudes from the patient's mouth like a fat transparent cigar. The tube is mated via lengthy corrugated hose to a large machine that provides a mixture of vaporized anesthesia, nitrous oxide, and oxygen, keeping the patient asleep and ventilated. You gingerly slide next to the anesthesiologist, moving into the small space amid an organized jumble of IV tubing, pressure lines, and a rolling forest of infusion pumps. From this vantage point, the patient's only visible body part is his head, and you watch as the anesthesiologist slips a transesophageal echo probe into the patient's mouth. Unlike the endotracheal tube positioned in the airway, this much longer ultrasound transducer is destined for the esophagus, which lies behind the heart; it provides inside-out surveillance of cardiac function during the operation.

At the table you count four gowned participants. A surgeon's assistant beside one leg has inserted an endoscope under the skin and is working to remove an eighteen-inch-long segment of vein through a one-inch incision below the knee, a bit of magic that eliminates the long scars and swollen legs common to bypass surgery patients a decade ago. A scrub nurse positioned near the waist presides over a broad back table filled with a gleaming menagerie of elegant stainless-steel instruments. Across the room, the perfusionist sits behind the heart-lung machine, its pump temporarily idle. You step onto a small platform and peer over the screen to watch the surgeon and first assistant open the chest with a sternal saw, a pneumatic-powered tool with a jagged reciprocating blade that slices effortlessly through the hard breastbone with a loud and angry growl, reminding you more of wood shop than science lab. An adjustable metal retractor is then wiggled into the breach and the chest is winched open revealing the beating heart still shrouded in its translucent pericardial sac.

In 1896, the English surgeon Stephen Paget published a textbook of thoracic surgery and began the chapter titled "Wounds of the Heart" with the following passage:

> Surgery of the heart has probably reached the limits set by Nature
> to all surgery: no new method, and no new discovery, can overcome
> the natural difficulties that attend a wound of the heart.

Paget's assessment reflects a view universally held by surgeons of his day. Thirty years earlier, during the American Civil War, there were sixty thousand limb amputations but not a single repair of a wound to the heart. From the time of Hippocrates, until the eve of the twentieth century, the heart was thought untouchable.

In September 1896, the same year that Paget's textbook was published, a twenty-two-year-old gardener was taken to the State Hospital in Frankfurt, Germany, after being stabbed over the heart. Two days after admission, the patient's condition deteriorated, prompting an evaluation by Dr. Ludwig Rehn, a prominent surgeon, who diagnosed a rapidly increasing hemothorax (collection of blood in the chest). To determine what was bleeding, Rehn opened the patient's chest and, ominously, found blood exiting from a tear in the pericardial sac. He then took the unusual step of opening the pericardium. As cardiac surgery was thought to be undoable and even an attempt unethical, there was usually little reason to enter the protective fibrous shell that encases the heart. Rehn later noted, "The sight of the heart beating in the opened pericardial sac was extraordinary." A 1.5 centimeter gash in the right ventricle was clearly visible, dark blood pouring from the wound with every cardiac contraction. Knowing that his patient was going to bleed to death, Rehn attempted to close the hole, explaining in his report, "Though one would have liked to have had time to carefully consider the problem, it demanded an immediate solution." Timing his movements to the end of diastole, when the heart rises and briefly pauses after it fills with blood, Rehn succeeded in placing three silk sutures through the right ventricular wall, completely sealing the wound. The patient survived his ordeal after a lengthy hospitalization, becoming the first recipient of successful cardiac surgery.

In a review of Rehn's landmark operation and the cases that followed, published in 1902 in the *Boston Medical and Surgical Journal* (the forerunner to the *New England Journal of Medicine*), Dr. Harry Sherman wrote:

# Bypass

The road to the heart is only 2 or 3 cm in a direct line, but it has taken surgery nearly 2,400 years to travel it . . . During most of this time surgery stood still.

In the years that followed Ludwig Rehn's taboo-breaking first cardiac operation, surgeons around the world became increasingly intrepid, frequently without success, in their attempts to repair a heart stricken with a congenital or acquired malady. All were hindered by a common problem: how do you keep a patient alive while you work on his or her heart?

Early in 1931, Dr. John Heysham Gibbon, a twenty-seven-year-old surgical research fellow at Harvard, watched as a middle-aged woman recovering from gallbladder surgery lost consciousness and died from a massive pulmonary embolus. He later wrote:

During that long night, helplessly watching the patient struggle for life, the idea naturally occurred to me that if it were possible to remove continuously some of the blue blood from the patient's distended veins, put oxygen into that blood and allow carbon dioxide to escape from it, and then inject continuously the now red blood back into the patient's arteries, we might have been able to save her life . . . and performed part of the work of the patient's heart and lungs outside the body.

For Gibbon's idea to work, he would need to devise a method not just to replace the blood pressure–producing left ventricular pump, but also solve the much more complex bioengineering problem of moving oxygen and carbon dioxide into and out of the blood. Eventually Gibbon's epiphany would lead to development of the heart-lung machine, but it would take a quarter-century to achieve as his and other groups vied to be the first to artificially support a patient's circulation during heart surgery.

• • •

In the first half of the twentieth century, there were very few people with more worldwide fame than the legendary aviator Charles Lindbergh. Lindbergh is best known for his landmark transatlantic flight in 1927, but the Medal of Honor winner was also a vocal isolationist, Nazi sympathizer, eugenicist, and inventor. Lindbergh's sister-in-law, Elisabeth Morrow, suffered from mitral stenosis, a narrowing of the mitral valve (the valve that separates the left atrium from the left ventricle) caused by rheumatic fever, which in the 1930s was a fatal disease because there was no way to support a patient long enough to open the heart and repair the valve. Determined to solve the problem, Lindbergh teamed with Dr. Alexis Carrel, a vascular surgeon and Nobel Prize winner (and later also a notorious eugenicist), and jointly they developed an apparatus capable of keeping an organ alive for days. Lindbergh and Carrel appeared together on the June 13, 1938, cover of *Time* magazine with their glass pump, which worked well in the laboratory but was never used clinically in humans.

Dr. C. Walton Lillehei, a surgeon at the University of Minnesota, developed a daring method to support children undergoing congenital heart surgery by connecting the child's circulation to a parent with the same blood type. The idea for this approach came from Lillehei's surgical resident, Dr. Marley Cohen, who noted that his pregnant wife was the oxygenator for their fetus. In Lillehei's "cross-circulation" technique, used in a few dozen patients in the mid-1950s, the child's venous blood was pumped to the parent lying on an adjacent table, whose lungs oxygenated the blood before returning it to an artery in the child. The technique was groundbreaking but not adequate for adult surgery, and there were real risks to the parent. Dr. Willis Potts, surgeon-in-chief at Children's Memorial Hospital in Chicago, referred to it "as the only operation that carried a potential mortality of 200 percent."

In Detroit, Dr. Forest Dodrill, a surgeon at Wayne State University, collaborated with engineers at General Motors Research to develop a mechanical pump capable of supporting the circulation of an adult. The resulting stainless-steel and glass device, the Dodrill-GMR mechanical heart pump, had multiple cylinders from which blood circulated and, perhaps not surprisingly, bore an uncanny resemblance to a Cadillac V-12 automobile engine. The device was intended to temporarily replace either the right or left ventricle and was first used in 1952 to support a patient for fifty minutes while Dr. Dodrill repaired a mitral valve.

Following his patient's death from a pulmonary embolus in 1931, Dr. John Gibbon spent the next twenty-two years working to develop a heart-lung machine at Massachusetts General Hospital, the University of Pennsylvania, and finally Jefferson Medical College in Philadelphia. As early as 1935, Gibbon, working with his wife, Mary, demonstrated the ability of his invention to keep a cat alive, but achieving this in larger animals remained elusive because they could not build an oxygenator large enough to provide sufficient gas exchange. In a human lung, gas exchange occurs in the alveoli, where red blood cells pass through small vessels separated from air by one-cell-thick walls. An adult has almost half a billion alveoli in the two lungs with, collectively, approximately 750 square feet of surface area. A variety of novel approaches to creating an oxygenator were conceived, including one group that used isolated monkey lungs. Gibbon's team finally discovered that creating turbulence in a thin film of blood increased the efficiency of gas exchange, and they could produce this by layering blood over vertical stainless-steel screens suspended in a plastic case infused with oxygen. Gibbon's design, produced with engineering and construction support provided without charge by IBM, was first used in a patient in 1952, but because of an erroneous preoperative diagnosis, the patient died in the operating room.

On May 6, 1953, Dr. Gibbon operated on Cecelia Bavolek, a Wilkes College freshman whose heart was failing because of a congenital hole in the wall separating her right and left atria (referred to as an atrial septal defect). To repair the defect, Gibbon connected the eighteen-year-old patient to his heart-lung machine, which supported her entire circulation for the twenty-six minutes it took him to sew closed the hole in her heart, successfully accomplishing the world's first surgery using cardiopulmonary support. Two months later, Gibbon attempted two more open heart repairs using his machine, but after the death of both children, he abandoned the procedure he pioneered and never again performed heart surgery.

In 1968, in recognition of his remarkable work, Gibbon received the prestigious Albert Lasker Clinical Medical Research Award. The award states:

> Untold numbers of people who would otherwise have remained incapacitated, or died because of previously incurable heart disease, are now living. . . . The vast impact of Dr. Gibbon's discovery on medical science exemplifies the way in which new knowledge, gained from a single research project, can trigger a chain reaction of inquiries leading to additional knowledge, and ultimately to the prevention or cure of human diseases.

Dr. Gibbon died in 1973 at the age of sixty-nine, ironically from a heart attack. At the time of his Lasker Award, he concluded a review of the development of the heart-lung machine with the following prescient passage:

> I would say that unquestionably it has proven its worth and has become a necessity in the armamentarium of the cardiac surgeon. It is used all over the world. It is used in the surgical correction of all congenital defects of the heart. Its employment is necessary for the replacement of diseased valves in the human heart with plastic prostheses. It is essential for the transplantation of the human heart, whatever may be the future of that extraordinary procedure. I believe also that we can look forward to the day it will be used to enable surgeons to replace a hopelessly diseased heart with an intracorporeal blood pump.

• • •

In the 1960s, armed with the ability to operate on a motionless heart and with detailed coronary images now obtainable following Mason Sones's serendipitous discovery a few years earlier, surgeons became increasingly interested in "revascularizing" the heart, providing the muscle with new sources of blood. Early attempts at tunneling a new vessel into the muscle itself, like drip irrigation (referred to as the Vineberg procedure) or slicing open the arteries to peel out the obstructive plaque (endarterectomy), yielded mixed results. By the mid-1960s a new technique to directly suture new blood vessels onto the diseased coronaries, thereby "bypassing" atherosclerotic obstructions, was developing simultaneously in several centers around the world.

Controversy surrounds the question as to who performed the first coronary bypass operation, but two of the earliest were Vasilii Kolesov, a surgeon from St. Petersburg, and Michael DeBakey, from Baylor in Houston, who both performed cases in 1964. When Kolesov published his initial results of coronary artery bypass surgery in the *Journal of Thoracic and Cardiovascular Surgery*, it was accompanied by an editorial warning readers:

> The opinions concerning the management and surgical treatment of angina pectoris as expressed in this paper by Professor VI Kolesov are at variance with the concepts of many surgeons in the United States.

Skepticism about coronary artery bypass graft (CABG) surgery would soon dissipate, and by 1996 the number of CABG operations performed per year in the United States would reach its peak of 190,000.

The beating heart lies suspended in a cradle of pericardium, illuminated in the bright white light of the overhead surgical spots, exposed and vulnerable, inexorably pushing its contents into the aorta with a movement more like the wringing of a towel than the squeezing of a ball. The surgeon inserts hollow cannulas the thickness of a thumb into the aorta and right atrium, ties them securely in place with heavy suture, and couples them to several feet of clear plastic tubing stretching across the room to the heart-lung machine. When clamps are removed, the circuit fills with color as the conduit sewn into the patient's right atrium drains blood back to the heart-lung machine, its four centrifugal pump heads now spinning at 3,500 RPM, every minute transforming eight liters of dark venous blood into its crimson oxygenated form before returning it under pressure into the patient's aorta.

You watch as the heart suddenly stops beating, the intentional result of an injection of a solution appropriately named cardioplegia. The scene in the room is remarkably calm; the players perform with a confident nonchalance born of skill and repetition. Using suture the diameter of a human hair, the surgeon sews to the aorta one end of a segment of the vein harvested from the leg and the other end to a vessel on the surface of the heart, now lying cool and still in the chest. This "bypass" graft is replicated for other regions of the heart, including one in which an artery from the wall of the chest is used as the conduit for new blood flow.

About forty-five minutes later, the "revascularization" is complete, and warm blood is allowed to enter the muscle through the newly constructed pathways. You watch as the dormant heart starts to beat again, its contractions becoming progressively more forceful until the heart-lung machine is no longer needed, the culmination of a procedure twenty-five hundred years in the making.

On August 19, 1988, the day after George Herbert Walker Bush accepted the Republican Party's nomination for president of the United States in the Louisiana Superdome with a speech invoking "a thousand points of light," Dick Cheney was wheeled into an operating room in George Washington University Hospital for heart surgery.

In a March 1989 letter to Senator Sam Nunn, chair of the Armed

# Bypass

Services Committee, Dr. Allan Ross explained his rationale for recommending bypass surgery for Cheney:

> Continued conservative management was contemplated, however follow-up exercise testing demonstrated ischemia (albeit at a respectable treadmill work load). After careful consideration, I advised the Congressman that in my opinion, although bypass surgery was probably not strictly required for longevity purposes (the usual surgical indication), it was advisable, in view of his lifestyle. Specifically, I felt that activities such as high altitude downhill skiing, backpacking, etc., would push him to his physiological limits and would be more safely undertaken if he had the bypass procedure.

Ross did not believe surgery would necessarily improve Cheney's longevity because the artery supplying the front (anterior) wall of Cheney's heart, the left anterior descending (LAD), did not have significant narrowing. Absent a significant blockage in that critical vessel, sometimes indelicately called "the widowmaker," bypass surgery is usually no better than medical therapy in improving survival.

Dr. Benjamin Aaron performed Cheney's surgery. Aaron, who came to GW in 1979 as chief of cardiac and thoracic surgery after spending twenty-two years in the Navy, received international recognition in 1981 when he removed an attempted assassin's bullet from President Ronald Reagan's left lung. The number of surgeons who have operated on a president of the United States is small, and Aaron is the only surgeon to ever operate on both a sitting president and a future vice president.

Cheney's surgery was performed using cardiopulmonary bypass, allowing Aaron to work on a still target. Using a section of saphenous vein removed from Cheney's left lower leg and both internal mammary arteries lying under the chest wall, Aaron performed a quadruple bypass, grafting the right coronary artery (the vessel responsible for the heart attack one month prior), the circumflex branch (the culprit in the

1978 and 1984 heart attacks), and the LAD and diagonal vessels on the front wall of the heart (arteries with only moderate disease). One day following surgery, Cheney was taken off the respirator, the next day he transferred out of the intensive care unit, and he was discharged from the hospital on August 26, 1988, postoperative day seven.

In his March 1989 letter to Senator Nunn, Dr. Ross summarized Cheney's progress.

> His recovery has been excellent and he has been advised to continue unrestricted professional and recreational objectives. Furthermore his formerly significant high cholesterol levels have been completely reversed on medical therapy. His pharmacological regimen is free of any side effects that would affect his judgment or behavior. The Congressman is presently fit to accept any position requiring the highest intellectual behavior and physical performance.

CHAPTER 7

# Post-Op

## VICE PRESIDENT CHENEY

In January 1989, as Congress was reconvening, the House Republican leadership met with President-elect George H. W. Bush. We held regular weekly leadership meetings in room H-227 of the Capitol, but this one was very special because the new president came to the House for that first meeting, a thoughtful gesture by the man we were about to inaugurate as the forty-first president. As the meeting broke up, the president elect, whom I'd first met when he was a young congressman from Texas and I was working for his colleague, Bill Steiger of Wisconsin, twenty years before, took me aside to ask me how my health was. I told him the bypass surgery had gone remarkably well, that I'd had no further problems or complications, and that I'd finished out my year, four months after the surgery, skiing ten thousand feet up in the Rockies. At the time I didn't attribute any special significance to his question. I just thought it was George Bush being George Bush, always thoughtful and considerate of others.

After winning the election, Bush began to put together his cabinet. One of the choices he made was to nominate former senator John Tower of Texas to be secretary of defense. Initially there was a general consensus that Tower could be easily confirmed. For many years, he had served on and been chair of the Senate Armed Services Committee, the committee that would have to approve his confirmation. Furthermore, no senator nominated for a position in the executive branch had ever been denied confirmation by his former colleagues.

But this time would be different. During the confirmation process, questions were raised about Senator Tower's fitness to serve based on reports of womanizing and drinking, and in early March, the Senate voted not to confirm Tower to be secretary of defense. A majority of the members of the Armed Services Committee opposed his nomination.

The Tower vote was scheduled for Thursday, March 9, and that morning before the vote, I received a phone call from John Sununu, President Bush's chief of staff. John asked me to go to the White House after the vote and meet with him and General Brent Scowcroft, the president's national security adviser, to discuss what the administration's next move should be. I agreed to the meeting, assuming they wanted to consult with me because I had previously been in their situation, recruiting cabinet members for President Ford, and because I was a senior member of the congressional leadership.

We met in Sununu's office, the same one I had during the Ford administration twelve years before. They began by asking if I had any recommendation for someone to serve as secretary of defense. I offered a recommendation, which was quickly rejected. Then Brent said, "What about you? Would you consider taking the job?" This was not a question I had expected. After a general discussion of the subject, I indicated I would have to think about it and discuss it with my family. We agreed that if I decided I wanted to pursue the matter further, I would call John the next morning and he would arrange for me to talk directly with the president.

That evening at home as Lynne and I discussed the possibility of my becoming secretary of defense, I received a phone call from my old friend Jim Baker who had just been tapped for secretary of state. Jim urged me to accept the defense job and indicated he had recommended me. I must admit I was intrigued with the proposition. I had an abiding interest in national security issues. I had held George Bush in high regard since I first met him in 1969 and believed he was going to be a good president. Jim, Brent, and I had been friends since we had all worked together for President Ford, and I liked the idea of the three of us working together in the top national security positions in the new administration. On the downside, if I accepted the post, it would most likely mean the end of my career in elective office. I had devoted the previous ten years to working my way up to the number-two position in the House GOP leadership and could look forward to becoming the leader when Bob Michel retired. But the job of secretary of defense was enormously important to the nation and very attractive in its own right. I would be responsible for some four million men and women: two million active duty, one million reservists, and one million civilians. I would be second to the president in the chain of command if we were called on to use force. As secretary I would be responsible for overseeing a larger portion of the intelligence community than the director of the Central Intelligence Agency. As a statutory member of the National Security Council, I would be involved in all of the major national security issues of the time.

I decided that Thursday evening that I was definitely interested in taking the next step, and on Friday morning I called Sununu. We agreed that I would meet the president at noon in the family quarters of the White House.

Our meeting was held in the president's private office on the second floor of the residence, where the cabinet used to meet before the West Wing was built. As I walked in I noticed the famous painting on the wall. It's called *The Peacemakers*, and it shows President Lincoln meeting with General Ulysses S. Grant, General William Tecumseh Sherman, and Admiral David Porter at City Point, Virginia, just before the end of the Civil War. My great-grandfather, Samuel Fletcher Cheney, had served throughout the war as a captain in the Twenty-First Ohio, a volunteer infantry regiment. In 1864–1865 he had served under General Sherman and been with him in the siege of Atlanta and on the March to the Sea. In May 1865, after the war ended, he had marched in the Grand Review, a great military parade in Washington. I wondered to myself what he would have thought about his great-grandson meeting in the White House with the president to discuss becoming secretary of defense.

After the president greeted me warmly, we covered a wide range of topics, including his priorities for the Defense Department. We talked about procurement reform, Central America, arms control issues, and the Soviets. I wanted to make sure he knew about my misspent youth. I had flunked out of Yale twice and twice been arrested for driving under the influence in my early twenties. I had the impression that he already knew about these episodes. He assured me he did not believe they would create any problem for my confirmation. (The FBI had known about them before I was cleared to work at the White House in the Nixon and Ford administrations.)

One subject that didn't come up was my health. It had occurred to me by now that George Bush's question in January about how I was doing may have had a motive I didn't suspect at the time. He was already thinking of me for the Defense Department, and by way of friendly inquiry at the GOP leadership meeting had satisfied himself that I was up to the job.

Scowcroft and Sununu joined us for the latter part of the meeting, and then I returned to my office on Capitol Hill. Less than an hour later, the president called and offered me the defense position, and I readily accepted. That afternoon we announced the nomination from the White House briefing room.

The entire process of confirmation from announcement to final vote in the Senate took only one week, near record time, from March 10 to 17. The hearing before the Senate Armed Services Committee was warm and friendly. I was introduced by my colleagues from Wyoming, Senators Alan Simpson and Malcolm Wallop. I had worked with many of the members over the years when I was at the White House and in Congress. The chairman, Sam Nunn of Georgia, arranged to have my misspent youth discussed in closed session. Senator John Glenn of Ohio asked how I had been able to "clean up my act" as a young man, and I explained that I had gotten married and given up hanging out in bars.

The committee was interested in the status of my health. My cardiologist, Dr. Allan Ross, submitted a letter to the committee summarizing my history of coronary artery disease. He wrote that I had undergone successful coronary bypass surgery in August 1988 and that my high cholesterol level had been successfully treated with lovastatin, a new cholesterol-lowering drug. He reported that I had "no functional limitations whatsoever, and a prognosis not substantially different from men of the same age group without such a previous cardiologic history." He added, "Finally and additionally, he takes no medication which should be expected to influence his mood or intellectual performance. I see no medical reason for him not to perform well in the highest and most sensitive of public offices." Both the Armed Services Committee and the entire Senate voted unanimously to confirm my nomination to be the seventeenth secretary of defense.

Of all the jobs I've held, if I had to choose just one as my favorite I would have to say secretary of defense. There are several reasons that my time at Defense stands out in memory. The US military is one of the finest institutions in the world, and it was a very special privilege to lead it from 1989 to 1993 as the Soviet Union collapsed, the Cold War ended, and we rolled back Saddam Hussein's aggression in the Persian Gulf. If I were asked to design a commander in chief for that set of circumstances, he would look a lot like George H. W. Bush: combat veteran from World War II, director of the CIA, ambassador to China and the UN, and vice president. He was a great boss. He made clear what he expected, set clear objectives, then trusted the members of his national security team to get the job done. When one of us had to make a tough or controversial decision, he would give his complete support and never second-guess. I feel proud and privileged to have been a part of his national security team.

I am certain that everyone who ever served as secretary of defense will tell you that his time at the Pentagon was special, but the period from 1989 to 1993 was undeniably so because of all that we had to deal with as the Cold War ended. The president had to manage a very delicate situation with the Soviet Union as the Berlin Wall came down, Russian forces withdrew from Eastern Europe, Germany was reunified, the Soviet Union imploded, and there was an attempted coup in Moscow.

All of these developments had major ramifications for the Defense Department and the US military. The liberation of Eastern Europe led to a surge of interest from nations that once belonged to the old Warsaw Pact in joining NATO. At the same time, the commitment the United States had maintained throughout the Cold War, to have ten divisions deployed in Western Europe within ten days of a decision by NATO to mobilize against a Soviet invasion, was no longer necessary. For decades we had maintained several army divisions forward-deployed in Europe and more at home ready to deploy. We now were able to plan to reduce our overall force structure by 25 percent, which included cutting the army from eighteen to twelve active divisions and closing a number of bases at home and abroad. After a complete review of our nuclear inventory and strategy within the Department of Defense, we enabled the president to take the initiative to put forth bold proposals to reduce our tactical and strategic nuclear forces, which President Mikhail Gorbachev and the Russians then matched.

The rapidly changing circumstances also required dramatic new thinking about our national security strategy. We shifted from focusing on having to fight an all-out global war with the Soviets to a strategy of being able to defend the regions of the world where vital US interests were at stake. We also needed to maintain the quality force we had inherited from the Reagan administration, in terms of both personnel and equipment. At the same time, we had to persuade the Congress that while budget cuts were in order, they had to be done in a manner that wouldn't do long-term damage to our military capabilities. The Congress had to be persuaded to avoid a meat-axe approach that would sacrifice essential items; their thinking was sometimes driven more by political considerations than military requirements.

In the midst of all these changes in our strategic situation, Saddam Hussein, president of Iraq, invaded Kuwait in early August 1990. With little notice and within a matter of hours, Iraqi forces swallowed up Kuwait and were poised on the border between that country and Saudi Arabia. If Saddam continued south and occupied the eastern portion of the Saudi Kingdom, he would control a significant percentage of the world's oil production and reserves. Saudi Arabia and many of the other Gulf countries looked to the United States as the guarantor of their security. The Iraqi aggression generated the first major crisis in the post–Cold War world and placed significant demands on President Bush and his national security team.

On the first weekend of the crisis, the National Security Council met at Camp David to review our options, including a review with senior officers of our capabilities if we found it necessary to use military force. That Sunday, the president sent me to Saudi Arabia and Egypt to consult with King Fahd and President Mubarak and to seek from them permission to begin deploying US forces to the region. King Fahd agreed to our use of bases in the kingdom but wanted a commitment that we would send enough forces to do the job and that we would leave when it was over, which I gave him. I called the president afterward, and he authorized me to begin the deployment of a force that eventually exceeded five hundred thousand troops. President Mubarak agreed to grant us overflight rights and approved sending our nuclear-powered aircraft carriers through the Suez Canal. Mubarak was very angry with Saddam and volunteered to send two Egyptian divisions to serve alongside the Americans. With the leadership of President Bush, the enormous capability of our military, and support at home and abroad, Operation Desert Storm was a great success.


The period from August 1990 to March 1991 was one of the most intense of my career. It was a special privilege to be part of the Bush national security team and to be responsible for the men and women of the US military. They were superb. From the standpoint of my health, these years marked a period that was relatively trouble free. I am sometimes tempted to call them the "golden years," when my medical condition had significantly improved as a result of my quadruple bypass and the availability of cholesterol-lowering drugs.

I left the Defense Department in January 1993 and the following summer took an eight-thousand-mile road trip. The ultimate objective was to meet some friends for a week of fly-fishing for steelhead on a remote section of the Dean River in British Columbia. En route, I stopped for speeches in West Virginia, Ohio, Colorado, and Wyoming. For the first time in a long time I was alone—no staff and no security. And I was driving.

I had a lot of time to think about what I wanted to do with the rest of my life and particularly about running for president. By then, I had worked for three presidents—Nixon, Ford, and George H. W. Bush—and watched a fourth, Reagan, up close as part of the House Republican leadership team for eight years. I had served as White House chief of staff and done well in one of the toughest and most difficult assignments as secretary of defense in wartime. I believed I knew what was needed in a president and that I had the experience and knowledge to do the job well.

As secretary of defense, I had not been in a position to be active politically. By tradition, the defense secretary stays away from partisan political activities. I made a decision as I returned to private life that I wanted to get involved in the 1993–1994 election cycle. As a midterm election and because of a lot of good work building the party, 1994 looked like a potentially good year for congressional Republicans.

In an effort to help the cause, I participated in approximately 150 campaign-related events around the country in that cycle. I also took advantage of the opportunity to test the waters to ascertain whether I should run for president in 1996. I established a political action committee (PAC) to finance my travels and contribute to a select number of candidates. David Addington and Patty Howe, who had previously worked on my staff at the Pentagon and in Congress, signed on to run the PAC.

The year 1994 turned out to be a great one for the GOP. We took back control of the House of Representatives for the first time in forty years, and Newt Gingrich, who succeeded me as GOP whip when I left to take over the Defense Department, was elected Speaker of the House.

At the end of 1994, our family gathered for Christmas as we always did at our home in Jackson Hole. We spent time that holiday discussing the topic of my possible candidacy for president in 1996. In the end, I decided not to run.

While I liked the idea of being president, I didn't like what would be involved in running. I did not relish the idea of the significant amount of time I'd have to devote to fund-raising. I also didn't like the loss of privacy that would be involved for my family and me. And of course my heart disease factored in. While I had experienced no heart incidents since my bypass surgery six years earlier and believed there was no limit on my physical ability to do the job, I was concerned that my history of heart disease could become an issue in the campaign. If that occurred—if I were perceived as having lost as a result of my health—I would be permanently labeled as "the guy with the bad heart." That could severely limit my future possibilities.

I was fifty-three years old and had had a great twenty-five years in public life. I was still young enough to have a second career in the business world. So as 1995 began, I announced that I had decided not to be a candidate for president in 1996.

When I left the Defense Department in 1993, I went on the lecture circuit, making speeches across the country, and I joined a number of corporate boards. I became a director of Union Pacific, Morgan Stanley, Procter & Gamble, and US West. Having spent most of my career in academia and government, service on the boards of some of the most important and successful companies in America gave me a whole new perspective on our economy and the private sector.

In January 1993, as we were making the transition from the Bush to the Clinton administration, our daughter Liz was married to Phil Perry in Wyoming. Lynne and I took advantage of the opportunity to make a down payment on a home in Jackson Hole, our favorite part of the world and part of my old congressional district. We planned to live in Jackson full-time and enjoy private life. There was no better place to pursue two of my favorite activities, skiing and fly-fishing, and I could travel from there to fulfill my speaking commitments and board responsibilities.

But within a few years, our plans took a detour. In September 1994, I was invited to join a group of men for a trip to a salmon camp on the Miramichi River in New Brunswick, Canada. One of the eight fishermen there was Tom Cruikshank, then chairman and CEO of Halliburton, a Fortune 500 company and one of the largest energy services and engineering and construction companies in the world. Some months later, I received a phone call from Tom indicating that he was preparing to retire and that after an extensive search for a replacement, the company hadn't yet found anyone. He wanted to know if I would consider becoming Halliburton's CEO. I agreed to fly to Dallas to meet with the board of directors and explore the possibility. In August 1995, we announced that I would begin full-time with the company on October 1 and after a ninety-day transition period would become chairman and CEO on the first of January 1996.

When the Halliburton board recruited me, I made it clear that I had no further political aspirations. I'd had a great twenty-five years in public office and had no desire to return. I was committed to spending the remainder of my working career at Halliburton, which was a great company. In 1996, it had 100,000 employees operating in 130 countries around the world. We built offshore oil platforms in the North Sea and the Gulf of Mexico and provided energy services to major oil companies worldwide. We built a new baseball stadium for the Astros in Houston and a railroad across the Australian Outback from Alice Springs to Darwin. I had put public life behind me.

My mother had died in 1993 of a stroke after nearly ten years of battling Parkinson's disease. She had refused to give in to the Parkinson's, insisting on doing all the things she had always done, including cooking for my dad. When she began falling occasionally, she started wearing knee pads, like a basketball player, so that when she fell, she could land on her knees and get right up and keep on working.

During my time at Halliburton, my father, who was living in an assisted living care facility in Casper, died. He was still able to get around unassisted and drive his own car, although he was increasingly display-ing the symptoms of congestive heart failure. Periodically he would ac-cumulate excess fluid in his body and would then enter the hospital for a few days so they could administer doses of Lasix intravenously and "dry him out."

He had begun to get his affairs in order. He "had his sale," an old Nebraska saying for getting rid of all the items accumulated over a life-time. First, he told my sister, Susan; my brother, Bob; and me to take anything we might want, and then he brought in someone to run the sale. Early on the day of the sale, my sister found him sitting alone in the garage, among the belongings of his lifetime, with tears streaming down his face. I had never seen my dad cry, but coming to terms with the end of his life was understandably overwhelming.

I had told him not to worry about his sale—that we would take care of everything at the appropriate time. But he was determined to take care of it himself. After the sale was over, he put the house on the market and sold it.

A few days after Dad's sale, I was back in Dallas on a Saturday when I decided to call him. He had checked back into the hospital for another round of "drying out." When I called, I got a busy signal. At that same moment, we later discovered, my brother and sister also tried to call him. Bob also got a busy signal, but Susan got through. Later that afternoon, I received a call from the hospital in Casper telling me that Dad had died shortly after Sue talked to him.

As the family gathered in Casper for the funeral, I thought about the last time Dad and I had been together. A few weeks before his death, I'd been in Casper closing up a house Lynne and I had owned and rented out for many years to the parents of some friends. As I was packing up to close down and sell the house, Dad appeared. He had driven over to spend some time with me while I worked. Dad was not someone who engaged in idle chatter, but that afternoon we talked for nearly two hours.

Among other things, we talked about the fact that Congress had passed legislation naming the federal building in Casper after me. He liked knowing that the building where he had worked for many years as the state administrative officer for the Soil Conservation Service was to be named after his son, probably especially because his name was also Dick Cheney. He didn't live long enough to be there for the formal ceremony, but he took pride in knowing it was going to happen.

As he left that afternoon, I walked him across the street to his car, an old Buick. Dad never bought a new car in his life, no matter how much money he had. He said you could get a perfectly good car without paying for a new one. Until the day he died, he was saving money every month of his life, a habit he acquired when he saw the pain his parents lived through during the Depression.

When Dad died, I was fifty-eight. I had already survived three heart attacks and quadruple bypass surgery. Since that surgery in 1988, I had lived trouble free for more than a decade, and two things made me optimistic that I had a lot of years ahead. First, my dad had lived to be almost eighty-four, despite having serious coronary artery disease. Second, I had already been the beneficiary of amazing medical advances and was hopeful there would be more ahead.

## CHAPTER 8

# Fitness to Serve

## VICE PRESIDENT CHENEY

In fall 1999, Lynne and I hosted a fund-raiser at our home in Dallas for the literacy program sponsored by Barbara Bush. George W. Bush, governor of Texas, attended and during the evening asked if there were some place where we could talk privately. I took him into the library and closed the door. He asked me if I would be willing to take on a major role in his campaign for the presidency. I supported Bush and was prepared to do what I could to help him get elected, but I also had a full-time commitment to Halliburton and a significant position in the campaign simply wasn't possible.

A few months later, once the primary campaign had gotten under-way, Joe Allbaugh, one of the governor's top aides, came to see me in my office in Dallas and asked if I would be willing to be considered as a candidate for vice president. I said no; I was not interested. I told Joe that I thought I was a bad choice from the campaign's standpoint. My home state of Wyoming is one of the most Republican in the country and has only three electoral votes. I told Joe that if Governor Bush couldn't carry Wyoming without me on the ticket, they had bigger problems. I made the point that because I was in the oil business and Governor Bush had previously been in the oil business, a Bush-Cheney ticket would be a ripe target for the Democrats. I also pointed out that I had a history of coronary artery disease—three heart attacks and qua-druple bypass surgery. Joe didn't argue with me. He took my answers on board and reported back to the governor.

What I didn't tell Joe, because I wanted to be polite, was that I had absolutely no interest in being vice president; I thought it was a terrible job. President Ford had told me on more than one occasion that the eight months he spent as vice president were the worst months of his life. I knew from personal experience that Nelson Rockefeller hated the job. The city of Washington is full of people telling stories about the irrelevance of the post. The only reason to take the job is to run for president, and I had decided not to do that several years before. Finally, I was very happy as chairman and CEO of Halliburton, and it paid a lot better than government work.

A few days after Joe's visit, Governor Bush called me directly and asked if I would help him find a vice-presidential candidate. I readily agreed. It was an important assignment, and it was something I had done before for President Ford in 1976. It was also a short-term commitment that would not last beyond the national convention. I would not have to leave Halliburton to do it.

I pulled together a small team of key people to help review and screen the potential candidates. I had learned over the years that while there are a great many who want to be vice president, only a few meet the very high standards to qualify. First and foremost, the individual has to be capable of serving as president if something happens to the incumbent. Second, the candidate has to add to the overall political attractiveness of the ticket. Third, you want to avoid the train wreck of picking someone whose background or personal life contains embarrassing episodes or information.

The first list we put together numbered twenty-five or thirty prospects. We prepared and sent out a detailed form asking for a wide range of information from those still on the list after I had personally contacted each one. Not everyone wanted to be considered. One potential candidate threatened never to speak to me again if I put his name on the list. There were a couple of people not on the list who contacted me seeking to be included. They explained that they had tough reelection campaigns and it would help them back home in their districts if word got around that they were under consideration. I promptly put them on the list.

We put together a file on each candidate who was seriously under consideration. We promised to maintain the confidentiality of their submissions, and when the process was complete, we returned all the materials they had submitted. As we went through this process, the list grew shorter. I personally interviewed a number of candidates. Throughout the process, I kept in regular contact with the governor. For each of our sessions, we prepared two notebooks, one for each of us—and he returned his to me when we finished.

On July 2, 2000, I went to the Bush ranch in Crawford, Texas, for a final meeting. We spent the morning reviewing the remaining candidates, a much shorter list than we had started with. Then Laura joined us for lunch. Afterward, the governor took me out on the back porch for some further conversation. It was a typical Texas July day, with the temperature well over 100 degrees. He looked me in the eye and said, "You know, you're the solution to my problem."

At that moment, it occurred to me that he had never accepted my "no" when Joe Allbaugh had asked if I was willing to be considered for vice president some months before. And I must admit that going through the search with him had a significant impact on me. I had seen up close how much time he had devoted to selecting a running mate. He had given a great deal of thought to what he wanted in a vice president. He wasn't making a conventional choice in terms of the Electoral College, or the GOP, or the expected impact on the popular vote. He had emphasized repeatedly to me that he wanted his vice president to be an important part of his team, someone who could help govern.

He had worked my "no" around to a tentative "yes." I told him I would consider it. I said I would see what I would have to do if he were to select me. I had obligations to Halliburton and would have to have a conversation with my directors.

I would also have to switch my voter registration from Texas to

Wyoming. Under the Twelfth Amendment to the Constitution, the electoral votes of a state cannot be cast for a president and vice president from the same state.

There was also the matter of my medical history. We would need to satisfy ourselves that there was no health problem that would prevent me from running or serving.

Finally, I emphasized that I had not been vetted in the conventional sense and that I needed a day when I could meet with him and lay out all the reasons I wasn't the right choice.

A few days later, I flew down to Austin and met with Governor Bush and campaign strategist Karl Rove at the mansion. We discussed the vice presidency, and Karl and I made essentially the same arguments against my candidacy, pointing out that I was not a good choice from a political standpoint. I underscored my misspent youth just as I had done with his father ten years before when I was under consideration for secretary of defense. I repeated that I had twice been kicked out of Yale and twice arrested for driving under the influence in my early twenties.

Finally, I focused on my history of coronary artery disease. I told him that I had to be aware at all times of my heart condition and that if I ever felt so much as a twinge, I would have to have it checked out immediately to determine whether I was having another heart attack. I said if it happened in the middle of the vice-presidential debate, I wouldn't delay until the debate was over. I would, without hesitation, seek the nearest emergency room for the appropriate tests. The governor took all this in, and we arranged to have his physician, Dr. Denton Cooley, talk to my cardiologist, Jonathan Reiner, about my fitness to run and serve as vice president.

It soon became clear that Rove and I hadn't been very persuasive. I received a call from the governor telling me that Dr. Cooley had reviewed my medical situation with Dr. Reiner and concluded that there was no health reason that I couldn't run for and serve as vice president. A few days later the governor posed the question formally, asking me in an early-morning call to be his running mate as the GOP candidate for vice president of the United States. That afternoon, Lynne, Liz, and I flew to Austin, and George Bush announced me as his choice for vice president on the GOP ticket.

I have never regretted my decision to accept his offer. I had been able to think of many reasons that it wasn't a good idea, but in the end, there were two basic considerations that I found persuasive. First, I fit the profile of what he was looking for in a running mate because of my previous experience, especially in national security matters. Second, I was persuaded it would be a consequential vice presidency. He made it clear I would be an important part of his team, not just a typical vice president relegated to attending funerals and fund-raisers. President Bush kept his word throughout our eight years in the White House. He did not always follow my advice, but he always gave me an opportunity to tell him what I thought on important issues. I was able to play a significant role because that is what he wanted.

Some of my critics have suggested that I "manipulated the process" to get selected as vice president. That proposition is simply not supported by the facts. If I had wanted to be vice president, all I had to do was say "yes" the first time it came up with Joe Allbaugh.

In the end, I agreed to become vice president because George Bush persuaded me I was what he was looking for and that my experience would be a valued addition to this ticket. When you are asked to do something on behalf of the country, you have an obligation to try to do it. Looking back now some thirteen years after I made that decision, I am deeply grateful for the opportunity I had to serve during those difficult and challenging years. And I owe President George W. Bush a deep debt of gratitude for having made that possible.

## DR. REINER

The pink "While You Were Away" note said simply, "Dick Cheney called."

A little annoyed to discover the message so late in the day, I asked my assistant, Yaa Oforiwaa, why she didn't page me when Cheney called hours earlier.

"He didn't want to bother you," she said.

For many years, Cheney's cardiologist had been Dr. Allan Ross, an internationally renowned clinician and researcher. Allan was chief of cardiology at GW when I began my fellowship in 1990, and he quickly became a mentor. Allan brought me into his research group when I was a first-year fellow and later, when I completed my training, he gave me a job. After Allan's retirement in 1998, Cheney's internist, Gary Malakoff, asked if I would assume Cheney's care. Gary told me that Secretary Cheney was now CEO of Halliburton, a Dallas-based company, but he still came to Washington periodically for checkups. I had met Cheney a few years earlier when he came in for a catheterization, and I told Gary I would be happy to see him.

Mr. Cheney's most recent clinic visit was in November 1999, at which time he seemed to be doing pretty well. In spring 2000, Cheney had been in the news a lot. He was vetting potential vice-presidential running mates for Governor Bush, and the press was speculating that an announcement was going to be made soon. The Veep sweepstakes is a quadrennial DC obsession, and the spotlight at the time seemed to be focusing on Pennsylvania governor Tom Ridge.

Yaa told me that Mr. Cheney needed to schedule a clinic appointment in the next week or so, but he wanted to have a stress test first.

*Why does Cheney need a stress test now?* I wondered.

I walked over to the clinic and tracked down Gary and asked him if Cheney was feeling all right. Gary told me that as far as he knew, everything was okay.

"Gary," I said, "I think Cheney is going to run for vice president!"


Stress testing has been used for decades as a noninvasive way to assess the adequacy of the heart's blood supply and is based on a fairly simple principle. Progressively vigorous exercise, usually walking on a treadmill with increasing pace and incline, results in a rise in blood pressure and pulse, and consequently increases the work required of the heart. If the blood supply to the myocardium is intact and unimpeded, the continuously monitored EKG reveals only a faster heart rate. If a coronary artery contains a narrowing restricting blood flow, characteristic changes are often evident in the EKG tracing and patients may also develop chest pain. Ironically, this abnormal result is called a "positive" test (positive for whom?) whereas a normal result is referred to as "negative."

If a patient has had a prior heart attack or has an otherwise abnormal baseline EKG, a standard stress test can be difficult to interpret, and myocardial perfusion imaging is often performed instead. At the outset of this procedure, commonly called a nuclear stress test, patients are injected intravenously with either the radioactive isotope thallium-201 or technetium-99m, agents that are avidly absorbed by the heart as long as the muscle is alive and the blood supply to it is unobstructed. Images of the heart are acquired while the patient lies under a gamma camera, essentially a digital detector of radioactive particles, a technology that was invented in the 1940s during work on the Manhattan Project. The patient then exercises, is injected with a second dose of radioisotope, and again is imaged under the camera. The entire process takes about two hours.

Normal heart muscle absorbs the tracer homogeneously, which the computer displays as color-enhanced, cross-sectional silhouettes, and the pictures at peak exercise should be similar to those obtained at baseline. If there is a blockage in one or more of the coronary arteries or the patient has had a prior heart attack, a defect is apparent in the digital images. A nuclear stress test is more sensitive and specific for detecting the presence of coronary disease than is a regular stress test, raising the precision of the exam. It does, however, expose the patient to a significant amount of radiation, about the same as a CT scan, equivalent to about 850 chest X-rays, enough to set off the radiation detectors at federal buildings like the White House. Still, for patients with a prior heart attack, known complex coronary disease, or women in whom the false-positive rate for a regular stress test is quite high, nuclear imaging, can be quite useful.

Dick Cheney arrived unaccompanied for his stress test at George Washington University Hospital on July 11, 2000. He was able to exercise for nine minutes on the treadmill (about average for a fifty-nine-year-old man) and had no chest pain. Not bad. The nuclear images, however, were a mixed bag. While the test was unchanged compared to the prior year's exam, with no signs of new ischemia, there was clearly evidence of significant damage from the old heart attacks involving both the lateral and inferior walls of the heart. Overall it was a stable but definitely abnormal test.

The next day, I stopped by Cheney's internist's office, and together Gary Malakoff and I walked over to the clinic to see Cheney. After brief pleasantries, Cheney almost matter-of-factly said, "It looks like I may be asked to run for vice president."

I think Gary might have actually said, "Oh my God!" but I forced myself to channel some of Cheney's preternatural calmness and tried to act as if patients tell me that all the time.

"What will you be able to say about my health?" Cheney asked.

I began by reviewing the results from the stress test and echocardiogram. I told Cheney that although the two studies clearly showed impairment of his cardiac function, a consequence of his three heart attacks, the results appeared to be stable when compared to tests performed a year earlier. It was a good sign that Cheney continued to lead an energetic life, with a very demanding job, and was able to ski at high altitudes and hunt, reassuringly without signs of clinical heart failure. I told Mr. Cheney that I felt his cardiovascular status was sufficient for what I could only imagine would be a remarkably fatiguing and stressful job, but although I thought he would do well, there was obviously no way I could predict the future. Cheney never really asked whether we thought he was physically fit to be vice president. I don't think he intended the meeting to be the political version of preoperative clearance. He simply wanted to know what we would be able to say. Before leaving, Cheney asked us to keep the news confidential until an announcement was made and told us that at some point, Gary and I would need to put together something in writing. At no time did he try to suggest what we would or wouldn't be able to talk about.

Five days later, on Monday, July 17, my assistant Yaa called the cath lab to tell me there was a Dr. Cooley on the phone from Texas.

"Dr. Denton Cooley?" I asked.

"Yes, Denton Cooley."

I didn't know Dr. Cooley personally, but I certainly knew who he was. Dr. Cooley was one of the pioneers of cardiovascular surgery, and at eighty years old, he was still one of the world's preeminent heart surgeons. Cooley's career had been filled with legendary accomplishments. He was the founder of the Texas Heart Institute and its chief surgeon, and in 1968, he performed the first successful heart transplant in the United States. The following year, he implanted the world's first total artificial heart, a gutsy attempt to save the life of a dying forty-seven-year-old man using an untested and unapproved device. In 1984, President Ronald Reagan presented Dr. Cooley with the Medal of Freedom, the nation's highest civilian award.

"Do you know what he wants to talk about?" I asked.

"He didn't say, but Dick Cheney called earlier and said it was okay for you to speak to him."

I moved to a phone where I could talk in private and called Dr. Cooley in Houston. He was cordial but got right to the point. He told me that Governor Bush had asked him to review Dick Cheney's medical history, and Cooley asked me to summarize it for him. After a quick, slightly uncomfortable flashback to medical school and my first day on cardiac surgery, I launched into a long, detailed, and comprehensive review of Cheney's history.

I told Dr. Cooley about Cheney's three prior heart attacks, the first at age thirty-seven and the most recent twelve years before, in 1988.

I discussed Allan Ross's decision to send then Congressman Cheney for coronary artery bypass surgery and the details of the operation performed by Dr. Aaron. Following surgery, Cheney had undergone cardiac catheterization twice in the 1990s, both of which I had participated in, revealing that two of his bypass grafts had closed. One of these grafts, the left internal mammary, was not functioning, likely because all of the blood flow to the front of the heart was going through the relatively little diseased, "native" left anterior descending coronary artery that the graft was intended to bypass. The second graft undoubtedly had failed because Aaron had attempted to bypass the artery that caused the 1984 heart attack, which he described in his op-note as an "unfilled, unused, and atrophied vessel." I went on to review the results of Cheney's recent stress test and echocardiograms and his lack of symptoms or congestive heart failure. After I had spoken uninterrupted for several minutes, Dr. Cooley asked me if Cheney was ever in cardiogenic shock.

Cardiogenic shock is a critical condition defined as the inability of the heart to provide the bare minimum amount of blood necessary for organ function. If it is not quickly rectified, death usually follows.

"No, sir," I replied.

"Well, then, I will call and reassure the governor," Cooley said, thanking me for my time before ending the call.

Governor Bush later said, "Dick had talked to his doctor and then I got Denton Cooley to call Dick's doctor to discuss the record, and I talked to Dick extensively about his health." Mr. Bush went on to say that when Dr. Denton Cooley told him Mr. Cheney "was suited to be the vice president, I felt that was good enough for me."

Later that day, I wrote a letter to Gary Malakoff that reviewed the events of the prior week and summarized what I thought about Dick Cheney's cardiovascular fitness to serve as vice president of the United States. I concluded the letter in this way:

Today I spoke with Dr. Denton Cooley after this was requested by Mr. Cheney. I reviewed Mr. Cheney's medical history essentially as

I outlined it to you above. Later I spoke with Mr. Cheney. During that conversation I clearly reviewed what I consider to be key elements of his cardiovascular status; that his heart shows the effects of at least 2 prior MI's, that his left ventricular performance is impaired but he has no symptoms c/w CHF [congestive heart failure] and has no angina. I stated that his risk of an adverse event is higher than a person of similar age without heart disease but that his short-term and long-term risk is not quantifiable. I also mentioned that his current vigorous lifestyle is in many ways very reassuring.

On July 25, 2000, the day that the Bush campaign announced that Dick Cheney was the governor's pick for vice president, Dr. Cooley released a statement from Houston in which he said, "In a recent checkup by Dr. Jonathan Reiner, he declared that Mr. Cheney is in good health with normal cardiac function."

While I did believe that overall Dick Cheney was in good health and I thought his cardiac history would not interfere with the duties of vice president, I knew that his heart function hadn't been normal in twenty-two years, and I had explained that to Dr. Cooley.

The newspapers and cable news outlets soon filled with uninvolved and uninformed medical pundits opining about Dick Cheney's chances of surviving his time in office. Without either a physical exam or record review, the *New York Times's* Lawrence K. Altman actually calculated the candidate's odds:

> Mr. Cheney's statistical chances of survival for the next five years are 94 percent, slightly lower than for Americans without heart disease, according to figures that a Duke University cardiologist, Dr. Eric Peterson, calculated by comparing Mr. Cheney's medical profile with those of other patients in a national registry of bypass operations kept at Duke.

*USA Today* quoted Dr. Lawrence Cohn, of Brigham and Women's Hospital in Boston, as saying that "if Cheney has scrupulously taken his medicine, watched his diet and exercised, 'he's golden.' " Other experts offered less rosy pronouncements. In the *New York Daily News*, Dr. Stephen Siegel, a cardiologist at NYU Medical Center, said, "Atherosclerosis is like incurable cancer—it's a disease you control, not cure." Craig Smith, chief of cardiothoracic surgery at New York-Presbyterian Medical Center in New York City, said, "The negatives are that he had early onset of coronary disease, which makes him more prone to have a recurrence."

Sometimes the determination of whether a patient is medically fit for a job is easy. Consider the case of a commercial pilot who came to see me several years ago after he began to have chest pain. The patient was an experienced 747 captain who flew long-haul, trans-Pacific routes for a major airline and had flown as recently as a few days before his clinic appointment. Because pilots fear being grounded, they tend to be notorious doctor-phobes, a fact that made this patient's visit all the more concerning. I ordered a stress test, which was grossly abnormal, and the cardiac catheterization that followed a few days later identified severe coronary disease. When we finished the procedure, I put a hand on the pilot's shoulder and told him I thought he was a very lucky guy, having dodged a huge bullet. Imagine developing a heart attack while strapped into the cockpit of a jumbo jet traveling at 550 miles per hour 38,000 feet over the Pacific Ocean or, worse, losing consciousness on final approach with 450 souls in the seats behind you. The good news was that his heart could be fixed, and I was confident he would do very well. The bad news was that because he was going to need bypass surgery, his days as an airline pilot were over. Federal aviation regulations disqualify pilots with angina, significant coronary disease, or a history of myocardial infarction and it would be difficult for him to regain his flight certificate. I told him that I was very sorry that he wasn't going to be able to fly, projecting how I would feel if I could no longer practice medicine. He told me not to worry; he was close to retirement and he would be fine.

I've been asked to clear Secret Service and FBI agents before they return to duty, foreign service officers prior to their overseas postings, as well as tour bus drivers, US marshals, and police officers; each of these occupations has well-codified health requirements. You can't get a driver's license if your vision is poor, enter the military if you fail the physical, or get security clearance without a background check. There are, however, no established medical fitness criteria for candidates for president or vice president of the United States.

On March 4, 1841, William Henry Harrison became the nation's ninth president, but his time in office would be very brief, ending only thirty-two days after his inauguration when he died after developing pneumonia. Following Harrison's death, Vice President John Tyler assumed the presidency, invoking for the first time in American history Article II, section 1 of the US Constitution, which states:

> In Case of the Removal of the President from Office, or of his
> Death, Resignation, or Inability to discharge the Powers and Duties
> of the said Office, the same shall devolve on the vice president . . .

Because eight of the thirty-seven vice presidents who followed Tyler were eventually elevated to the presidency, the essential medical qualification of a vice president is undoubtedly fitness to be president. How medical fitness is defined, who gets to define it, and how much the public has a right to know are more difficult questions.

During the 1960 presidential primaries, rumors began to circulate that Senator John F. Kennedy had Addison's disease, a serious and potentially life-threatening illness involving the adrenal glands, prompting the candidate's brother Robert F. Kennedy to declare:

> The Senator does not now nor has he ever had an ailment described
> classically as Addison's Disease, which is a tubercular destruction of

the adrenal gland. Any statement to the contrary is malicious and false.

While tuberculosis was not the cause of Senator Kennedy's adrenal insufficiency, he clearly did have Addison's disease, which was diagnosed in England in 1947 after Kennedy, then a Massachusetts congressman, collapsed during a visit to London. Senator Kennedy told the historian Arthur Schlesinger, "No one who has the real Addison's disease should run for the presidency, but I do not have it." Kennedy adviser Theodore Sorensen said, "He is not on cortisone. . . . I don't know that he is on anything—anymore than you and I are on." The candidate was, in fact, taking cortisone daily and had a steroid pellet surgically inserted under his skin every few months to replace hormones his adrenal glands could no longer sufficiently produce.

In 1992, the *Journal of the American Medical Association* published an interview with two of the pathologists who performed President Kennedy's autopsy after his assassination on November 22, 1963. While the Warren Commission report of the autopsy findings did not describe the adrenal glands, in the journal interview, Dr. J. T. Boswell, one of the principal Kennedy pathologists, stated that they could find no gross evidence of adrenal tissue and only scant cells on microscopic examination, consistent with the diagnosis of severe Addison's disease. In a follow-up editorial, the journal's editor in chief, Dr. George Lundberg, noted that in the 1960 general election, only 114,673 (0.17 percent) votes separated Kennedy from Nixon. Lundberg writes:

> The mental and physical health of a presidential candidate . . . is of great political concern to the electorate. But had the American people been told that one candidate had suffered for more than 13 years from an incurable, potentially fatal, although fully treatable disease and that there were potential serious adverse effects of treatment, would the election results have been different?

Herbert Abrams, professor emeritus of radiology at Stanford University and a member of Stanford's Center for International Security and Cooperation, has written extensively about presidential health and public disclosure. He notes that when the public votes, "it expresses its consent and endorsement at the ballot box. Such consent can only be informed if it is based on full disclosure." How much does the public have a right to know? Abrams likens the threshold for candidate disclosure to the informed consent process prior to medical procedures:

> When the public chooses a president, the risk that must be disclosed is any illness that may impede the candidate's capacity for decision-making for the nation, or render him disabled during the course of his tenure as president and thereby unable to serve.

Lawrence Altman, now a senior scholar at the Woodrow Wilson International Center in Washington, DC, who has spent much of his career relentlessly advocating for greater access to the medical records of political candidates, states:

> In my view, the public uses elections to hire its officials, expecting these employees to be able to serve their full terms without being inconvenienced except for minor ailments. Nevertheless, no ailment should disqualify anyone, even if ill or dying, from holding office. The choice is the electorate's.

Although in recent elections it has become increasingly common for the candidates' physicians to release statements outlining their patient's pertinent medical issues, cooperation, transparency, and veracity have varied over the years.

In spring 1944, as US and Allied forces were readying for the invasion of Europe, President Franklin Delano Roosevelt's health was declining. The president had developed influenza in December 1943 and had not rallied after that illness. On March 27, 1944, Dr. Howard Bruenn, a cardiologist from the National Naval Medical Center, examined the president. He found that the president appeared tired and gray, coughed frequently, and was significantly short of breath when he moved. The president's blood pressure was 186/108, and examination of the chest revealed rales (derived from the French *râle*, meaning "rattle," indicating the presence of fluid in the lungs). Dr. Bruenn diagnosed congestive heart failure and recommended one to two weeks of bed rest, codeine to suppress the cough, digitalis to strengthen the heart, and sedation. Admiral Ross McIntire, the president's physician, rejected the recommendations, citing in Bruenn's words the "exigencies and demands on the President." The president's condition remained unchanged over the next few days, and civilian consultants were brought in, one of whom was the prominent surgeon Frank Lahey, founder of Boston's Lahey Clinic. On April 4, the president felt better, but his blood pressure was now 226/118. In response to growing rumors about the health of the president, Admiral McIntire held a press conference and declared:

> When we got through, we decided that for a man of 62-plus we had very little to argue about, with the exception that we have had to combat the influenza plus the respiratory complications that came along after.

The public was never told that the president was struggling with congestive heart failure.

In a letter dated July 10, 1944, ten days before FDR accepted the nomination of the Democratic Party for a fourth term, Dr. Lahey wrote:

> On Saturday, July 8, I talked with Admiral McIntire in my capacity as one of the group of three, Admiral McIntire, Dr. James Paullin of Atlanta, Georgia, and myself, who saw President Roosevelt in consultation and who have been over his physical examination, x-rays, and laboratory findings concerning his physical condition. . . . I am recording these opinions in the light of having informed Ad-

miral McIntire Saturday afternoon July 8, 1944 that I did not believe that, if Mr. Roosevelt was elected President again, he had the
physical capacity to complete a term. I told him that, as a result of
activities in his trip to Russia he had been in a state which was, if
not in heart failure, at least on the verge of it, that this was the result of high blood pressure he has had now for a long time, plus a
question of a coronary damage. With this in mind it was my opinion that over the four years of another term with its burdens, he
would again have heart failure and be unable to complete it. Admiral McIntire was in agreement with this.

In November, President Roosevelt defeated New York's governor, Thomas E. Dewey, in an Electoral College landslide. Only a few
months into his fourth term, on April 12, 1945, President Roosevelt
died from an apparent cerebral hemorrhage, likely precipitated by his
uncontrolled hypertension.

Mr. Cheney asked Gary Malakoff and me to provide our own reports,
which the campaign released the same day as Dr. Cooley's. I intended
the statement to be a succinct and accurate description of Mr. Cheney's
medical history and his current status, not an exhaustive case presentation. No one from the Bush-Cheney campaign proffered any guidance
or guidelines for the documents, which were released to the public un-
edited. I wrote:

> Mr. Cheney has a remote history of an inferior wall myocardial
> infarction that occurred in the late 1970's. Cardiac catheterization
> following that episode revealed moderate coronary artery disease
> and he was managed medically for the next several years. A small,
> second, myocardial infarction occurred in 1984 and again in June
> 1988. Cardiac catheterization during that hospitalization demon-
> strated an increase in the extent of his coronary disease and he
> subsequently underwent successful coronary artery bypass graft

surgery at George Washington University by Dr. Benjamin Aaron. Following surgery, Mr. Cheney returned to his vigorous lifestyle and has been essentially asymptomatic for more than a decade. Recent nuclear stress tests have been stable, and unchanged, for the past several years. Recent echocardiography shows some left ventricular dysfunction consistent with the history and distribution of his remote myocardial infarctions.

Clinically, Mr. Cheney continues to lead an asymptomatic and extraordinarily vigorous lifestyle. He travels extensively for work, exercises 30 minutes per day several days per week on a treadmill, and engages in vigorous recreational activities such as hunting.

I knew that my statement would be carefully scrutinized, and for that reason, the 173 words took me most of an afternoon to write. Cheney had a complicated medical history, and the task of distilling twenty-two years of cardiac events into a few paragraphs of text intended for the general public was challenging. Ultimately I decided to simply summarize Cheney's salient history and his current status.

## CHAPTER 9

# Recount

## VICE PRESIDENT CHENEY

Presidential campaigns are about electing presidents. Rarely does a vice-presidential candidate matter to the outcome. There are two times, however, when he or she can make a real difference—for better or worse. The first is the acceptance speech at the party's national convention. The second is the nationally televised debate.

From the time my selection was announced, we had only eight days to prepare my convention speech. I had the help of three first-rate speechwriters: John McConnell, Matthew Scully, and Lynne. Lynne knows me better than anyone else, is a supremely skilled writer, and my toughest critic. I have always felt blessed to have her in my corner. We worked around the clock those first days, as we were also making our initial campaign stops, to prepare for a speech we knew the world, or at least the country, would be watching. I have made other important speeches since then, including my acceptance speech at the 2004 convention, but nothing will match the feeling of walking onto that stage in Philadelphia the night I was nominated for the first time. I had a great time delivering the speech to an applauding, cheering, chanting, foot-stomping crowd.

The rest of the launch of the vice-presidential campaign wasn't as smooth. When George Bush selected me to be his running mate in 2000, I'd already had more than twenty-five years of national political experience. As we say in Wyoming, this wasn't my first rodeo. I had run successfully six times statewide in Wyoming and had overseen

Gerald Ford's 1976 presidential campaign. Nevertheless, joining a national ticket as the vice-presidential nominee was a life-changing experience for my family and me. Among other things, it meant that I had to make the transition from being CEO of a major corporation with 100,000 people in 130 countries working for me to being a candidate for vice president where I wasn't in charge of anything except my personal performance on the stump making political speeches.

I hadn't been active in a campaign since 1994, and I hadn't been a candidate since 1988, so when we split off from the presidential campaign after a train ride through the Midwest with the Bushes, things got a little rocky. My first solo outing was to Florida, where I was to deliver a speech on education, specifically focused on our policy of using tax-exempt bonds to finance new school construction. Someone at campaign headquarters in Austin had produced the speech and scheduled the event at an elementary school.

I realized I was in trouble when I walked into a room full of third graders sitting cross-legged on the floor. There was a good deal of technical financial complexity in the speech. Wanting to do well and not wanting to cross headquarters in Austin on my first solo event on the trail, I decided to deliver it as written. Periodically I looked up from the text into the faces of the gathered eight-year-olds who were looking up at me completely perplexed. It was clear they were all thinking, *Who is this guy, and when is recess?*

Eventually we got the kinks worked out thanks to some wonderful campaign staff who became like family and to my actual family. Mary joined me on the road as my personal assistant, Lynne was my top adviser on everything from education policy to speech editing to what tie I should wear, and Liz oversaw my debate preparation. She was especially helpful during one of the high points of the campaign for me, my debate with Senator Joe Lieberman from Connecticut, the Democratic vice-presidential candidate. Joe and I had a good deal of respect for one another, and it showed in the debate, which was well received in most quarters.

Our grandkids accompanied us on the campaign planes, trains, and buses for most trips. They always helped us keep our perspective, and they made us laugh, which is important on a campaign. The conventional wisdom is that a career in politics and political campaigns can put strains on a family, but that was never the case for us. Campaigns have always been family affairs that have pulled us closer together, perhaps because we never lost when I was on the ballot. The 2000 campaign was the closest we ever came to ending our winning streak.

On Election Day, Lynne and I voted in our home polling place at the Wilson fire station in Jackson Hole. Then we took the campaign plane, loaded with staff, family, and a few friends, and flew to Austin to await the returns. En route we received the results of some early exit polls, which were not encouraging, but exit polls are notoriously inaccurate.

On arrival in Austin, I stopped by campaign headquarters to talk to our chief strategist, Karl Rove. Karl was optimistic and remained confident we would win. He was ultimately right, but it was one of the closest races in history. I'd been through a close election before. The day before the balloting in 1976, the Gallup organization had President Ford ahead by 1 percent. That evening the returns showed Governor Carter with a clear lead, but it was close enough that President Ford decided to wait until the next morning when all the returns would be in before making a concession statement. In 2000, Vice President Gore called Governor Bush to concede late in the evening and then changed his mind and withdrew his concession statement.

When we checked into the Four Seasons Hotel in Austin, we had planned to stay for one night and then fly to Washington. Instead, we ended up staying for ten days, and when we finally left for Washington, we still didn't know the outcome. As we went through the recounts and endless press analyses of "hanging chads," all we could do was wait. Most days we had conference calls with our man in Florida, Jim Baker, who kept the governor and me informed of the state of play. He sometimes asked for guidance on various legal issues. It was reassuring that every time the Florida votes were counted and recounted, we were ahead.

During the recount, Lynne and I accepted an invitation from the governor and Laura to join them for a night on their ranch near Crawford. We enjoyed the quiet time together with the Bushes, even though it was impossible to talk about much of anything other than the ongoing Florida contest.

Although there had been no official outcome to the election, I knew we needed to begin the transition. Under normal circumstances, a president-elect has the time from the election in early November until the January 20 inauguration to find and recruit a cabinet, fill thousands of jobs, and put together a legislative program. Many of the jobs require Senate confirmation, security clearances, full field FBI background investigations, financial reviews, and the resolution of potential conflicts of interest. Under normal circumstances, the task is challenging, and most presidents spend a good part of their first year in office operating with holdovers and acting personnel in many of the most important positions. In the situation we faced in 2000, it would be virtually impossible to run an effective transition if we waited for the final resolution of the Florida recount.

Governor Bush asked me to return to Washington and get things started. Fortunately I had the work of Clay Johnson, a longtime friend of the president, to build on. He had begun planning for the transition months before the election.

As long as the outcome of the election remained in dispute, the federal assets of office space and money set aside to support the transition weren't available to us. So we started our transition planning around the kitchen table in our townhouse in McLean, Virginia, just across the Potomac from Washington, DC. We raised money from private contributions and quickly found a supporter willing to provide space in an empty office building near Tysons Corner, Virginia. Our staff consisted mostly of unpaid volunteers.

I was in our townhouse in McLean on November 22 when I awoke in the middle of the night with chest discomfort. I had experienced similar instances over the years that proved to be false alarms, but if I had learned anything over the twenty-two years since my first heart attack in 1978, it was "When in doubt, check it out."

I woke Lynne and told her I was having chest discomfort and wanted to go to the hospital to have it checked. Then I alerted the Secret Service detail that had been set up in my garage since I'd joined the ticket. We climbed into their black Suburban for the drive to George Washington University Hospital in downtown Washington. We made good time, being about the only car on the road at 4:30 a.m.

Preliminary tests showed no increase in my blood enzyme levels, indicating there had been no damage to my heart and therefore no heart attack. Nonetheless, Dr. Reiner recommended that given my history and my chest discomfort, we should do a cardiac catheterization. That procedure showed that one of my coronary arteries had a 90 to 95 percent blockage. A stent was inserted to open up the artery, and I returned to my hospital room. Subsequent blood tests showed there had been a slight increase in my enzyme levels and that I had indeed suffered a very mild heart attack.

The fact that I was in the hospital in the middle of the presidential election recount generated considerable interest among the press. Journalists along with their cameras, lights, microphones, and satellite trucks gathered outside the hospital. Governor Bush was also getting questions down in Texas. Acting on the first set of test results, which had shown no rise in my enzyme levels, we had told the governor's staff that I had not had a heart attack, and this was the information he repeated to the press.

A short while later my doctors held a press briefing in Washington. In front of a packed room, they explained that my enzyme levels had been elevated, a clear message from their perspective that I'd had a heart attack. Unfortunately, the press pool missed the subtlety. Austin was concerned that we would be accused of a cover-up since the physicians had not actually said the words *heart attack*. At my family's request, the doctors convened a second press conference in which they said the key words, emphasizing, "This would be the smallest possible heart attack a person can have and still have it classified as a heart attack."

We had a unique Thanksgiving dinner in the hospital that year, with food brought in by friends and family and Secret Service agents gathered around. Shortly after that, I was released, and on December 12, 2000, the Supreme Court handed down its decision in *Bush* v. *Gore*. George Bush and I became the president-elect and vice president–elect of the United States.

## DR. REINER

November 22, 2000

A ringing phone in the middle of the night rarely brings good news. For me, the call usually comes from a wide-awake ER doc telling me that someone I am about to meet is having a heart attack.

I glanced at the clock as I reached for the phone: 5:00 a.m.

*I don't even think I'm on call tonight.*

"Jon, it's Alan."

It was Alan Wasserman, the chairman of the Department of Medicine at George Washington University. I could hear the urgency in his voice.

"Cheney is having chest pain. The Secret Service is bringing him in."

That was about all Alan knew.

"Okay, I'll meet you there," I said, and hung up the phone.

I hurtled out of bed, took a thirty-second shower, shaved, and jumped into a business suit like a firefighter rushing to catch the truck.

As I hustled out of the house, my wife, Charisse, gave me a kiss, told me to be careful driving, and said, "Do a good job. I know you will."

So early in the day before Thanksgiving, the roads were free of the usual choking morning traffic. I raced into Washington ignoring the speed limit; the Potomac River on my right not yet visible in the chilly predawn gloom.

Two weeks had passed since one of the closest presidential elections in US history, and the outcome was still uncertain. The previous night, the Florida Supreme Court had ruled in favor of Vice President Gore, allowing the swing state's recount to continue. The whole process had devolved into a bitter court battle involving scores of lawyers, with the presidency of the United States at stake. This was going to be a circus.

As I pulled off the Whitehurst Freeway and swung my car onto Washington Circle, I found network satellite trucks, black Secret Service Suburbans, and DC police cars everywhere. It was still dark, but the sidewalk across from George Washington University Hospital on Twenty-Third Street was starting to fill with camera crews, cables, and correspondents.

I parked, grabbed my white coat from my office across the street, and headed into the hospital, flashing my ID at the lobby checkpoint where the security had been beefed up. Cheney had initially been taken to the emergency room where a chest X-ray, EKG, and blood tests were obtained, but for security reasons he was quickly moved out of the busy and relatively open ER and brought to the more secure third-floor coronary care unit (CCU).

When I arrived in the CCU, Secret Service agents were posted outside Cheney's room and at other points in the corridor. I met Alan Wasserman, Gary Malakoff, and Dick Katz, GW's chief of cardiology, in the hallway, and they briefed me on what they knew.

Cheney had woken up around 3:30 a.m. with chest and left shoulder pain. He didn't have some of the other typical cardiac symptoms, such as nausea, sweatiness, or shortness of breath, but when his chest pain persisted, he wisely decided to come to the emergency room. Upon arrival, he was given a nitroglycerin tablet under his tongue, and it promptly relieved his pain. A nurse handed me Cheney's EKGs.

Think of an electrocardiogram as essentially a map of cardiac electrical activity. Contraction and relaxation of the heart are governed by a wave of electricity that takes about half a second to spread through the muscle. Injury to the heart causes characteristic EKG abnormalities.

When compared to prior tracings, Cheney's initial EKG showed subtle changes, particularly in the leads recording activity from the left side of the heart. A subsequent EKG had more pronounced abnormalities, quite characteristic of muscle injury.

"He needs to be cathed," I said.

The first casualty of a hospitalization is privacy, which is why I always knock before entering a patient's room. When I did, a familiar voice told us to come in.

When we entered the room, we found Cheney awake, pain free, and in good spirits. Lynne Cheney, whom I had not met before, stood on the right side of the bed, a monitor on the wall behind her displaying her husband's vital signs and EKG waveform.

I introduced myself to Mrs. Cheney and then asked the patient to describe, one more time, what happened during the night. Cheney said that he had been well the day before and had gone to sleep at his usual time. Sometime after midnight, he went down to the kitchen and made himself a snack. Eventually he went back to bed but was awakened a few hours later by chest and shoulder pain that persisted until he was given the nitroglycerin in the ER. I asked if he had noticed any similar discomfort in recent days, and he said no. Finally, I did a brief physical exam, listening with my stethoscope for any signs of congestive heart failure or new murmurs, which, reassuringly, I did not find.

I told Cheney that his symptoms concerned me, and I knew that to make a decision to come to the hospital on this particular night, he must have felt quite unwell. Furthermore, I noted that there were new abnormalities in the electrocardiogram, and coupled with the fact that his pain resolved promptly with the nitro, there likely was a new coronary lesion, but the only way to know for sure was to do a cath. At the time, Cheney's cardiac enzymes were not yet available.

I outlined what we might find during the procedure. I told Cheney that his pain was likely coming from a narrowing in one of his "native" (original) coronary arteries. I knew this because a prior catheterization in 1995 had shown that two of his bypass grafts were closed, and the

EKG changes pointed toward involvement of a region of the heart no longer supplied by a graft. I said that if we found a blockage and if the vessel could be treated, we would repair it during the same procedure. I also told Cheney that it was possible, but not likely, that this was a false alarm. Finally, I stated that I thought it was important that we treat him the same way we treat every other patient who is admitted with a similar clinical presentation and not try to take any shortcuts.

It is commonly believed that VIPs receive better medical care than the general public. While it is true that connected people are often immunized from some of the annoying facets of modern American health care (waiting interminably for a call to be returned, being told that the next available appointment is six months away, or getting stuck in an ER for hours), there is a potential downside to being a celebrity.

In 1964, Walter Weintraub published an article, "The VIP Syndrome," in which he described the hospital turmoil that frequently follows the admission of prominent or powerful patients and the poor outcomes that sometimes ensue. Weintraub and others have noted that when a well-known person is admitted to a hospital, there is a tendency to consciously or unconsciously alter the care that is typically provided, and it often has negative consequences. For example, in an attempt to spare a VIP inconvenience or discomfort, fewer tests may be performed, or conversely, in a desire to leave no stone unturned, every conceivable test will be ordered. The department chief may be called, when in reality the better choice is a different, sometimes younger, physician who has more experience treating the problem at hand. Numerous specialists may be consulted, each told only what they need to know, creating silos of care. There is a tendency to place a VIP in a more luxurious or more discrete hospital location, apart from where treatment is usually rendered, and the treating physicians may avoid using the intensive care unit because of the perceived undesirable atmospherics, even when that setting might be preferable.

I had cared for hundreds of patients with the same clinical presentation as Mr. Cheney, and the recommendation to proceed with cardiac catheterization was the standard approach. In fact, one week before

Cheney's hospitalization, a large clinical trial had validated this strategy, showing better outcomes in patients whose treatment included an early trip to the cath lab compared to those treated more conservatively. I told Cheney that I knew the cath might be politically awkward at that moment, but it was the correct thing to do, and I did not want political expediency to get in the way of doing what was right.

Mr. Cheney, who appeared remarkably calm, responded, "Nothing is more important," and agreed that the cath made sense. It would be hard to imagine a more inconvenient time to undergo an invasive procedure, but if Cheney had any anxiety or reluctance to proceed, it didn't show. I excused myself and left the room in order to make arrangements for the procedure.

In my absence, Mrs. Cheney asked Alan Wasserman, "Tell me, if this were you, would you let him perform this procedure?"

"As a matter of fact, I did."


In November 1976, Andreas Gruentzig, a thirty-seven-year-old German-born physician, visited the United States to present his research at the annual scientific sessions of the American Heart Association (AHA). He had moved to Zurich in 1969 and became interested in vascular disease, at the time called "angiology." Before that, the available methods for treating a narrowed leg vessel mostly involved surgical bypass or the less invasive Dotter technique, in which a series of increasingly larger-diameter rigid catheters were forced into the obstruction. Gruentzig understood that while this method could be effective in the large-caliber superficial femoral artery, which supplies blood to the leg, it could not work in small-diameter vessels and therefore would not be appropriate for use in the heart. Gruentzig had an idea to use a small inflatable balloon to crack open the obstruction, and he and his wife and some colleagues worked in his kitchen to develop a prototype. Because no such catheter existed anywhere, Gruentzig had to develop all the components, making it small enough to deliver into an artery through a puncture in the skin, with a way to inflate and deflate the balloon, and a balloon material strong enough to dilate the sometimes rigid and calcified plaques found in arteries. Gruentzig and his team eventually developed a catheter with a resilient polyvinyl chloride (PVC) balloon mounted on its tip, and in January 1975 he used it to dilate a narrowing in a patient's iliac artery, a large blood vessel in the pelvis.

A year and a half later at the AHA sessions, Gruentzig shared the results of his balloon technique adapted for use in the coronary arteries. The work, entitled "Experimental Percutaneous Dilatation of Coronary Artery Stenoses," described experiments in dogs and was delivered as a poster to a group of somewhat doubtful colleagues. Dr. Spencer King III, who would later go on to become a renowned interventional cardiologist, president of the American College of Cardiology, and friend and colleague of Gruentzig, remembered seeing the presentation and thinking, "this will never work."

Gruentzig's next step was to attempt his procedure, what is now called percutaneous transluminal coronary angioplasty (PTCA), in a live human heart. There are many considerations that go into planning a first-in-man procedure. What patient or lesion characteristics are ideal? Where should the procedure be performed? What could go wrong? The ideal patient would be someone with a relatively simple coronary narrowing suitable for treatment with a fairly crude, first-generation device. Because a lot could go wrong, Gruentzig decided to perform the first procedures in patients undergoing scheduled heart bypass surgery; should a major complication occur, it would happen in the very controlled environment of the cardiac operating room with a surgical team poised to react.

The risks were many. The inflated balloon could rupture the slender coronary artery, and if that occurred, blood would rapidly fill the pericardial space causing cardiac tamponade, a potentially fatal compression of the heart. During the dilation, fragments of atherosclerotic plaque could break off (embolize) and lodge downstream, blocking flow and precipitating a heart attack. The patient might not tolerate temporary occlusion of the coronary artery and could develop a dangerous ventricular arrhythmia or cardiac arrest. The balloon might burst, becoming trapped in the vessel, or fail to deflate, causing a heart attack. Since this procedure had never before been performed in a human, there was no way to anticipate all the risks.

Although Gruentzig could not find a surgeon in Zurich who would allow him to perform coronary angioplasty during their surgery, Dr. Elias Hanna, a cardiac surgeon in San Francisco, was amenable, and that is where Gruentzig successfully refined his technique prior to attempting the procedure in an awake patient not already destined for open heart surgery.

On September 16, 1977, Adolf Bachmann, a thirty-eight-year-old Swiss insurance salesman with severe chest pain, a tight narrowing in his left anterior descending coronary artery, and a strong desire to avoid cardiac surgery, was brought to Gruentzig's cath lab in Zurich. Gruentzig later described the index procedure:

> Early in the afternoon at a time when the anesthesiologist and the cardiac surgeon were available and no cardiac procedure was underway in the operating room, the patient came to our catheterization laboratory and was catheterized in the usual fashion. . . . The Chief of Cardiology, the cardiac surgeon, anesthesiologist, cardiology and radiology fellows were in the recording room to observe the procedure. The guiding catheter was placed in the left coronary orifice and the dilatation catheter was inserted. . . . The catheter wedged the stenosis so that there was no antegrade flow and the distal coronary pressure was very low. . . . To the surprise of all of us, no ST elevation, ventricular fibrillation or even extrasystole occurred and the patient had no chest pain. . . . After the first balloon deflation, the distal coronary pressure rose nicely. Encouraged by this positive response, I inflated the balloon a second time to relieve the residual gradient. Everyone was surprised about the ease of the procedure and I started to realize that my dreams had come true.

Several successful cases followed, and in November, Gruentzig presented a summary of his initial patients at the annual AHA meeting. Whereas one year earlier, his poster had been met with great skepticism, now his oral presentation was interrupted by a resounding standing ovation. Angioplasty and the field of interventional cardiology had been born, and physician and corporate interest in the new technique exploded.

Dr. Andreas Gruentzig and his wife, Margaret Anne, died on October 27, 1985, when the twin-engine Beechcraft Baron airplane he was flying crashed during a storm into a forest in Forsyth, Georgia.

Exactly ten years to the day after the world's first coronary angioplasty, Gruentzig's close friend and colleague, Dr. Spencer King III of Emory University, brought Adolph Bachmann back to the cath lab for a relook. The first coronary artery ever treated with balloon angioplasty was wide open.

Gruentzig was only forty-six years old when he died, but in his too-short life he changed medicine forever, and the technology he pioneered has touched the lives of millions of people.

Because of GW's location just seven blocks from the White House and its close proximity to the Capitol and virtually every other federal department, contingency plans are always in place for care of the nation's leadership, and GW Hospital has perhaps the only emergency room in the United States with a dedicated hotline to the Secret Service.

When Mr. Cheney arrived at the hospital, he was assigned an alias. His pseudonym, Red Adair, was not an attempt to hide his admission, which would have been impossible, but rather a standard procedure designed to help protect the privacy of his clinical data. (The real-life Paul "Red" Adair was a legendary Texas firefighter who became famous for putting out some of the world's worst oilfield and offshore platform fires.) A Secret Service command post was set up in the hospital administration suite, and a large medical school auditorium across

Twenty-Third Street was configured as a media briefing room following the long-standing, prudent practice of keeping the press out of the hospital.

As the East Coast was waking to breaking news, Dick Cheney was being prepped for cardiac catheterization. Prior to transporting him to the cath lab, I did a walk-through with an agent from his Secret Service detail so he could plan the deployment of his personnel. The Secret Service did not post anyone in the procedure room itself; instead they positioned their agents in the control room and hallways surrounding the suite. Over the years, I have been asked many times to allow a patient's family member, friend, or colleague to be present during a cath, but it's distracting to have a visitor in the room, and I don't allow it. I wouldn't want anyone kibitzing with the pilots when they are landing the plane I'm on, and I extend that same courtesy to my patients while I am working inside their heart.

I gave the staff in the cath lab a brief pregame talk, reminding them that this was a procedure we did several times every day and I knew we would provide this patient the same great care we gave to everyone else. My team didn't really need that reminder. I'm sure I intended it as much for myself as for them.

Cheney was transported by stretcher to the cath lab and helped onto the narrow padded table by Fernando Najera, a technologist, and Julia Mason, a nurse. I had met Fernando in 1990 on the first day of my cardiology fellowship, and he quickly became a friend. I've always admired his dedication to the care of patients with heart disease and his loyalty to GW. Fernando can do a surprisingly good rendition of the famous aria "Nessun Dorma," and despite the vagaries of my morning mood, he can always make me smile. Julia came to GW in 1998 after working in a cath lab in Saudi Arabia while her husband, a US State Department official, was stationed there. There isn't another health care professional with any title I have ever worked with whom I have relied on as much, or for whom I have more respect than Julia. The first thing I do every morning when I enter the cath lab is to check if Julia is working that day. Every physician knows that it is the nurses who really keep patients alive, and if I ever get sick, I want Julia to take care of me.

After settling the patient on the table, Julia gave Mr. Cheney Versed, an intravenous Valium-like benzodiazepine, and fentanyl, a narcotic. The cocktail is called, somewhat incorrectly, "conscious sedation," and it induces a sleepy, relaxed state with retrograde amnesia, the inability to remember what has just occurred. When I entered the room, Cheney appeared to be asleep, covered in a long, blue surgical drape, its two round circular cutouts exposing the skin of both groins.

I turned to my third-year cardiology fellow, Dr. Brian Rah, and handed him the needle.

"Really?" he said.

"Absolutely," I replied.

I run an interventional cardiology training program in a university teaching hospital and perform all of my procedures with a cardiology fellow. This wasn't the day to change my routine.

Brian easily entered the right common femoral artery, and together we advanced angiographic catheters to Cheney's heart.

Before the procedure, I had reviewed Cheney's images from the catheterization five years earlier, which I performed with Allan Ross. Now I was looking for what had changed.

The right coronary artery (the vessel that caused the 1988 heart attack) was still closed, but its right internal mammary artery bypass was wide open. The circumflex branch (the likely culprit of the 1978 and 1984 heart attacks) was also occluded, as was its bypass, both unchanged compared with the prior catheterization. When we injected dye into the left anterior descending (LAD) coronary artery, we found the problem: the LAD had been bypassed at surgery in 1988, but because the vessel had only moderate disease, the graft never properly developed and was closed, which we already knew. A large branch of the LAD called the diagonal coronary artery, supplying a significant segment of the front and side of the heart, had a tight new narrowing.

"Hey, Dick, do you see that?" I said, trying to get the attention of Dick Katz who was watching on a monitor in the next room.

"See what?" Cheney responded.

"Oh, I'm not calling you, Dick," I replied, embarrassed, and surprised that he was awake.

Cheney said, "You can call me Dick."

"No, sir," I said. "I'm talking to the Dick in the control room."

*Stop talking. You've just called at least one of them a dick.*

Over the intercom, Katz told me that he did see the diagonal narrowing and he agreed that it was likely the cause of Cheney's pain.

"I'm going to stent it," I said.

In February 1978, a thirty-two-year-old Argentinean physician attended the Society of Interventional Radiology meeting in New Orleans where Dr. Andreas Gruentzig was presenting his new angioplasty procedure. Dr. Julio Palmaz, who had come to the United States the year before to do a radiology residency at the University of California, Davis, listened as Gruentzig described some of the potential complications from angioplasty and how an artery could abruptly close. Palmaz started to think of ways to solve the problem and came up with the novel idea of placing a metallic scaffold inside.

Dr. Palmaz spent years creating prototypes of his new "stent," beginning with a meshwork of copper wire woven over a pencil in his home. He soon realized that to provide structural rigidity, the points where the wires crossed needed to be fixed, and eventually he crimped his sleeve of metallic meshwork onto an angioplasty balloon. When the balloon was inflated inside a tube, the stent expanded, becoming apposed to the wall, creating an internal scaffold.

While searching for ways to construct his device from a single piece of metal rather than woven stands of wire, Palmaz found a fragment of metal masonry mesh on the floor of his garage, the kind of material used to reinforce concrete or plaster. Two decades later, he described his discovery:

## Recount

It was total serendipity. . . . I looked at it and thought, "This looks like what I'm trying to do here." I grabbed it, cut out a small piece, then closed it by pushing it together and bouncing it on the table with a hammer. I realized that the staggered openings were staggered slots when it was closed. I thought, "Well, if I make this pattern in a tube, then, when a balloon expands, it will become a mesh." And it's made of a single material. This was the inspiration for the slotted stent.

Palmaz continued to work on stent designs but had difficulty funding his research. In 1985, now the chief of angiography at the University of Texas Health and Science Center in San Antonio, Palmaz met Dr. Richard Schatz, a cardiologist at nearby Brooke Army Medical Center. Schatz knew that a major risk of coronary angioplasty was abrupt vessel closure, a potentially catastrophic event that occurred in 5 to 10 percent of patients, typically caused by balloon-induced disruption of the arterial lining. Also, almost half the vessels treated with angioplasty renarrowed within a few months of the initial procedure, a phenomenon called restenosis. Schatz recognized the need for a technology that might reduce these events. Later that same year, Schatz met Phil Romano at San Antonio's Dominion Country Club. Romano, a prolific entrepreneur, was the founder of the Fuddruckers and Romano's Macaroni Grill restaurant chains, and despite the protestations of his lawyer and accountant, he agreed to invest $250,000 in the stent project. Palmaz, Schatz, and Romano formed a business entity they called the Expandable Grafts Partnership, and on March 29, 1988, they were issued US patent 4,733,665 for an "expandable intraluminal graft, and method and apparatus for implanting an expandable intraluminal graft." The patent abstract describes how the invention works:

An expandable intraluminal vascular graft is expanded within a blood vessel by an angioplasty balloon associated with a catheter to dilate and expand the lumen of a blood vessel. The graft may be a wire mesh.

Johnson & Johnson licensed the new stent in 1988 agreeing to pay the partners $10 million in addition to future royalties. With J&J pouring both money and intellectual resources into product development, clinical trials began for the Palmaz stent, now manufactured from tubes of stainless steel etched with staggered rows of rectangular slots that created diamond-shaped interstices when expanded. In 1991, the FDA approved the Palmaz stent for use in arteries supplying the leg, and in 1994 the Palmaz-Schatz stent was approved for use in the heart.

Cardiologists enthusiastically embraced the new technology, and the use of stents rose rapidly from 5 percent of interventional procedures in 1994 to almost 70 percent in 1997. In 2009, there were almost 650,000 hospitalizations in the United States involving the implantation of a coronary stent. Stenting made angioplasty safer, vastly reducing the number of patients requiring emergency surgery because of a procedural complication such as a coronary dissection or abrupt occlusion, and enabled increasingly complex lesions to be treated without the need for coronary artery bypass surgery.

Phil Romano's $250,000 gamble in 1985 would ultimately yield him well over $100 million.

When I see a patient in the clinic, I always start the appointment by asking about work, family, a recent trip—something personal. No one looks in the mirror and sees a "fifty-eight-year-old white male with atrial fibrillation" or a "seventy-two-year-old female status post LAD stenting," and when they come to see me, I want them to know that I don't see them that way either. I once received a card from a patient in whom I had recently repaired multiple coronary arteries. Taped inside was a vacation photo of the patient with his wife, and their two small children, everyone huddled close together in a happy family tangle of sunglasses and smiles. In little kid handwriting, his seven-year-old son wrote, "Thanks for fixing my dad's heart," a poignant reminder of how much there had been to lose.

In the cath lab, I try to make all of that disappear and focus instead on the technical tasks: the artery to be punctured, the lesion to be crossed, the stent to deploy. I gazed down the table at Cheney and tried not to think about who he was, or his family waiting down the hall, or the election, and I consciously avoided looking through the leaded glass window at the control room filled with anxious medical center leadership.

My colleague Dr. Conor Lundergan joined me after a hurried drive from his home in Maryland, some of it on the shoulder of the road, and together we again reviewed the images looping on the video displays suspended from the ceiling. Conor agreed that we should fix the large diagonal, and I gave Julia a "shopping list" of equipment I wanted, most of which she had already set aside.

I told Cheney that we had identified the problem and were going to take care of it. Although he appeared to be sleeping, he immediately acknowledged what I said and responded, "Good."

*Take a deep breath; you've done this thousands of times.*

I inserted a guide catheter (essentially, a one-meter-long, steel-reinforced, hollow tube with a shaped tip, roughly the diameter of a soda straw) into the sheath in Mr. Cheney's right femoral artery and maneuvered it with the aid of fluoroscopy to the origin of his left main coronary artery. I then advanced a thin (.014-inch diameter) guide wire through the guide catheter into the left anterior descending coronary and out into its diagonal branch, the culprit for Cheney's chest pain.

A diseased coronary artery is a slender structure that flexes in concert with the underlying beating heart and is filled with ragged outcroppings of calcified plaque, creating a moving three-dimensional environment. Manipulating a device inside an atherosclerotic coronary is like crawling through a tight cave filled with stalactites and stalagmites while the cave jumps up and down.

Without too much difficulty, we succeeded in wiggling the soft tip of the wire beyond the tight coronary narrowing into the relatively less diseased vessel segment downstream, step one in repairing the artery. Next we loaded the back end of the wire into the central lumen of the balloon, like threading a needle, except the eye is about the same diameter as the thread, and then we slid the balloon over the wire into the coronary. With a bit of coaxing, the balloon slipped into the tightly restricted section of the diagonal. The inflation device, a large syringe with a screw-in plunger, filled with diluted X-ray dye, was connected to the balloon, and as we twisted the plunger clockwise, the 2.5-millimeter balloon expanded inside Dick Cheney's coronary artery.

I checked the hemodynamic monitor and his pulse, blood pressure, and rhythm were all fine. I looked to my left down the table, and Cheney was sleeping.

*So far so good.*

After about a minute of dilation, the balloon was deflated and removed, and another set of pictures revealed a still narrowed, but somewhat improved, appearance of the vessel, step two.

The final part of the procedure was delivering and then expanding a stent in the diseased segment, a task that is sometimes easier said than done. Although a lot of engineering has gone into increasing stent flexibility, the metallic device has an intrinsically rigid architecture, and in order to pass it through an angulated vessel, either the artery or the stent has to bend. The more inflexible either structure is, the harder it is to deliver the device to the intended target.

We watched on the monitor as the stent entered the left main and then the LAD. It's not so easy to see the actual stent, but the balloon on which it is crimped has visible markers at both ends, identifying the leading and trailing edges of the device. With a bit of effort, we were able to get the stent to make the ninety-degree turn into the diagonal, but there was a second acute bend to negotiate, and the stent would go no farther.

I backed the stent off a few millimeters and tried again. No luck. We removed the stent and re-dilated the artery with a balloon. Still, the stent would not pass. We changed to a different type of stent, but that too would not make the second turn into the short segment with the worst disease.

I don't usually perspire much during a case because the rooms are kept cool, and I've performed these procedures so many times, but the scrubs under my protective lead were soaked by now. As hard as I tried to tell myself that this was just another angioplasty, the growing crowd in the control room, the Secret Service outside the door, and the camera trucks outside the hospital were constant reminders that while the medicine might have been routine, nothing else was. Although the success rate for coronary interventions is very high, it's not 100 percent, and occasionally a lesion can't be fixed. There's no shame in that. But in this particular case, to paraphrase NASA's Gene Kranz, "failure was not an option."

We had long since passed the two-hour mark, and I looked over again to see how Cheney was doing. I turned to Julia and asked her if we had any juice.

"Sure," she said, as she went to the refrigerator outside the room, returning quickly with a small round container of apple juice, a flexible straw protruding from its foil cover.

"Here you go," she said, offering Cheney the juice.

"Not him, Julia, me," I said.

"Oh," she said, pivoting away from the patient with a nervous laugh.

Sometimes it's best to press the pause button. When an initial attempt to solve a problem fails, there's a natural tendency to try the same approach over and over again, creating an endless, unsuccessful loop. I could feel some frustration beginning to fester, and I was also really thirsty. It was time to stop for a moment.

Julia slipped the straw under the side of my mask, and I downed the cold liquid in a single slurp.

*Okay, let's try something else.*

After the brief time-out, we reentered the vessel with a different balloon in a slightly different place, hoping that the inflation would alter the internal geometry of the artery just enough to allow passage of the stent. Now when we advanced the stent, it slid into position, and when it did, I could sense the collective sigh of relief. After a half dozen clockwise turns on the inflation syringe, the stent was finally deployed. We were done.

I took off my gown and gloves and told Mr. Cheney what we had found and what we were able to do. As I left the room, I told the Secret Service agents that we would be bringing him back to his room in a few minutes, and they immediately began talking quietly into the microphones clipped discreetly inside their jacket cuffs.

It was now after noon and while we were in the cath lab, Governor Bush had made a brief statement in Austin in which he said, "Dick Cheney is healthy. He did not have a heart attack." The governor's statement had been based on the first set of cardiac enzymes drawn shortly after Mr. Cheney's arrival at the hospital, which were negative. The second set of enzymes, however, obtained a few hours later when we started the cath, specifically the highly sensitive troponin assay, was mildly elevated, indicative of a small heart attack. Governor Bush had not been told these results before he made his statement.

Alan Wasserman, Conor Lundergan, Gary Malakoff, and I went to talk with Mrs. Cheney who was waiting in an office in the hospital's administrative suite. I told Mrs. Cheney that the findings were quite similar to the cath five years earlier with the exception of the diagonal, which we were able to repair with a single stent. We talked about the mildly elevated cardiac enzymes and her husband's very favorable prognosis. There was some discussion as to who would brief the media, and ultimately it was decided that Dr. Wasserman would do it.

At about 2:30 p.m., Alan addressed the media.

As I think everyone is aware, Secretary Richard Cheney came to the George Washington University Hospital emergency room with chest pain . . . early this morning.

Neither his initial EKG nor his blood work indicated that he had a heart attack. After consultation with his internist, Dr. Gary Malakoff, director of the division of internal medicine, Dr. Jonathan Reiner, cardiologist and director of the cardiac catheterization laboratory and Dr. Richard Katz, chief of cardiology, and when a second EKG showed minor changes, a decision was made to perform a cardiac catheterization. The results of the catheterization showed an increased narrowing in a side branch of artery, specifically the diagonal branch of the left anterior descending artery. The rest of his coronary anatomy is completely unchanged from a previous study performed in 1996.

A decision was made to place a coronary stent in that area that showed some additional narrowing. After placement of the stent, the artery now appears normal. Mr. Cheney has returned to his hospital room and is doing well.

While there is no evidence of any new heart muscle damage on either the heart catheterization or the follow-up electrocardiograms, a second set of cardiac enzymes tests was minimally elevated. He is in good condition and will be at bed rest for the remainder of the day as a standard protocol in procedures such as this. We expect a short hospital stay and expect that Mr. Cheney will be back to normal functions without limitations in a brief period of time.

Alan took a lot of heat for his statement. While he clearly stated that the second set of cardiac enzymes was elevated, he hadn't used the lay term *heart attack*. I was present throughout the hospitalization, and no one in Mr. Cheney's family or the Bush campaign at any time tried to edit our disclosure or obscure the fact that there had been a small heart attack. In fact, to ensure that we were being fully transparent, we held a second press conference two hours later in which I participated. Before Alan introduced me, he passed out copies of Mr. Cheney's cardiac enzymes and explained them more fully:

The first value was obtained at approximately 8 a.m., and the values are completely normal. The second set of values were obtained, were available to Dr. Reiner sometime after noon today, while he was in the catheterization laboratory. The second set of values show an elevated level, a minimally elevated level that shows that there was a very slight heart attack. The third set of values shows that the levels have basically tapered off and have not continued to increase.

It is generally accepted that plaque rupture is the typical trigger for an event such as Mr. Cheney's. Inside the vessel, a cholesterol plaque becomes abraded, or "ruptures," allowing a clot to develop and changing a lesion that the day before may have been only moderately narrowed into a much more significant blockage. Sometimes very minute pieces of clot can break off, lodge downstream, and cause the small enzyme elevations (small heart attacks) like Mr. Cheney's. Angioplasty and stent placement can seal these roughened areas inside the artery and prevent these events from becoming much larger, clinically more significant heart attacks. I don't think any heart attack is insignificant, but Mr. Cheney's heart attack was small, and I described it at the press conference in the following way:

> We have biochemical markers that enable us to determine whether or not there has been any damage at all to the heart muscle. And over the last several years . . . we've had some new tools, much more sensitive markers which weren't available several years ago which enable us to detect extremely small levels of heart muscle damage. . . . Two or three years ago we would simply—based on the biochemical data available then, we would simply have classified the event as just angina. But because we have more sensitive markers, we can detect extraordinarily minute elevations in these markers of heart muscle damage. So, you know, we've really had to rethink what a heart attack is.

Mr. Cheney's hospitalization was brief and his recovery uncomplicated, but in an editorial a few days after Mr. Cheney was discharged, the *New York Times* said Americans "have reason to be concerned by the failure of Mr. Cheney's aides and doctors to inform the public fully and promptly about his true condition," an insulting allegation that was simply wrong. The *Times* went on to say, "Wednesday's bumbling performance may not fall into the category of deliberate misinformation, but it did not cover anyone with glory."

Despite the tumult in the press, I was proud of the care provided to Mr. Cheney at GW, what the *Wall Street Journal* called, "aggressive, invasive treatment with cardiology's state-of-the-art technology."

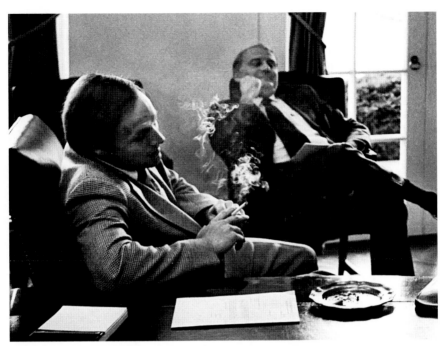

Meeting with presidential counselor Jack Marsh in my West Wing office in 1976. The White House used to give out free packs of cigarettes emblazoned with the presidential seal. *Official White House Photo by David Hume Kennerly*

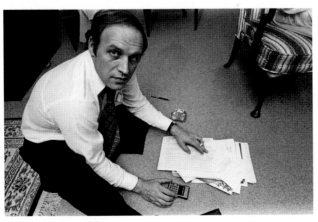

On the floor of my West Wing office with a calculator and election returns from the 1976 New Hampshire primary. *Official White House Photo by David Hume Kennerly*

Late on election night 1976, when Bob Teeter and I met with President Ford and Senator Jacob Javits, one of Ford's closest friends, and delivered the news to the president that it looked like we had lost the 1976 election. All the votes weren't in yet, and we decided to wait until the next morning to concede the election. *Official White House Photo by David Hume Kennerly*

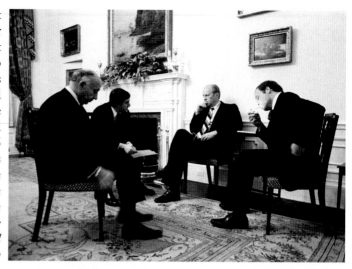

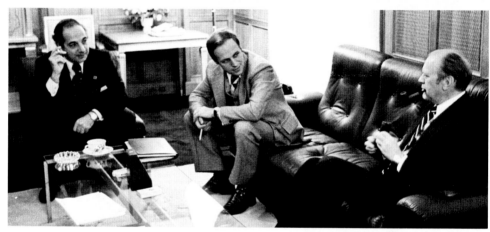

On the road during the 1976 campaign with President Ford and press secretary Ron Nessen. *Official White House Photo by David Hume Kennerly*

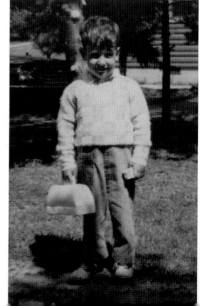

Dr. Reiner, circa 1964.

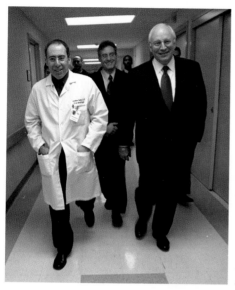

With Dr. Jonathan Reiner and
Dr. Alan Wasserman, leaving
GW Hospital, March 6, 2001.
*Official White House Photo by David Bohrer;*
*Presidential Materials Division, National*
*Archives and Records Administration*

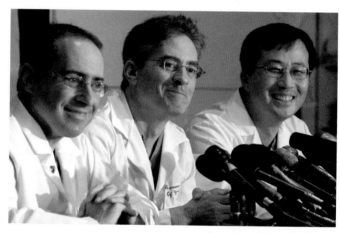

Drs. Jonathan Reiner, Alan
Wasserman, and Sung Lee at
the press conference after the
ICD implant, June 30, 2001.
*Getty Images/Greg Whitesell*

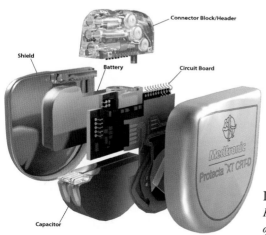

Internal components of an ICD.
*Reproduced with permission*
*of Medtronic, Inc.*

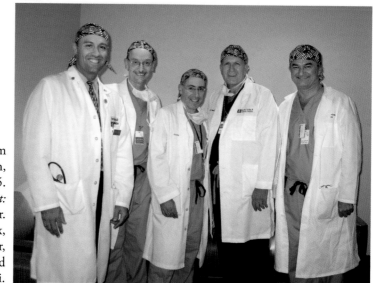

Popliteal aneurysm repair team, September 24, 2005. *From left to right:* Dr. Ryan Bosch, Dr. Anthony Venbrux, Dr. Jonathan Reiner, Dr. Barry Katzen, and Dr. Peter Gloviczki.

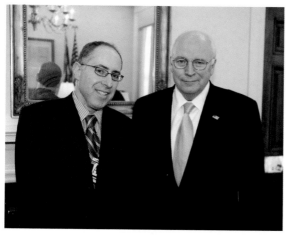

In my West Wing office, April 2008. *Official White House Photo by David Bohrer; Presidential Materials Division, National Archives and Records Administration*

In the West Wing, April 2008. *From left to right:* Dr. Cindy Tracy, Dr. Ryan Bosch, Dr. Jonathan Reiner, and Col. (Dr.) Lewis Hofmann. *Official White House Photo by David Bohrer; Presidential Materials Division, National Archives and Records Administration*

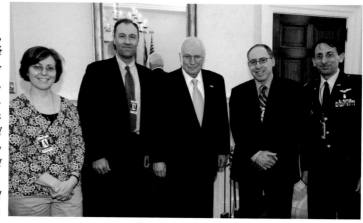

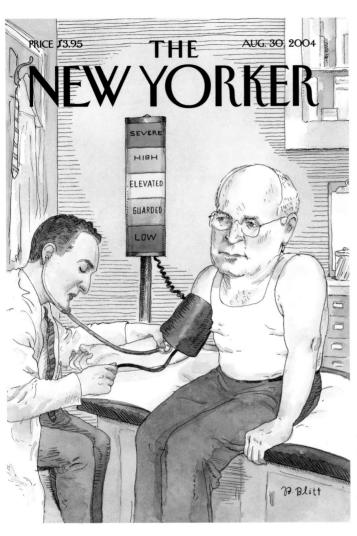

Cover of *The New Yorker*
from August 30, 2004.
*Copyright © 2004.*
*Originally published in*
The New Yorker. *Reprinted*
*by permission.*

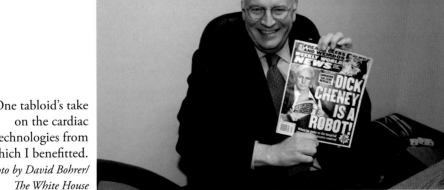

One tabloid's take
on the cardiac
technologies from
which I benefitted.
*Photo by David Bohrer/*
*The White House*

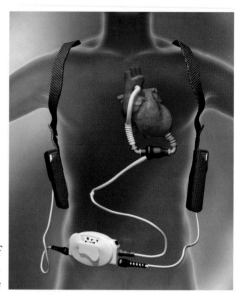

Schematic diagram of
HeartMate II LVAD system.
*Photograph courtesy of Thoratec Corporation*

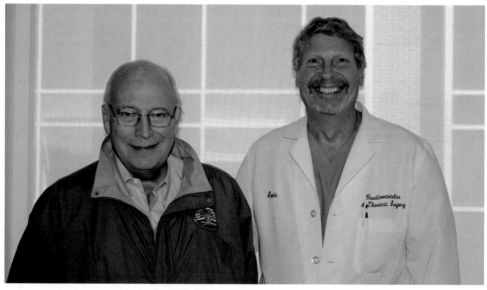

With my surgeon Dr. Alan Speir
at Inova Fairfax Hospital four
days after the heart transplant.
*Photograph courtesy of Liz Cheney*

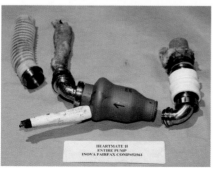

Components of the explanted VAD.
*Photograph courtesy of Thoratec Corporation*

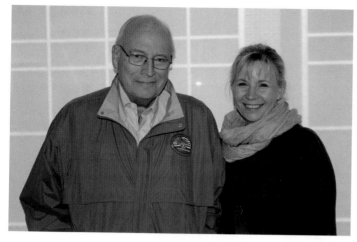

With Liz at Inova Fairfax Hospital four days after the heart transplant. *Photograph courtesy of Alan Speir, MD*

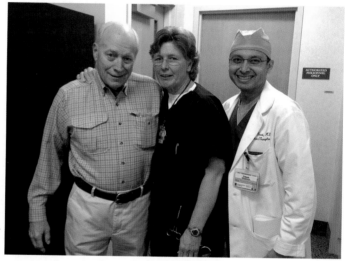

With Dr. Shashank Desai and Pat Rakers, my ICU nurse, one year after the transplant. *Photograph courtesy of Jonathan Reiner, MD*

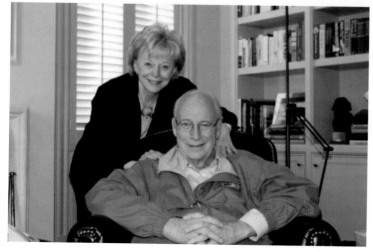

With Lynne at our home in McLean a few hours after I was released from the hospital following my transplant operation. *Photograph courtesy of Kara Ahern*

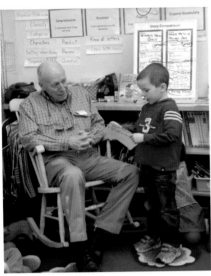

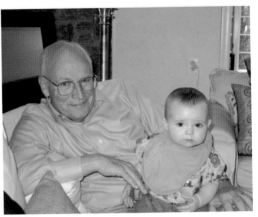

In the spring of 2013, my grandson Richard asked me to be his kindergarten show-and-tell. I was happy to oblige. The teacher said I was the most exciting show-and-tell since the morning a little girl brought her cow to class. *Photograph courtesy of Liz Cheney*

This picture of me with my youngest grandchild, Sarah Lynne Cheney, was taken in May 2010, shortly before I went into end-stage heart failure. I was much more sick than I knew or looked at the time. How lucky I am that now I have the chance to watch her grow up. *Photograph courtesy of Heather Poe*

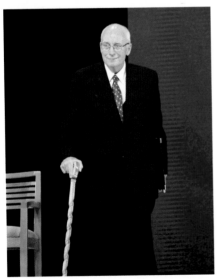

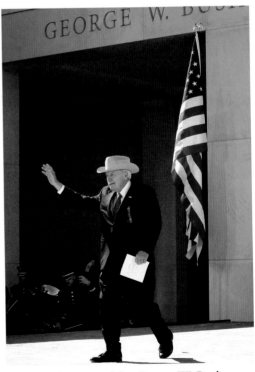

At the ceremony for the Bush Library groundbreaking on November 16, 2010, my first public appearance after the LVAD surgery. There were audible gasps when I walked onstage. *AP Photo/ LM Otero*

At the dedication of the George W. Bush Presidential Library and Museum in April 2013, a little more than a year after my transplant. *Getty Images/Alex Wong*

## CHAPTER 10

# White House Calls

## VICE PRESIDENT CHENEY

When I took the oath of office as vice president of the United States on January 20, 2001, I had been living with coronary artery disease for twenty-two years. I had survived four heart attacks, the last occurring just months before, and quadruple bypass surgery. Medical advances such as cholesterol-lowering drugs and stents had improved my life expectancy and justified my doctors' view that I was capable of serving as vice president. Without those advances, I would have long since been forced to retire and may not have survived at all. While I had not sought the second-highest office in the land, I had been chosen by the president, nominated by my party, and elected to serve. I was honored to do so.

One of my first acts after being sworn in as vice president was to sign a letter resigning the vice presidency. I had asked David Addington, my longtime assistant and legal counsel, to review all of the procedures and authorities having to do with the continuity of government. What were the procedures, for example, if the president became ill or incapacitated? What about the vice president? How would we make sure the government could continue to function if we were attacked and either the president or vice president was unable to carry out his responsibilities? My most important responsibility as vice president was to be prepared to take over in the event something happened to the president. I wanted to be fully briefed on everything that would be involved in such a transition.

After David completed his review, he came to see me. Looking over the Constitution and relevant statutes, he had discovered a potential problem that could be significant especially in my case.

The Twenty-Fifth Amendment to the Constitution specifies a procedure for temporarily removing a sitting president if he is unable to perform the duties of the office. The vice president convenes the cabinet and puts the question of the removal of the president to a vote. If a majority of the cabinet concurs, the vice president becomes acting president, and the Speaker of the House and the president pro tem of the Senate are notified.

The Twenty-Fifth Amendment also made provision for the president to appoint a vice president if there was a vacancy in that office. Nixon used it to appoint Gerald Ford when Spiro Agnew resigned. Ford used it to appoint Nelson Rockefeller when he became president upon Nixon's resignation. There is no provision for replacing a vice president who becomes incapacitated, however. This is especially problematic since only the vice president can convene the cabinet to initiate the procedure for replacing a president. There is also the possibility that in the case of a president's death, a nonfunctioning vice president would replace him. As a constitutional officer, the vice president cannot be fired. He can resign or be removed only through the impeachment process.

At least once in our history, we have seen a president disabled: Woodrow Wilson suffered a stroke in October 1919 with seventeen months left in his second term of office. Given my medical history, I thought it was important to make a provision for the possibility that my abilities might be impaired by a stroke or a serious heart attack that would leave me still in office but unable to carry out the duties of vice president.

The solution we came up with was for me to sign a letter of resignation dated March 28, 2001, just sixty-seven days after we were inaugurated. I addressed it to the secretary of state, the standard form for such a letter from a president or vice president, and printed it on my official stationery. I gave the signed letter to David Addington with very clear instructions that he was to hold on to the letter and if the need ever arose, he was to present it to the president. It would then be up to the president to decide if and when to forward it to the secretary of state. Once it was submitted to the secretary, the office of vice president would be vacant, and the president could appoint a successor using the provisions of the Twenty-Fifth Amendment. The only other person I told about this arrangement was President Bush. I thought it was important that he know about it.

When Governor Bush asked me to be his running mate, he made it clear that it would be a consequential post. I would be a full member of his team and help govern the nation. From our first week in office, he was a man of his word. California had been experiencing rolling brownouts, and Alan Greenspan, chairman of the Federal Reserve and an old friend of mine from the Ford administration, was greatly concerned that the power shortages could spread to other parts of the country and cause significant problems in the economy. After we talked about the matter in my West Wing office, we went together to see the president, and our meeting led to the creation of an energy task force to develop a new national energy policy, which the president asked me to chair.

He also asked me to take on the task of conducting a review of a number of studies that dealt with the problem of "homeland security." My national security background had been an important reason for his selecting me, and with his approval, I embarked on a series of visits to the Central Intelligence Agency, the National Security Agency, the Defense Intelligence Agency, and other parts of the intelligence community. I'd had a special interest in intelligence matters since my days on the House Intelligence Committee and as secretary of defense, but after eight years in the private sector, I needed to catch up.

As vice president, I also served as the president of the Senate, which after the 2000 elections was evenly divided, with Republicans and Democrats each holding fifty seats. My tie-breaking vote placed the

Republicans in the majority and allowed them to select the chairs of each committee. My Senate colleagues invited me to attend the weekly GOP policy lunch, which I did whenever I was in Washington.

House Speaker Denny Hastert and Ways and Means Committee chairman Bill Thomas approached me with a unique suggestion. They were old friends from our days together in the House and said they looked on me as a "Man of the House." For that reason, they wanted me to have an office on the House side of the Capitol as well as the Senate side. Given the opportunity to choose one of two offices that were traditionally occupied by the chairman of Ways and Means, I chose one right off the House floor near the Democratic cloakroom. For the first and only time, the vice president had been given offices on both the Senate and House sides of the Capitol, and they turned out to be great locations for me to work with senators and representatives on important issues before the Congress.

In 2001 and again in 2003, President Bush called for major tax legislation, and I worked with the congressional leadership to get it passed. In 2003 both the House and the Senate passed major tax bills but were deadlocked when it came to convening a conference to rewrite the two versions. Emotions were running high among Republicans in both chambers, especially between the chairmen of the House Ways and Means Committee and the Senate Finance Committees. Senate Majority Leader Bill Frist and House Speaker Denny Hastert asked me to intervene and broker a deal. I worked with Congressman Bill Thomas and Senator Chuck Grassley and we crafted an agreement acceptable to both. I then cast the tie-breaking vote to get the bill passed by the Senate.

While I was vice president, my daily health care was primarily the responsibility of the White House Medical Unit (WHMU). Some view the WHMU and the idea of around-the-clock medical care for the president and vice president as unjustified perquisites of office. In fact, they are an integral and vital part of the White House operations, just as are the Secret Service and the White House Communications Agency. The nation has a significant stake in the health and well-being of the president and vice president once they are elected and sworn in, and helping to ensure that well-being is the job of the medical unit.

Traditionally the director of the WHMU, always a physician, has the president as his patient. The vice president's physician is the deputy director. In my case, that was Lewis Hofmann, an Air Force lieutenant colonel, later promoted to full colonel. Lew oversaw a team of nurses, physician's assistants, and other doctors who played an important role in my care. I was extraordinarily fortunate to draw Lew for that assignment. He is a top-notch physician. He was always discreet, worked endless hours, and traveled over a million miles with me on Air Force Two during my time in office. He played a vital role in dealing with all my health issues during that time. He remains a good friend today, and I consult him from time to time even though we are both now civilians. Perhaps Lew's greatest contribution was his ability to adapt to my special requirements.

I had made the decision after my 1984 heart attack to pick a doctor and a hospital where I would go for all matters related to my coronary artery disease. I had also developed the habit over the years that I wouldn't sign up for any procedure or prescription for any kind of medical problem without first checking with my cardiologist. My heart always came first, and I wanted Dr. Reiner and George Washington University Hospital to continue the role they had played before I was elected. As a former member of the Board of Trustees of the Mayo Clinic, I was also eligible for ongoing care at the clinic, and from time to time, I sought medical advice from experts there. Instead of relying solely on White House doctors and Bethesda Naval Hospital for my care, which is the conventional arrangement, I wanted to make certain that I continued my previous relationships.

Lew Hofmann worked effectively to put together a team approach that included everyone in my annual checkups, and he saw to it that the appropriate people were involved any time their area of expertise was needed. From my perspective as the patient, the process was flawless.

Whenever I traveled, even if it was just the short distance from the White House to the vice president's residence, I was accompanied by an entourage that included not only the Secret Service but also one of my military aides with the "football," which is actually a briefcase containing the codes necessary to execute our nuclear options, which I carried as a backup to the president. In addition, there would be my chief of staff or one of a handful of senior assistants trained in his responsibilities. And always Dr. Hofmann or one of his designated representatives from the WHMU would be in the motorcade. The traveling party expanded when I traveled outside Washington, DC, or overseas, but there was always twenty-four-hour coverage by the WHMU.

In 1993, when I left the Defense Department and joined the private sector, Lynne and I had purchased a home in Jackson Hole at the foot of the Tetons. This had always been our favorite part of the world, a place we had intended to honeymoon after our wedding in 1964. Unfortunately, I'd been hospitalized with food poisoning shortly before the wedding and had no health insurance. The money I'd saved for a honeymoon went to pay medical bills. But over the years, we'd been able to spend a good deal of time in Jackson with our family. It is home to one of the world's greatest ski mountains and some of the best trout fishing anywhere. And, of course, it had been part of my congressional district for the ten years I served in the House of Representatives.

When I returned there as vice president, I skied at first, although not as hard as I once had because of a football injury to my right knee. Still, I loved to get out on the slopes, especially with the family's newest skier, my granddaughter, Kate. A few years into my time as vice president, however, I gave it up. The knee problem and my history of heart disease led the doctors to recommend I stop taking the risk of flying downhill on a pair of skis.

Luckily, no one suggested I should give up fishing, which I usually do on rivers, using a drift boat. There is room for only three in a boat—two fishermen and a guide. Thus the Secret Service and my usual entourage had to get their own boats, and we always ended up with a flotilla. A local police boat was normally in the lead, followed by vessels carrying two agents in wet suits who were rescue swimmers. They were on call in case I fell into the river. Next was my boat, followed by a boat carrying my lead Secret Service agent and another rescue swimmer.

Behind that, normally out of sight, were additional boats with my military aide, doctor, and a medical assistant; a representative from the White House Communications Agency; additional agents; and more law enforcement officials. Depending on the landscape, there were also sometimes Secret Service agents on horseback on the banks of the river. And there were usually helicopters stationed nearby, operated by a military unit that could respond in minutes if a crisis occurred. The WHMU and the Secret Service always made arrangements with the closest hospital in case I needed emergency care.

During my first fishing trips as vice president, the boat in front of mine was rowed by a Secret Service agent. That created problems because the agents didn't know the river and would often row right through the best fishing holes, which would ruin it for the fishermen. Once we substituted guides for agents rowing in that lead boat, the fishing improved.

There were times when I had to place or receive secure calls from the river, and the WHCA personnel were there to set up the necessary satellite communications. Every year I took one trip that involved camping out overnight in a rugged remote canyon on the South Fork of the Snake River. Even there, my CIA briefer would arrive in the early morning with the president's daily brief so I could stay abreast of events around the world.

In the eight years I was vice president, I never fell into the water, and I never had a medical crisis on the river. On one occasion, I witnessed the team in action when a friend fishing with me developed chest pains. I flagged down my lead agent and told him to contact the doctor. Within a matter of minutes, we were surrounded by most of my entourage, including a helicopter overhead. A medical technician administered an EKG to my friend while he was still in the drift boat.

Fortunately, he was not having a heart attack. But I was very impressed with the rapid, professional response. It was reassuring to see firsthand the capabilities of the team that was there should I ever need them.

Another occasion when the WHMU rendered great service was when I accidentally shot one of my companions on a South Texas quail hunt. Major Kenneth Baron, who had accompanied me on that trip to the Armstrong Ranch, immediately stepped up and took charge of providing first aid. The ambulance that was standing by in case I needed care was summoned to transport my friend, Harry Whittington, to the hospital. The major stayed with Harry and his wife, Mercedes, through the night at the hospital in Corpus Christi and did everything possible to make sure Harry got the care he required. Harry Whittington couldn't have been kinder and more understanding about the accident. He was more worried about the flak I was going to receive in the press than he was about his own injuries. He was right about the flak. For years afterward, this incident was fodder for the late-night comedians. Years later, when I was going through my own medical crisis with end-stage heart failure, one of the kindest and most thoughtful letters I received came from Harry.

## DR. REINER

When I was a boy growing up in Brooklyn in the 1960s and 1970s, physicians made house calls. They didn't call it "concierge" care and patients didn't have to pay $2,000 for "special access"; it was simply the way medicine was practiced. Dr. Morris Steiner, our doctor, lived above his office in a beautiful turn-of-the-century Victorian house on East Nineteenth Street, a few blocks from our apartment. When my sisters or I got sick, he came to see us, bringing with him his seemingly bottomless leather doctor's bag from which he would pull stethoscope and prescription pad, tongue depressors and otoscope, penlight, the occasional lollipop, and much wisdom.

Thirty-five years later and now with a stethoscope tucked in my own bag, I walked the five blocks from my office on Pennsylvania Avenue to the northwest gate of the White House. Almost six weeks had passed since Chief Justice William Rehnquist swore in President Bush and Vice President Cheney on the west front of the Capitol, and Dr. Lew Hofmann, a physician from the WHMU, arranged for us to make a house call.

The WHMU is part of the White House Military Office, a group of US military agencies with about twenty-three hundred people who supply support services to the president; they include the White House Communications Agency, the Presidential Airlift Group, the White House Transportation Agency, and Marine Helicopter Squadron One.

I first met then Lieutenant Colonel Hofmann, an Air Force doctor specializing in family and aerospace medicine, shortly after the 2001 inauguration, when he became the vice president's full-time White House physician. Lew was recruited to the WHMU in 2000 after spending three years with the Ninety-Sixth Medical Group at Eglin Air Force Base in Florida. When Dick Cheney took the oath of office and became the forty-sixth vice president of the United States, Lew became his doctor and, like me, he would spend the next 2,922 consecutive days and nights on call for his patient.

When Gary Malakoff and I arrived at the White House, Lew was waiting for us on the corner outside the security checkpoint, smiling warmly and dressed in civilian clothing. The military makes an effort to decrease their visibility while working at the White House, and most members of the WHMU wear their uniforms to work only one day per week.

I passed my driver's license to a uniformed Secret Service officer inside a security booth and waited as he checked my name in his computer. He then handed me a plastic White House visitor pass suspended from a beaded chain, emblazoned with a large black "A [appointment]."

Gary and I placed our bags and phones in an X-ray scanner before walking through a magnetometer. After retrieving our belongings, we waved our visitor passes in front of a detector labeled with a small

White House icon, and an indicator light on a turnstile changed from red to green, the gate issuing a loud metallic *thwack* as it unlocked, granting us access to the White House grounds.

Our appointment with the vice president was scheduled for 6:00 p.m. (18:00 in the parlance of our new colleagues), but Lew asked us to arrive at 5:30 so that we could meet for a few minutes in the medical unit before going over to the West Wing. I think Lew, who had not worked with us before, wanted to be sure that we would not be late and would be ready when the vice president's assistant, Debbie Heiden, called to tell us to come over.

On the way to his office, Lew gave us a brief tour of the Eisenhower Executive Office Building where the medical unit is based, his appreciation for its history very apparent. The building opened in 1888 to house the State, War, and Navy Departments, the original occupants immortalized in the scrollwork of hundreds of beautiful brass door-knobs. The essential role of the WHMU is to provide comprehensive health care to the president and vice president of the United States as well as their families wherever they go. It is staffed by six physicians, six nurses, and seven physician's assistants, recruited equally from the Army, Navy, and Air Force (with an additional physician's assistant from the Coast Guard).

Administrative offices for the WHMU and a sizable medical clinic that includes treatment rooms, X-ray, EKG, and emergency medical capabilities are located on the ground floor. In Lew's words, "Pretty much we could do the first ten minutes of what could be done in an emergency room while waiting for the ambulance to come."

Lew Hofmann later described the rationale for the WHMU clinic:

First, the purpose of the OEOB Clinic is to provide what we referred to as "Care by Proxy." This means that if we are able to keep everyone in the staff running at best efficiency—from the Chief of Staff right down to the janitors—it enhances the ability of the President and Vice President to be efficient in their duties. When a staff member becomes ill, the advantages of our clinic are: (1) a visit might only take the patient away from work for thirty minutes or so—including prescription—whereas leaving the complex for an appointment elsewhere could use up half the day or more; (2) we are uniquely qualified to advise the patient on whether to remain at work or go home; (3) with the availability of physical therapy in the clinic, patients are able to obtain these needed treatments with minimal interruption of their day—otherwise they likely would have chosen to forgo the treatments and experienced negative immediate and future quality-of-life consequences.

We exited the office building and walked across West Executive Avenue and into the West Wing through a white-canopied entrance bearing the presidential seal. With Lew Hofmann leading the way, we paused momentarily at the Secret Service desk just inside the doorway and entered a stairway on the left heading for the first-floor office of the vice president of the United States. When we entered the suite, Debbie Heiden, the vice president's executive assistant, greeted us warmly. After just a few minutes, she told us we could go in and pressed a hidden button that unlocked a heavy mahogany door.

When we entered the office, Vice President Cheney was sitting at his desk, a large historical map decorating the wall behind him.

"Good afternoon, Mr. Vice President," Gary and I said, almost in unison, as we shook Cheney's hand.

The office was large, with a desk at the north end flanked on both sides by two flags and a fireplace on the opposite wall. A blue couch with adjacent armchairs and a Chippendale-style butler's tray table sat in the middle of the room under a brass chandelier. Portraits of Thomas Jefferson and John Adams, both former vice presidents, hung on the walls separating the tall windows.

Although many of the checkups to follow would be conducted in this striking space, on this day I wanted to get an EKG, which would be easier to acquire in an exam room. Therefore, Lew had arranged for us to use the office of the physician to the president, Dr. Richard Tubb, located in the White House residence.

It's a short but very interesting walk from the West Wing to the executive mansion. We turned right as we left the suite into a corridor lined with photos of the new administration and formed an unlikely, rapidly moving procession of the vice president, his Secret Service detail, and his three doctors. As we turned a corner, I noticed an open door with only a velvet rope barring entry. I was pretending that this was just another day at work, but when we walked past the open Oval Office, my head spun around like the tourist I was trying so hard not to be. We continued down the hallway, past the cabinet room, and left the building into the West Colonnade, the open columned walkway bordered on one side by the Rose Garden that connects the West Wing with the residence.

The physician to the president, usually also the director of the WHMU, has a separate office on the ground floor of the White House adjacent to the Map Room, in what was originally servants' quarters, with two examination rooms and a beautiful view of the South Lawn. The vice president entered one of the exam rooms, and a WHMU nurse obtained an EKG that showed Cheney's old inferior wall MI and other chronic changes. I noticed that the vice president had quite a few extra beats (premature ventricular contractions). I asked about any new symptoms, we reviewed his medications, and I did a focused cardiovascular examination. In my note summarizing the visit, I wrote:

Impression:

Symptomatically is doing very well. Has lost a significant amount of weight (was 220 lbs in 9/00). I discussed at length the importance of obtaining a Holter monitor to evaluate whether he has NSVT [Non-Sustained Ventricular Tachycardia] (defined as a triplet or more) which would place him at a higher risk of having sudden death. If the vice president does have NSVT this would then warrant an EP [electrophysiology] study. If inducible he would then require an ICD [implantable cardioverter defibrillator]. Mr. Cheney has agreed to schedule the placement of a Holter.

As the thallium chronically shows lateral wall ischemia (secondary to closed SVG) and this territory is similar to diagonal I do not think, in the absence of symptoms, a follow-up thallium will be helpful at this time.

Overall, I thought the vice president was doing well, but to help us further quantify Mr. Cheney's risk I wanted him to wear a Holter monitor, which would continuously record his heart rhythm for twenty-four hours.

On Monday morning, March 5, 2001, only four days after our White House visit, Debbie Heiden called and asked if I had a moment to speak with the vice president.

"Of course," I said.

A moment later, the vice president was on the line. Calmly, almost matter-of-factly, Mr. Cheney reported that he was having some chest pain.

*Chest pain? I just saw you a few days ago and you were fine.*

The first episode occurred two days before, on Saturday, after about thirty minutes of exercise. The vice president described the discomfort as a "burning" that lasted about five minutes and dissipated without any treatment. The second episode occurred the next day at rest after Mr. Cheney awoke from a midafternoon nap and was relieved by a nitroglycerin tablet. Over the weekend, the vice president and Mrs. Cheney had moved into the newly renovated official residence at the Naval Observatory on Massachusetts Avenue, and on Sunday evening he felt well enough to attend a seventy-fifth birthday party for Alan Greenspan, the chairman of the Federal Reserve. It was now Monday morning, and the vice president had developed another episode of chest burning, this time after showering. Again, nitroglycerin relieved it. At the time of the call, Mr. Cheney said he felt fine.

We spoke about the possibility that we might need to repeat the cardiac catheterization, and I told the vice president that I would arrange for an EKG to be performed by the WHMU. At 2:45 p.m. Vice

President Cheney walked over to the clinic in the White House residence for an EKG. On his way back to the West Wing, he had more chest pain, and when he called me to report his symptoms I told him we should repeat the catheterization.

"Where should I go?" he asked.

"There's going to be no way to keep this quiet," I said, stating the obvious.

"Don't worry about that."

"Just go to the emergency room," I said. "I'll meet you there."

He told me he was on his way.


Unique logistics accompany a hospital admission for the vice president of the United States. The first necessity is to identify secure and private accommodations, ideally a location without much through traffic, where access can be limited to authorized personnel. It's helpful to provide family members with an adjacent but separate room, which can be used for meetings with staff or as a lounge while the patient is resting or needs some privacy. The vice president travels with a military aide who carries the "nuclear football," electronic gear for communicating with military leadership during a national emergency, and if the vice president will be in the hospital overnight, the aide needs a place to stay. The Secret Service deploys a large number of agents and tactical personnel in and around the hospital, and a conference room is typically provided for their use as a command post. The patient also needs a pseudonym, security needs to be configured to keep the press and paparazzi out of the hospital, and the same as it would be for anyone, the patient must authorize the release of any health information.

George Washington University Hospital is only six blocks from the White House, so I hung up the phone and quickly dialed the emergency room to tell the attending physician on duty that the vice president was about to walk through their door. Next, I called the cath lab and told Julia that we were going to recath Cheney as soon as everyone was ready. I informed the hospital administration of the plan and also let Alan Wasserman know what was happening and asked him to inform medical center leadership. Finally, I called Charisse and told her I wouldn't be home for dinner. By the time I finished making the calls, Vice President Cheney was in the emergency room.

The introduction of coronary stents in the 1990s made angioplasty a dramatically safer procedure. A balloon exerts its therapeutic effect by fracturing a coronary's atherosclerotic plaque and also literally stretching the vessel. Sometimes the "cracks" created in the plaque can obstruct the flow of blood, and the scaffolding properties of a stent greatly reduce this risk. Stents also prevent the stretched arterial wall from recoiling and renarrowing the vessel over time.

The Achilles' heel of stenting is a biological process called restenosis. After a stent is expanded, it becomes embedded in the arterial wall, and over the next several weeks, tissue begins to cover the metallic struts. A small amount of tissue growth is desirable, as it "heals" the vessel and reduces the likelihood that a clot will form within the foreign body. In 20 to 30 percent of patients who receive a stent, however, the tissue growth progresses unchecked, resulting in significant renarrowing of the stented vessel segment, typically occurring within the first six months following stent implantation and often resulting in a recurrence of the patient's symptoms. In 2000, when Dick Cheney's stent was implanted, there were about 1,025,000 coronary angioplasty or stent procedures performed in the United States, about 25 percent of them for treatment of restenosis.

Almost four months had passed since we implanted the stent in Vice President Cheney's diagonal coronary artery, and because the odds favored restenosis as the cause of his symptoms, it was likely that we would need to do another angioplasty. I asked Dr. Alan Wasserman to join me in the cath lab. Alan had practiced interventional cardiology for many years before becoming chairman of GW's Department of Medicine, and I welcomed his wise counsel.

Following a brief stop in the emergency room, the vice president was brought to the cath lab, and Julia again assisted him onto the padded table. Shortly after Cheney's procedure in November, this lab had been gutted and replaced by a latest-generation system manufactured by Philips, the huge Dutch multinational company, and we had only recently resumed using it for cases. In the old cath lab, images were recorded on 35mm movie film. This new room did away with the quaint celluloid and stored the much better quality images in a state-of-the-art digital archive.

After Julia prepped and sedated Mr. Cheney, I used our X-ray system to guide a catheter to the heart. When we injected contrast into the coronaries, we quickly found that the four-month-old stent had a very tightly narrowed restenotic segment, undoubtedly the cause of the vice president's pain.

*Okay, no problem. This can be fixed.*

Without difficulty we passed a wire beyond the obstruction, and over the wire we slid an intravascular ultrasound catheter (IVUS) into the narrowed stent. An IVUS catheter has a miniaturized ultrasound transducer small enough to fit inside a coronary artery and uses high-frequency sound waves (ultrasound) to create detailed, inside-out images of a vessel's architecture. The study demonstrated that although the stent was well expanded, we could see a very short segment of bulky restenotic material inside it.

We removed the IVUS catheter and easily positioned a balloon within the narrowing. After leaving the balloon inflated for about a minute, I stepped on the foot pedal to reactivate the fluoroscopy.

The screen was blank.

I stepped on the pedal again, but still there was no image on the monitor.

My technologist, Fernando Najera, announced that the system was frozen and needed to be rebooted, a process that takes about five minutes.

*That's really great. I have a balloon inflated inside the heart of the vice president of the United States and my brand-new million-dollar cath lab doesn't seem to work.*

"Okay, reboot it," I said as I deflated the balloon and removed it without being able to see what I was doing. It was a risky maneuver, but the balloon had to come out.

After five minutes, Fernando said, "Okay, try it again."

Still nothing.

"Reboot it again, Fernando."

After waiting what seemed like much longer than five minutes, I again depressed the foot pedal. The screen was still blank.

Forgetting for a moment whom I had on the table, I shouted a profanity and then, remembering, hoped he was asleep.

"Get Philips on the phone," I said, and also asked the staff to set up the lab next door. If we were going to finish the procedure, it was looking as if we were going to need to move Cheney to a different room. Cath labs are complicated systems, and they do crash occasionally, but this time we had the vice president of the United States on the table. This couldn't have come at a worse moment.

Fernando rebooted the lab one last time and miraculously, perhaps aided by several silent Hail Marys from Julia, the system came back online. With a functional cath lab, we injected the coronary and found that the vessel looked much better. After one more balloon inflation, we were done.


The procedure had taken less than an hour to complete, and Alan and Gary Malakoff and I walked upstairs to hospital administration to brief Mrs. Cheney. When we entered the suite, there were a lot of people around. The CEO of the hospital, Dan McLean, was there, as was the medical director, Dr. Richard Becker, and Dr. John "Skip" Williams, the dean of the medical school. There were university and hospital media people, some staff of the vice president and Mrs. Cheney, and, of course, the Secret Service.

I make it a practice to talk to family members immediately after finishing a procedure because I know how hard it is to wait to hear about a person you love, and I usually prefer not to discuss these very personal details in a busy place. As Alan and I sat down, I could tell that Mrs. Cheney was also not comfortable with the large assembled crowd, and she politely but firmly asked everyone else to leave. They moved quickly, as if a fire alarm had gone off, but Dr. Williams, who in addition to being dean of the medical school was also the university's vice president for medical affairs, was reluctant to go. As Alan and I averted our gaze, Mrs. Cheney again excused Dr. Williams, who said, "These guys work for me."

Without hesitating, Mrs. Cheney smiled and said, "That's okay. This is about my husband," and she calmly ushered the dean to the door.

The fact was that I didn't work for Skip, I worked for Alan, but at that moment, there was no question who was in charge in that room.

With the suite cleared, we told Mrs. Cheney about the restenotic stent and the good result we were able to get with repeat angioplasty. We told her that there was no evidence the vice president had suffered a heart attack and that we thought he would be fine.

Mrs. Cheney called Mary Matalin, counselor to the vice president, and over a speakerphone discussed how we would handle the press conference. The initial release of information concerning the November heart attack hadn't gone well, and no one wanted a repeat of that. I argued for immediate full disclosure, and without any debate, it was agreed that Alan would make a brief statement and then I would answer the media's questions.

No classes in medical school cover the essential skills for holding a press conference, but the experience in November taught me a lot. If the press thinks you haven't been forthright, they will sense blood in the water and react like sharks. I do believe doctors should be advocates for their patients, but it's best to leave the spinning to others and focus instead on explaining the medicine, and presenting the facts and the best estimate of the outlook.

Alan began by making a brief, crystal-clear statement about the procedure and the vice president's condition and stated unequivocally that there was no evidence of a heart attack. Then, still wearing our scrubs, we answered questions for forty minutes until no one had anything left to ask.

During the press conference I described the cause of restenosis in the following way:

> This is a specific response to injury from the stent . . . what we know is that when an artery is stented . . . the stent itself initiates a series of events, normal events—response-to-injury events which in about 20 percent of patients results in renarrowing. . . .
>
> Picture a garden hose that starts to fill with sediment. Cut the hose in half and you'd see the hose itself is the same size it always was but the effective channel inside the hose is narrowed.

I tried to explain that clinical events such as Vice President Cheney's occur from time to time in patients with heart disease and I didn't consider it a crisis:

> The vice president clearly has chronic coronary artery disease, and he has probably had it for many decades, although it was first discovered when he had his first heart attack in the 1970s. And this is what coronary artery disease has become. It's become a chronic disease, affecting millions of people in this country.

When asked about what could happen next, I replied:

> I wish I could predict the future. I think there's a very high likelihood that he can finish out his term in his extremely vigorous . . . capacity.

The next morning I arrived early, and the coronary care unit nurse told me the vice president had spent an uneventful night. I reviewed the morning EKG and some labs and was pleased to note that his cardiac enzymes remained normal, meaning he had not had a heart attack. The agent posted at Cheney's door greeted me with "Morning, Doc," and after knocking, I found the vice president alone and in good spirits, reading a newspaper and watching TV, having already eaten his breakfast. I pulled up a chair and described again what we had found at cath and what we were able to do.

The vice president was remarkably relaxed. "It sounds like you had a little trouble with the equipment yesterday," Cheney said with a slight smile.

*I guess he wasn't asleep after all.*

While we spoke, the *Today* show ran an update on the vice president's condition, and we stopped talking to listen to NBC's Tim Russert. Russert was wondering whether Cheney should resign, and he said that the vice president might have to make a choice between spending the last days of his life in office or spending them with his family.

In 2001, about one in five patients who received a stent would develop restenosis similar to the vice president's, and in most instances it was more an annoyance than a crisis. If Mr. Russert's comment bothered the vice president, he didn't show it. I was angry, but Cheney just laughed. I told Mr. Cheney that I was confident he would be fine and that I would tell him if I ever thought he was not capable of serving as vice president.

Over the next couple of days, the newspapers and broadcast media weighed in about Mr. Cheney's fitness to serve.

The *Los Angeles Times* published an editorial:

Cheney comes across as an unflappable fellow, the sort who keeps a cool head and steady hand when the stress is great. . . . But daily stress and a very high workload of essential duties are not a prudent combination for a man with Cheney's health history. Cheney's doctor insisted he could be perfectly capable of finishing his term "in his fully vigorous capacity." Yet there is a difference between vigor and capacity.

*US News & World Report* speculated about who might replace the vice president:

White House officials concede there's a contingency plan in case Cheney can't continue in office. Bush confidants say any list of possible replacements would include Secretary of State Colin Powell, governors such as Pennsylvania's Tom Ridge, and other Washington gray beards like Defense Secretary Donald Rumsfeld. In the meantime, Bush has barred aides from speculating because he considers it macabre.

Arianna Huffington wasn't just ill informed; she was outright nasty:

The question remains: Is the vice president on a suicide mission—or just unable to overcome his type-A addiction to the adrenaline highs of his lofty position? After his last heart attack, he was asked if he was worried about having another one. "I don't operate that way," he replied. No, you just put the gun to your head and see if the next chamber is the one with the bullet.

After Mrs. Cheney arrived, the vice president changed into a suit, and Alan and I accompanied them to the entrance to the hospital where the motorcade was waiting. As we walked through the lobby, I stopped to allow Mr. Cheney to leave the hospital alone, but he paused and motioned to me to join him. A barrage of clicking camera shutters greeted us as we passed through the door. The vice president turned to shake my hand, and the photo of that moment made the front page of newspapers around the country.

Lew Hofmann arranged for Gary and me to return to the White House two weeks later. We planned to see the vice president in the residence clinic, and Lew met us at the gate and walked us over. As it would be a little while until the vice president arrived, we were told to make ourselves at home in Dr. Tubb's office. Brigadier General Richard Tubb (also called Dick) had graduated from the Air Force Academy before going to medical school at the University of Wisconsin, and his office, just a few steps from the elevator leading to the president's quarters, contained a mix of mementos, including a classic doctor's bag and a ceremonial sword, reflecting his dual careers as physician and military officer. While I waited, a medical unit staffer suggested that I look out the window. The ground-floor office faces the South Lawn, and just as I parted the drapes, I watched as Marine One, a green Sikorsky VH-3D helicopter, landed, returning President Bush to the White House.

When the vice president arrived, he looked well. He said that he had resumed exercising with a recumbent bike and elliptical trainer, and his weight was down a few pounds. Since the angioplasty two weeks earlier, there had been no chest pain, shortness of breath, or other symptoms. We spoke about the possibility that the stent could narrow again, and I told him that although there was a risk of that, I thought it was likely he would do well. During the press conference, I had quoted a 40 percent chance of restenosis, the textbook answer, but because Cheney's specific lesion involved such a short segment of the stent, I thought it was probably half that. Mary Matalin had asked me about this a few days after the hospitalization, and I told her that I was intentionally lowering expectations, but I thought the vice president would do very well. Before the visit ended, I reminded the vice president that we still wanted him to wear a Holter monitor to continuously record his heart rhythm for twenty-four hours, and Lew said he would arrange for it.

In June, Lew obtained a Holter monitor (essentially a small recorder with a few EKG leads) from Bethesda Naval Hospital, and the vice president wore it over a weekend. During that interval, the monitor recorded quite a few isolated premature beats, a benign finding, but on two occasions four of these extra beats came one after another at a very fast rate, an ominous rhythm called ventricular tachycardia.

It had been known for many years that some patients with chronic heart disease die suddenly as a consequence of ventricular fibrillation (V Fib), essentially a chaotic electrical storm that causes the heart to quiver (fibrillate) ineffectively. In 2001 we knew that the risk of developing V Fib was inversely related to how well the heart contracts. A normal heart ejects about 60 percent of the blood that fills the left ventricle after each beat (ejection fraction 60 percent). The lower the ejection fraction (EF), the greater the risk of sudden cardiac death. The threshold for increased risk seemed to be around 35 percent, which is about what we estimated the vice president's ejection fraction to be. Other risk factors for developing sudden cardiac death included a prior (resuscitated) cardiac arrest (which the vice president had never had) and the identification of ventricular tachycardia by Holter monitoring (which we had just found).

Mr. Cheney's Holter monitor recorded more than 130,000 heartbeats over the thirty-four hours he wore it. Although only eight beats (.006 percent), lasting a total of about four seconds, were concerning, that was enough to identify the vice president as being at higher risk for a potentially fatal arrhythmia.

When we decided a couple of months earlier to have the vice president wear the monitor, a colleague had questioned the wisdom of the decision.

"Why look for trouble?" he asked.

To me, the answer was clear: sometimes what you don't know can kill your patient. Now that we had the data, I knew that Vice President Cheney was going to need a defibrillator.

Mordechai Friedman, a Polish Jew, was born in Warsaw in 1924. When he was a teenager, his name was changed to Mieczyslaw (Michel) Mirowski in an attempt to shield him from the fierce anti-Semitism that would soon become genocide. On September 1, 1939, German troops invaded Poland, the opening act of World War II, and the beginning of a five-year brutal occupation that included the methodical murder of most of Poland's Jewish population. Of the 3.3 million Jews living in Poland prior to the war, only 350,000 would survive to see the war end.

Three months after the German invasion, Mirowski, sixteen years old, left Warsaw, never to see his family again, and traveled east through wartime Soviet-occupied Poland, Uzbekistan, and the Ukraine.

After the war, he attended medical school in Lyon, France, and upon graduation went to Israel, where he worked for a while before moving to Mexico and the United States for training in cardiology. In 1963 he returned to Israel to practice cardiology and met Dr. Harry Heller, who would become his friend and mentor. Mirowski later said:

> In 1966, my old boss, Professor Harry Heller, started having bouts of ventricular tachycardia. He was repeatedly hospitalized and treated with quinidine and procainamide (the leading antiarrhythmic drugs of the time). My wife asked me why I was so concerned. "Because he will die from it," I told her. And he did, two weeks later while at dinner with his family.

Heller's death prompted Mirowski to start thinking about solutions for sudden cardiac death. The 1960s saw the introduction of coronary care units, where high-risk patients were monitored and treated rapidly should a lethal arrhythmia, such as ventricular fibrillation, occur. Mirowski wondered whether the large defibrillators stationed in CCUs could be miniaturized and implanted like a pacemaker in an ambulatory patient. Mirowski said:

> I talked to some cardiologists who knew more about such devices. They all told me that defibrillators couldn't be miniaturized. In those days, a defibrillator weighed 30 to 40 pounds; it was preposterous to reduce it to the size of a cigarette box. But I had been challenged by the problem, initially because of the death of a man I admired very much, but also because people told me it couldn't be done.

Mirowski moved his family to the United States in 1968 and accepted a job as the director of the CCU at Sinai Hospital, a community hospital in Baltimore, where he met Dr. Morton Mower, with whom he would collaborate to build the world's first implantable defibrillator. Mower later described the focus of the research:

> The initial goal set was a battery operated, automatic defibrillating device to be tested in animals, capable of monitoring in a standby mode and recycling in the event more than a single shock would be required in a particular episode.

A defibrillator, which sits atop a hospital "crash cart," contains a power source, usually a big battery that is continually charged through an AC outlet, a large capacitor, and the familiar paddles (now more commonly adhesive patches) that are used to transfer the energy to the patient for resuscitation. Before a defibrillator can deliver a shock, the capacitor must first be charged with several hundred joules of electricity, a process that takes several seconds. Crucially, Mirowski realized that a conventional defibrillator expends a lot of energy overcoming the resistance imposed by the skin and subcutaneous structures and that the heart could be defibrillated with much less energy if a shock was delivered from leads positioned inside the heart.

Mirowski and colleagues constructed prototypes, sometimes with components ordered from electronic catalogues and even scavenged from a camera flash. Soon they began laboratory tests on dogs. In 1972 Mirowski met Dr. Stephen Heilman, the CEO and founder of Medrad, a Pittsburgh-based manufacturer of angiographic injection devices. Heilman described his meeting with Mirowski:

> More memorable for me was Michel himself. He was intense. His speech was enriched by the expressive movement of his eyes. I knew that he had had contact with several languages and peoples as a result of being Jewish and living in Europe during World War II. His dedication to the project particularly impressed me. . . . I sensed in him a deep intelligence and a dedication that stood out. By the end of lunch we had agreed to collaborate on this exciting idea.

There were those, however, who derided Mirowski's implantable defibrillator, among them Dr. Bernard Lown, a world-famous cardiologist (and later winner of the Nobel Peace Prize), who more than a decade earlier had added greatly to the science of resuscitation with his significantly improved design for an external defibrillator. In a 1972 editorial in *Circulation*, the journal of the American Heart Association, written with Dr. Paul Axelrod, Lown wrote:

> Experience teaches that a rigid solution to a biologic problem is usually no solution. If the patient with such an implanted device is found dead, numerous questions will loom including the gnawing doubt that electrocution may have been a factor. . . . In fact, the implanted defibrillator system represents an imperfect solution in search of a plausible and practical application. In the absence of a clearly defined clinical purpose, what then energizes such undertakings by a number of groups? The rationale for some current bioelectronic development is best exemplified by Edmund Hillary's reasons for climbing Mt. Everest, "Because it was there." The same holds for some electronic gadget manufacture: "It was developed because it was possible."

Mirowski and colleagues responded to Lown's criticism:

> The authors' overcautious and negative attitude to the approach under investigation seems certainly premature at this experimental prototype stage. Would it not be more appropriate to postpone disqualification of this new way of approaching a major cause of mortality, however imperfect it may seem to be, until it faces the test of clinical trials?

Dr. Barry Maron, at the time a researcher at the National Heart Lung and Blood Institute, described Mirowski's reception as "a graphic illustration of the medical establishment against a guy who had no big name."

Undeterred, Mirowski and colleagues continued their research, and on February 4, 1980, at Johns Hopkins Hospital in Baltimore, a fifty-seven-year-old woman with a prior heart attack and multiple episodes of sudden cardiac death requiring defibrillation received the world's first implantable defibrillator. When the report of the initial implants was published in the *New England Journal of Medicine,* it was accompanied by an editorial with a decidedly different tone from Lown's eight years earlier:

> Although considerable additional work is needed to perfect the diagnostic and therapeutic capability of this device, it is a potentially important therapeutic contribution. . . . Viewed optimistically, this is yet another in an impressive series of contributions toward progress in the monitoring and identification of important ventricular arrhythmias and in their pharmacologic and electrical correction.

In 1985 the FDA approved the implantable defibrillator for commercial use. Since that time, millions of patients around the world have received the device during an outpatient procedure that takes about an hour and can be accomplished through a three-inch incision under the collarbone. Today implantable cardioverter defibrillators (ICDs) are used in patients who have survived cardiac arrest or those with high-risk features such as severely decreased heart function or certain inherited disorders.

On June 25, 2001, Gary and I went to the White House to discuss the results of the Holter monitor with the vice president. Lew arranged for us to meet in Dr. Tubb's office, and we asked Dr. Sung Lee, a cardiac electrophysiologist with our group at George Washington, to join us. We told the vice president that the monitor recorded a few brief episodes of ventricular tachycardia, and in the context of his prior heart attacks and impaired left ventricular function, this finding identified him as being at higher risk of developing a potentially fatal arrhythmia. I told the vice president that the risk could be reduced with the implantation of an ICD, and Sung described the procedure and the technology in great detail.

I acknowledged that the vice president had unique medical coverage in that Lew or one of his people was always nearby with an external defibrillator, but I reminded him that there were times when those precautions would be inadequate, for instance, when he was alone in his office or sleeping or showering. The ICD would be a 24/7 internal sentry. I told the vice president that if he received an ICD but never needed it, the decision to place it would still be correct.

Mr. Cheney asked Sung Lee some questions about the procedure itself and device durability, and finally said, "It makes sense."

Mary Matalin called a few days later to talk about the ICD and how the public announcement would be made. She told me that she cried when the vice president told her what we were planning to do. I reassured her that he was going to do well and that the device would protect him.

The plan was to bring the vice president to George Washington University Hospital early in the morning on Saturday, June 30. She said the vice president was going to make the announcement himself, in the White House briefing room on the Friday before the procedure, and they wanted me to join him there to answer questions from the press.

"That's a bad idea," I said.

"The president's people really want you to do it," she replied. "You're going to have to give me something to convince them."

"Tell them that if I have to field questions before the procedure, I almost certainly will be asked, 'What can go wrong?' "

"What can go wrong?"

"We can put a hole in a lung, or a hole in the heart, or cause severe bleeding," I responded. "After the procedure on Saturday, when there are no complications, no one will ask us what could have happened but didn't."

"Done," Mary said.

Instead of having me answer questions prior to the procedure, the White House released a statement I wrote. In it, I described the findings on the Holter monitor that prompted this procedure and stated that we were going to first do a test to verify that the vice president was indeed at risk, and if the test was abnormal, the vice president would receive an ICD:

> The electrophysiology study scheduled for June 30 involves the analysis of waveforms acquired from wires passed into the heart through the veins accessible at the top of the leg. This test will help assess Mr. Cheney's future risk of developing a sustained cardiac arrhythmia and determine if an implantable cardioverter defibrillator should be placed during the same procedure. An implantable cardioverter defibrillator (ICD) is a small electronic device, roughly the size of a small pager, weighing less than 80 grams, that is placed under the skin of the upper chest and has the capacity to continuously monitor and analyze a patient's heart rhythm. The ICD's main function is to interrupt rapid heart rhythms. If the ICD detects an arrhythmia, it can terminate the abnormal rhythm with either a pacemaker function or the delivery of a low-energy electrical shock. The device, which is designed to last 5–8 years before needing replacement, is placed with the aid of local anesthesia and intravenous sedation. Patients are usually discharged from the hospital later the same day and may return to work the next day.

Vice President Cheney's motorcade arrived at George Washington University Hospital early the next day, and we escorted him to the cath lab, where Sung Lee again reviewed the planned procedure, as well as its risks and alternatives, and the vice president signed the informed consent.

Sung was a graduate of the Medical College of Virginia and had completed a residency in internal medicine at the University of Maryland before spending four years as a research fellow at the National Institutes of Health. I was a few years ahead of Sung when he came to do his fellowship at George Washington University Hospital and was glad that he accepted a job with our group when he finished his training. He is a smart, easygoing guy with a warm spirit, but in the electrophysiology (EP) lab he is all business.

I'd sat down to talk with Sung the day before Cheney's procedure because he looked uncharacteristically nervous.

"What are you worrying about?" I asked.

"The press conference," he said a little sheepishly.

"The press conference?" I said, laughing. "I'll take care of that; you just concentrate on not killing the vice president."

With the vice president asleep on the examination table, Sung introduced a catheter into a vein in Mr. Cheney's leg and maneuvered it to the heart. Without much difficulty, Sung was able to induce ventricular tachycardia by stimulating the heart with three premature impulses, additional evidence that the vice president was prone to this arrhythmia. Outside the hospital, this heart rhythm could lead to death, but in the controlled environment of the electrophysiology lab, Sung quickly terminated the dangerous rapid rhythm.

I picked up a phone in the lab and called the control room on the other side of the glass to tell Alan Wasserman that we had found what we were looking for and Sung was going to implant the ICD. From the table, Sung said he might try to induce the arrhythmia one more time, and when I relayed that to the control room, Alan said, "Tell Sung if he tries to do that again I'm going to have the Secret Service shoot him." When the laughter subsided, the tension in the room had abated noticeably, no doubt just what Alan had intended.

Sung infiltrated lidocaine under the skin near the vice president's left collarbone and then made a small incision. A large vein, the subclavian, courses under the collarbone, and Sung promptly found it with a needle. He then passed two thick wires into Cheney's heart, anchoring one in the right atrium and the second larger lead in the right ventricle.

Sung worked quickly but not hurriedly, and next made a small pocket under the skin for the ICD.

The 2.75-ounce device, less than half the size of a deck of cards and the price of a small Lexus, is the direct descendant of Michel Mirowski's original invention and a triumph of bioengineering. Inside the smooth, sealed titanium enclosure sits a sophisticated programmable computer for rhythm analysis and treatment customization, a pulse generator for pacing, and capacitors for defibrillation. The battery will last on average about six years, when the entire ICD has to be replaced.

A few days prior to the procedure, before it was announced that we were going to implant a defibrillator in the vice president, I'd asked Sung to acquire an ICD still sealed in its original packaging and lock it away. A manufacturer's representative typically attends all defibrillator implants and will select a device from a giant bag of mobile inventory at the time of insertion. For this case, however, I thought it would be safer to choose a random ICD before anyone knew for whom it was destined.

Using a special screwdriver, Sung tightened the leads securely into the device before slipping it under the skin. Because the ICD is intended to treat ventricular fibrillation, the only way to know for sure that it will work is to induce the lethal arrhythmia in the lab and watch the device administer a shock. The vice president, who had been groggy but arousable after getting IV sedatives during the procedure, was given a dose of propofol, a short-acting hypnotic that induces sleep very quickly but dissipates rapidly when it is discontinued. With the patient asleep, a programming command was given to the ICD, which a moment later induced ventricular fibrillation.

We looked at the monitor and watched as the vice president's EKG suddenly changed from its slow, stable rhythm to a fast and chaotic pattern that, left untreated, would kill him in a few minutes. We watched as the ICD recognized the arrhythmia and charged its capacitor. The process took an excruciatingly long fifteen seconds. The device is programmed to check again for the arrhythmia before delivering its energy and, still detecting it, the ICD delivered a low-energy shock. There was a muffled *pop,* and Vice President Cheney shuddered under the sterile drapes. All eyes turned to the EKG monitor, which demonstrated that Cheney was still in V Fib. The device recharged, and while we waited for the ICD to deliver a higher-energy shock I saw Julia instinctively move closer to the external defibrillator, the backup plan in case the second ICD shock also failed. Again Cheney jerked a little with the shock. This time, the monitor showed that he had been successfully restored to a normal rhythm. Satisfied that the higher-energy setting would defibrillate the vice president, Sung grabbed a needle driver and suture and began to close the small wound as everyone in the room congratulated him on his cool performance. Julia called Sung a "rock star." I couldn't agree more.

I waited for Sung to finish, and together we walked over to tell Mrs. Cheney that all was well. The vice president's family was waiting in a secure area that during the week served as a small postprocedure recovery room, but had been dressed up for the occasion to function as a family lounge with a couch, food, TV, and Internet access. Sung and I were in good spirits when we entered the room, but right away it was apparent that Mrs. Cheney was not.

In 2001, ICD therapy was unknown to most of the public, and even within the cardiology community, it was still very much a cutting-edge technology that had yet to be fully embraced. It's easy to convince a patient who survives sudden cardiac death of the merit of a small implantable device that can prevent another episode, but it's a much harder task when the patient seemingly is well. Gary, Sung, Lew, and I had discussed the rationale for our recommendations in depth with the vice president when we met with him earlier in the week, but we had not met with Mrs. Cheney, and I think she clearly still had some questions about the need for the procedure. Now that the device was implanted, Mrs. Cheney was concerned about the safety of the ICD in the unusual environment in which the vice president lived, worked, and traveled.

Mrs. Cheney had done her homework and knew that ICDs could be affected by electromagnetic interference (EMI). Weak electromagnetic fields are emitted from all electrically powered equipment, but some types of gear emit significantly more EMI, which can mimic ventricular fibrillation and induce the ICD into inappropriately delivering a shock. Medtronic, the manufacturer of the vice president's new implant, lists antenna and large radio transmission equipment as significant sources of EMI. Mrs. Cheney reminded us that the vice president's limousine, residence, helicopter, airplane, and the White House itself were filled with high-power radio transmission gear, and she wanted to know how we knew it was going to be safe for her husband.

The truth is I didn't know. I had been focusing on the treatment algorithm (low ejection fraction + ventricular tachycardia = ICD) but had neglected to fully consider the unique considerations that might accompany this patient's job. It was a humbling moment, one that I was determined never to repeat.

Sung and I located John Naylor, the representative from Medtronic, who had been present during the implant, and explained Mrs. Cheney's concerns. John got on the phone, and over the next several days, company engineers swept the vice president's residence, offices, and vehicles for EMI. To our great relief, they found no areas that would be a safety concern.

## CHAPTER 11

# Treating the Vice President

## DR. REINER

The summers in Washington are long, but on this early September morning, the cooler air and crystalline light offered a whispered promise of the fall to come. I had an appointment at the White House with Vice President Cheney later in the day, so I dressed in a dark suit, a bit more formal than usual, and headed off into the dense DC morning traffic.

It had been about three months since Sung Lee implanted the defibrillator. Lew Hofmann had arranged for one of the WHMU nurses to draw blood from the vice president early in the morning and messenger it up to the lab at Bethesda Naval Hospital that day, so the results would be available when we met with him. We planned to arrive about fifteen minutes before our 5:00 p.m. appointment and review the labs with Lew before we saw Cheney.

At 9:00 a.m. a small crowd gathered around a television mounted on a wall in the hospital's first-floor radiology waiting room.

"What's going on?" I asked.

Someone said that a small plane had crashed into the World Trade Center in Lower Manhattan. I stood with a growing group of patients and staff and watched as smoke poured from the North Tower.

*There is always something happening in New York.*

I remembered the story of the B-25 bomber that struck the Empire State Building at the end of World War II. On that day, there had been dense fog in New York, but on this morning, there wasn't a cloud in the sky. A few minutes later, United 175 hit the South Tower, setting that building ablaze. The crowd of hospital staff and visitors stood in silence as the buildings burned; there were screams when they fell.

"Nothing will ever be the same," I said to no one in particular.

It wasn't long before we heard that the Pentagon had also been hit. From the upper floors of our office building, we could see smoke billow from across the river, and rumors began to circulate that another plane was headed for DC. The White House and the Capitol were evacuated, and the streets filled with thousands of people, some running, all trying to get out of town. I called Charisse and told her to go pick up the kids from school. Charisse asked me to come home, but I told her that the hospital had mobilized for casualties, and I was going to stay. Even if I wanted to leave, there was gridlock everywhere and no way to get out of town.

I heard from Lew in midafternoon. He was with the vice president; they were okay and soon to be on the move. He told me he would be in touch when he could.

Lew called again later. Despite the chaos of the day, the vice president's blood had somehow made it to the lab in Bethesda and the results were back. The blood had been drawn early in the morning, and after everything that had happened during the day, I had forgotten all about it. Lew told me that the vice president's potassium level was a potentially lethal 6.9.

"Say that again, Lew."

He did, and I told him that it must be an error. He said that's what he thought, but the lab had verified the result.

A high blood concentration of potassium is called hyperkalemia, and a level that high is a medical emergency because it can lead to cardiac arrest. Lew asked if the vice president's defibrillator would protect him, and I told him if the vice president really was hyperkalemic, it would not.

I asked Lew if there was any way to repeat the potassium test that night, and he told me that it was possible, but it would take a couple of hours to get the blood to a lab. I did not ask Lew where they were going; it wasn't something I needed or wanted to know. Many years later, I learned that to ensure the continuity of government, the vice president was taken to Camp David, the presidential retreat in the Catoctin Mountains of Maryland. On the helicopter ride from the White House, Lew passed a note to the vice president informing him that we needed another sample of blood.

"Not tonight, Lew. You can have it in the morning," the vice president responded.

The back cover of Vice President Cheney's memoir, *In My Time,* features a solemn photograph taken aboard Marine Two, the vice-presidential helicopter, as it left the South Lawn of the White House on September 11. The image, taken by White House photographer David Bohrer, depicts the vice president and Mrs. Cheney in an intensely personal moment. Just visible in the vice president's hand is the note from Lew Hofmann alerting Mr. Cheney to our concern about his blood.

## VICE PRESIDENT CHENEY

On the morning of September 11, 2001, I was at work in my West Wing office with John McConnell, my speechwriter, when my assistant, Debbie Heiden, called in to report that an airplane had struck the World Trade Center in New York. I turned on the TV and a few minutes later saw the second hijacked aircraft strike. I placed a phone call to the president, who was in Florida, and we agreed this was clearly a terrorist attack and discussed what he was preparing to say to the press.

As colleagues on the White House staff gathered in my office, the door suddenly burst open, and Jimmy Scott, one of my Secret Service agents, came rushing in and told me we had to leave immediately. He placed one hand on my left shoulder, and with the other hand he grabbed the back of my belt and propelled me out the door. When we reached a tunnel underneath the White House, we stopped as more agents joined us and additional weapons were taken out of a locker. At that point, Scott told me they had evacuated me from my office because of a report from the control tower at Washington Dulles International Airport that an aircraft, believed to have been hijacked, was headed for the prohibited air space over Crown (the code word for the White House). This plane was American flight 77, which had struck the Pentagon. There was a small black-and-white TV set in the tunnel as well as a secure phone, which I used to call the president. I told him that Washington was under attack as well as New York and recommended that he not return to the White House until we could ascertain the extent of the attack. The Secret Service made the same recommendation.

After the call we proceeded down the tunnel to the Presidential Emergency Operations Center (PEOC), where I would spend most of the rest of the day. Norm Mineta, secretary of transportation, joined me there and was instrumental in working with the Federal Aviation Administration in getting all of the aircraft down out of the sky that day. Initially we had reports of six hijacked aircraft and many inaccurate reports of car bombs, explosions, and other incidents.

One of my major concerns was to "preserve the continuity of government." In the event that an attack should take out both the president and vice president, it's crucial to make certain that potential successors are safe and secure. On 9/11, I worked to arrange for the movement of Speaker Hastert to a secure location, since he was next to me in the line of succession.

At one point shortly after I arrived in the PEOC, an Air Force officer came into the room and said that a plane believed to have been hijacked was headed for Washington and was just eighty miles out. He wanted to know if they were authorized to shoot it down. Based on a conversation I'd had previously with the president, I gave the order to take it out. A short time later, we received a report that a plane had gone down in Pennsylvania. Initially we believed one of our aircraft had shot it down. It was sometime later that we learned that the courageous passengers on United flight 93 had taken it down. If it hadn't been for their bravery, flight 93 would most likely have been flown into the Capitol or the White House.

Later that day after the president returned to the White House, he convened a meeting of the National Security Council and addressed the nation. That evening, Lynne and I flew by helicopter to Camp David, where we spent the night. I sat up until the early morning hours watching television coverage of the events of 9/11 and thinking about the policies we would need to pursue to make certain we didn't get hit again.

The events of 9/11 marked a sea change in terms of our priorities and policies and fundamentally changed the focus of our administration. Before 9/11, terrorist attacks such as the assault on the World Trade Center in 1993 and the attack on our embassies in East Africa in 1998 were treated as law enforcement problems. The FBI would investigate, capture the suspects, bring them to trial, and if convicted they would serve their terms in US prisons. But 9/11 changed the paradigm. The destruction of the World Trade Center, the attack on the Pentagon, and the murder of nearly three thousand Americans was an act of war, worse than the Japanese attack on Pearl Harbor.

Our main priority for the remaining seven and a half years we were in office was to make certain the terrorists were never able to launch another mass-casualty attack against the United States. We were especially concerned about an attack using weapons far deadlier than airline tickets and box cutters, such as biological or chemical weapons or even a nuclear device. Using the president's constitutional authority as commander in chief and the congressional authorization to use military force to capture al Qaeda, we implemented a number of programs designed to provide the intelligence we needed to prevent further attacks.

The two most important programs were the Terrorist Surveillance Program (TSP) and enhanced interrogation techniques. TSP permitted us to intercept contacts between al Qaeda terrorists overseas and their associates inside the United States. According to General Keith Alexander, director of the National Security Agency, this program has allowed us to intercept some fifty attacks targeting the United States and friends overseas. The enhanced interrogation program was instrumental in our ability to develop vital intelligence about al Qaeda. In 2004 the CIA produced a report concluding that Khalid Sheikh Mohammed, the mastermind of 9/11, had been the "pre-eminent source on Al Qaeda." KSM was subjected to these techniques more than any other high-value detainee. Both programs have generated considerable controversy, but they both produced valuable intelligence we needed to keep the country safe. The record speaks for itself.


For the twelve years prior to my election as vice president, I had no significant incidents involving my health. I experienced the one heart attack during the Florida recount, but it was a minor event, barely qualifying to be called a heart attack. For the eight years I was vice president, however, there were events that indicated my coronary artery disease was progressing. I never believed that the disease inhibited my capacity to do my job. I basically dealt with each problem as it came up, relying on my doctors to keep track of how I was doing physically and to let me know when I needed to make changes in my regimen or my medications. I did not sit in my office wringing my hands, worried about when the next heart attack would occur.

After my first heart attack in 1978, I felt a strong sense of fragility in the period immediately after I was released from the hospital. I worried that if I moved too suddenly, I might trigger another event. As I reengaged in that first political campaign, I frequently recalled

Dr. Rick Davis's advice that "hard work never killed anybody." As I grew stronger and was able to take on more and more responsibility in the campaign, I no longer worried about that next attack. I assumed my lifestyle changes had solved my problem.

By the time I began my service as vice president I could look back on twenty-two years of living with heart disease. I had accomplished a lot in spite of my condition and was confident going forward that I could continue to do the same. The key was to deal with my health separately from my job and never to let one interfere with the other. I didn't want worries about my heart disease to keep me from focusing on the requirements of my job. And I didn't want the job to be an excuse for not doing something that needed to be done to deal with a health problem.

As we approached the 2004 reelection campaign, I raised with President Bush the possibility of my stepping aside so he could appoint someone else to serve as vice president in his second term. This wasn't related to my health, but rather because I felt strongly that the president should have the opportunity to make a change if he thought it would strengthen the ticket. I believed, as the incumbent vice president, that it was my responsibility to make it easy for President Bush to select someone else if he wanted to do so. The first two times I brought the subject up, I felt President Bush had not really focused on it. So I went back a third time and he agreed to think about it. A few days later, he came back to me and said that he wanted me to continue on the ticket, which I was honored to do.

## DR. REINER

When Lew Hofmann redrew the vice president's blood early in the morning on Wednesday, September 12, he had more on his mind than just potassium. The repeat labs were normal, and ultimately we deduced that the high potassium was simply the result of the prolonged delay in processing the sample, which ensued following the evacuation of the White House. This is the note that he sent to the vice president:

*September 12, 2001*

*Mr. Vice President*

*I am very pleased to report that your repeat potassium was NORMAL! Both Dr. Reiner and Dr. Malakoff share my joy. . . .*

*Find enclosed your dose of Cozaar and K-Dur for today. Additionally, there is a packet of doxycycline antibiotic for protection from anthrax infection as we discussed this morning. Dr. Malakoff is fairly certain that he has given you this medication in the past without adverse effect. You should take one tablet twice per day for three days. Should the threat persist beyond then, I will provide another packet of medication. . . .*

*Lewis A. Hofmann, MD*
*White House Physician*

In the days and weeks following September 11, people in Washington, New York, and other cities around the country wondered whether, and when and how, the next attack would come. National Guard Humvees were posted around DC, including on the sidewalk in front of our clinic, antiaircraft batteries were positioned on the National Mall, and police stationed at strategic locations brandished automatic weapons. Within this new reality, the White House Medical Unit took steps to protect the president and vice president from potentially weaponized biological agents.

In a note to the vice president on September 15, Lew wrote:

We began the prophylaxis in an uncertain threat environment in order to provide protection, flexibility, and reassurance to you. . . .

Monitoring has been in place for several days, and no evidence of chemical or biological attack has been identified. . . . The risk of taking the medication is very small compared to the severity of illness that would be caused by exposure to anthrax. Therefore until the threat landscape becomes more clear, I recommend continuing the doxycycline.

A few days later, letters containing anthrax spores were mailed to two US senators and several media outlets, resulting in the deaths of five people, prompting Lew to change his advice for the vice president:

> Dr. Tubb has recommended anthrax vaccination for the President, and I recommend the same for you. . . . I am writing to you as your White House Physician rather than as a biological warfare expert. . . . My recommendations are specific to your situation only, and cannot be generalized to large groups, forces or populations. They should also be placed in the context of intelligence reports you may have received to which I am not privy.

In his book *The White House Physician,* Dr. Ludwig M. Deppisch calls the WHMU "an apolitical, professionally focused, tightly structured, military-staffed health maintenance organization," but in post-9/11 America, the fuller scope of the medical unit's mission became apparent.

In October, Lew Hofmann again updated the vice president:

> I would like to close by sharing with you that the White House Medical Unit took the lead several years ago in preparing for bio/chemical terrorism. On September 11th, in an uncertain environment, we took broad measures to defend against attack. . . . As we have discussed, you are now effectively immunized against anthrax and the antibiotics you are taking should protect you from plague and tularemia. We have an effective plan in place to treat an attack with botulism, and we stand prepared with vaccination to prevent you from smallpox infection if you are exposed. Please advise me if you require additional information, and I truly appreciate the opportunity to serve.

As if the concerns about a possible attack with anthrax, smallpox, botulism, tularemia, and plague weren't enough, in September 2001, a dead crow that tested positive for West Nile virus was found on the grounds of the vice president's residence in Washington.

Several weeks later, I met Lew and two of his White House colleagues for an early lunch a few blocks from my office at Mr. K's, an elegant Chinese restaurant that for years was a favorite haunt of lobbyists and K Street lawyers. When we arrived, the restaurant was eerily quiet.

"Do you have a reservation?" the maître d' asked.

We didn't. He didn't seem to notice that his restaurant was completely empty. After some head scratching and flipping back and forth in his reservation book, he sat us alone in a large formal dining room, the tables set with golden flatware and porcelain chopsticks rests.

It had been about a year since I first met Lew Hofmann, and he was quickly becoming a close friend. Lew's specialty is family medicine, which, the American Academy of Family Physicians states, "encompasses all ages, both sexes, each organ system and every disease entity," an excellent background for a doctor who may be called on to treat trauma, tonsillitis, or ventricular tachycardia. Despite rising to one of the most prestigious postings in military medicine, Lew managed to maintain a sincere humility, an admirable and uncommon trait in Washington.

Over lunch, the conversation veered toward some of the biological threats that had been in the news. I was curious whether the smallpox vaccine administered to everyone born before 1971 would still offer protection. Lew said that the best estimate was that the old vaccination would probably not keep you from getting the disease but might prevent you from dying of it.

Other tables were starting to fill with customers, and as we continued our not-so-light lunchtime conversation, a man I recognized approached our group. It was the prominent Washington lawyer Bob Bennett, who had represented President Bill Clinton. Bennett had been sitting at a nearby table with his brother, William Bennett, the former secretary of education, and he looked a little annoyed.

"Listen, guys," he said without a smile. "I can hear your conversation, and I really don't want to."

Such was the mood in Washington in the wake of the attacks, and for the vice president, bioterrorism countermeasures became an unexpected adjunct to his cardioprotective regimen that included aspirin, Plavix, and Lipitor.

When my home phone rang on a Saturday morning in late December 2001, the caller ID was blank. Expecting to hear a telemarketing pitch, I reluctantly answered the call, and when I did, a familiar voice on the other end said, "Hi, Jon, it's Dick Cheney."

The vice president was in Jackson, Wyoming, and was calling to report that he had been short of breath the previous night. He described the sensation as feeling that he wasn't able to take a full breath, but he denied experiencing any chest pain or difficulty with exertion and hadn't noticed any change in his weight. Unable to sleep, the vice president had gotten up and read for a while, but when he went back to bed, he still felt short of breath and didn't sleep for the rest of the night. When we spoke in the morning, he said he felt okay and thought his symptoms were similar to an episode a few years before that at the time we thought was altitude sickness.

Altitude sickness is a common constellation of mostly annoying symptoms such as headache, nausea, and insomnia that may occur at elevations higher than eight thousand feet. High-altitude pulmonary edema (HAPE), by contrast, is a potentially life-threatening condition involving fluid retention in the lungs, encountered unpredictably by otherwise healthy climbers and skiers, also usually occurring at altitudes above eight thousand feet. Untreated, extreme forms of HAPE can lead to death.

I thought it was probable that Cheney's symptoms were altitude related, but it was also possible that he was developing early signs of congestive heart failure (CHF); it was really impossible to tell for sure over the phone. Fortunately, the vice president traveled with medical support, and I was able to speak with Captain Thomas Waters, a White House physician's assistant, who examined Mr. Cheney. Together we surmised that the altitude was probably to blame, but in view of the vice president's known cardiac dysfunction, we prescribed a low dose of Lasix, a diuretic, which would help if the symptoms were due to CHF.

I told the vice president that I would call later to check on him, but after I hung up, I realized that I had neglected to ask for the phone number in Jackson.

"Why don't you press star six nine?" my wife, Charisse, suggested.

"Don't be ridiculous. I'm sure that's disabled."

Surprisingly it wasn't, and when I called later that evening, I was glad to hear that all was well. Although I still thought the thin mountain air was probably the cause of the breathlessness, Jackson is only about a thousand feet higher than Denver, and I was left with a lingering concern that Mr. Cheney's symptoms might have represented some early heart failure.

For much of Mr. Cheney's first term in office, he felt well, and our visits during those years were largely uneventful. The usual protocol for a patient with an ICD includes a quarterly evaluation during which the device is "interrogated" using an external programmer roughly the size of a large laptop computer, and during those visits, we always performed a quick history and physical examination. Often Lew Hofmann arranged for us to see Cheney in the vice president's West Wing office, usually at the end of the day, and he would pre-position a programmer in an inconspicuous corner of the suite. We tried to keep these visits brief, assuming that the vice president had more important things to do than spend time with a handful of doctors. Typically Gary Malakoff, Sung Lee, and I would make the ten-minute walk to the White House together, and after Sung left for private practice in Maryland in 2004, Dr. Cindy Tracy, GW's new head of electrophysiology, a nationally renowned electrophysiologist, took Sung's place in what Lew called "the three amigos."

We made a conscious effort to be discreet, never wearing white coats or openly carrying medical equipment. On her first trip to the White House, Cindy met us on the street still dressed in operating room scrubs.

"Cindy, you can't wear scrubs," I said.

"Why not?" she asked, looking surprisingly surprised.

"Because, we're going to the *White House*! Also, if the press spots scrub-wearing doctors entering the West Wing, they'll think Cheney's having another heart attack."

"Okay," Cindy said, and ran back to the hospital to change.


Most of the vice president's staff was situated in the Eisenhower Executive Office Building next door to the White House, but the vice president worked out of the West Wing in a small suite of offices staffed by a few aides led by Debbie Heiden, his longtime assistant. Debbie was the only member of the vice president's staff entrusted with any detailed knowledge of his personal medical history. She was also clearly the gatekeeper.

I looked forward to the White House visits, in part because of the singular venue, but more and more because I enjoyed seeing the vice president. I didn't really know him that well and had seen him only a few times before he decided to run in 2000, but over his two terms in office, I would spend dozens of hours with him at the White House, his residence, our offices, and the hospital.

My father used to say that it's one thing to have a disease, but quite another to let the disease have you, and clearly heart disease didn't have Dick Cheney. Each time Cheney faced a serious health crisis, he seemed to respond not by slowing down but by doing just the opposite and taking on increasingly demanding jobs. After the heart attack in 1978, he was elected to Congress, eventually rising to a leadership position in the House. Ten years later, after another heart attack and bypass surgery, Cheney served as secretary of defense, managing the military during the Gulf War and the collapse of the Soviet Union. Another decade later, after another MI, he became the vice president of the United States. The man managed to live an extraordinarily full life despite having had to live with an extraordinarily aggressive disease for a very long time.

In June 2001, when Vice President Cheney met with the White House press and announced that he was going to undergo testing the next day that might lead to the placement of an ICD, a reporter asked him if he was worried that his coronary disease might be getting worse. The vice president's candid answer that day is a glimpse into how he has lived his life.

> Well, no, I've—it's obviously a question I asked my doctors, in terms of what this might signify going forward. But as everybody knows, my history of coronary artery disease goes back to 1978. My entire career in politics, in elective office, in Congress, in the Defense Department, eight years in the private sector, now as vice president, it's all taken place after the onset of coronary artery disease. It's something you live with. And it's my great good fortune that the technology's gotten so good, that it's kept pace with my disease, if you will, so we've been able to manage it through the years. And as I say, if there were any inhibition on my ability to function, if it were the doctors' judgment that any of these developments constituted the kind of information that indicated I would not be able to perform, I'd be the first to step down. I don't have any interest in continuing in the post unless I'm able to perform adequately, and the doctors have assured me that is the case.

About once a year, the vice president underwent a series of comprehensive examinations that took days to plan. Our goal was to create an efficient, tightly choreographed schedule that condensed the maximum number of clinical evaluations into the smallest amount of time. Lew and I called it "kabuki theater" because there was quite a bit of stagecraft involved in coordinating the various consultants, and we generated timetables that would make NASA flight controllers look like slackers.

For a visit in July 2005, we assembled the following schedule:

Naval Observatory
Timeline for the Vice President's Evaluation
July 16, 2005

08:00 Arrive George Washington Hospital
      Proceed to Radiology Suite
08:05 Arrive CT Scan
      Change into Examination Attire
08:10 Intravenous Line Placement
08:15 Vascular CT Scan Leg Arteries and Aorta
08:30 Return to Arrival Attire
      Proceed to Ultrasound Suite
08:35 Arrive Ultrasound Suite
      Ultrasound of Neck Arteries
09:05 Proceed to Endoscopy Suite
      Change into Examination Gown
      Anesthesia Preparation and Monitor Placement
09:20 Commence Deep Sedation
09:25 Upper Scope
09:45 Complete Upper Scope
      Reposition for Lower Scope
      Colonoscopy
10:35 Recover from Deep Sedation
      Return to Arrival Attire
11:05 Synthesize Examination Findings
      Recommendations to Enhance Future Health
      Answer Questions
11:35 Depart Endoscopy Suite
      Proceed to Motorcade

The ability to coalesce, into a single morning, multiple tests that would usually be separated by several days is a perk not typically available to the general public, but very helpful for a patient who must travel with a large protective detail. The vice president had been due for a screening colonoscopy and upper endoscopy, and the relative quiet of a Saturday morning was the ideal time to do it. Patients with unusual security requirements can create significant disruptions in the normal work flow of a hospital, and using off-hours is often easier for both the hospital and the patient.

That day, the vice president was also scheduled to undergo a CT scan to evaluate his aorta and the arteries of his legs. An earlier ultrasound had identified the presence of aneurysms (abnormal dilatations) in the popliteal arteries, behind Cheney's knees, and we wanted to learn more about these. A localized weakening in a vessel wall can result in an aneurysm, and if it develops in the aorta or the brain, the principal risk is rupture, which can be devastating. An aneurysm in a popliteal artery doesn't usually rupture, but the clot that forms in the dilated sac can embolize and threaten the leg downstream.

The CT scan revealed that the aneurysm behind the vice president's right knee was large, measuring more than 4 centimeters, about the size of a golf ball, and it contained a lot of clot. The aneurysm in the left leg was a little smaller but still fairly big. Popliteal aneurysms are typically seen in patients with atherosclerosis, almost always in men, and left untreated, they can begin to shed small clumps of clot, causing gangrene of the lower leg and foot, a disaster. In the mid-1990s, a report from the Mayo Clinic showed that many of the popliteal aneurysm patients who suddenly developed symptoms (e.g., cold and painful foot or toes) would ultimately require an amputation. It was clear that both legs needed to be repaired before something bad happened. The only question was how.

In 2005, the standard approach to repairing a popliteal aneurysm was surgery to open the back of the leg, excise the diseased vessel segment, and then restore arterial continuity with a bypass composed of either a vein from the patient or a synthetic vascular graft. The surgery usually required general anesthesia and a few days in the hospital. Overall, vascular surgery is considered a high-risk procedure, in large part because it is frequently performed on patients who also have heart disease, and I thought Vice President Cheney was particularly high risk for surgery.

Although Cheney had not had any recent angina or overt episodes of congestive heart failure, I knew that he was delicately balanced. Earlier in the summer, an echocardiogram estimated his ejection fraction at 25 to 30 percent, somewhat lower than when he took office. Surgery to repair the aneurysm was going to require the harvesting of a vein, but surgeons had used the vein from his left leg during the coronary bypass surgery in 1988 and it wasn't clear how much of the remaining vein in the right leg would be usable. A synthetic graft was less desirable. Anesthesia places a stress on the heart, as does the tachycardia that may result from pain or blood loss, and the surgical procedure itself makes it more likely that blood will clot, not a good thing for a patient with severe coronary disease. To make matters worse, Cheney was going to need *two* operations.

I consulted Dr. Anthony Venbrux, GW's director of interventional radiology, an internationally renowned physician who had come to George Washington University Hospital five years earlier after spending the first part of his career at Johns Hopkins. Tony is a brilliant radiologist and a truly gifted teacher, and one of the kindest people I have ever known. He proposed a new, less invasive method to treat the aneurysms. The procedure, called endovascular repair, would involve placing a Gore-Tex–covered stent inside the vessel (an "endograft") to connect the relatively normal upstream and downstream arterial segments, thereby functionally excluding the aneurysm. The potential advantage of this technique was that it could be performed without general anesthesia, would not require the surgical excision of a vein, and should be safer. Also, recovery would be quicker, and if all went well, it might be possible to treat both legs during the same procedure.

The major negatives of this approach were its newness and the scarcity of long-term safety and efficacy data.

Tony told me that Dr. Barry Katzen, the founder and medical director of Baptist Cardiac & Vascular Institute in Miami, was one of the world's experts in this technique, and Tony said he would reach out to him and solicit his opinion without disclosing the identity of the patient. Barry agreed that endovascular popliteal aneurysm repair was a very reasonable option, particularly for high-risk patients, and that although it was relatively new, the evolving data were very favorable.

Tony subsequently drafted a long document, basically a medical brief, in which he outlined the rationale for his proposed strategy to repair the vice president's aneurysms with endografts:

> There are several clinical factors to consider regarding management of the bilateral popliteal aneurysms in this patient. Clinical comorbidities include significant cardiac history with previous harvesting of greater saphenous vein for CABG from one of the lower extremities. The patient also has had coronary artery interventions and placement of a pacemaker. The desire to preserve the remaining saphenous vein for potential future cardiac surgery is an important consideration. . . . Recognizing the lack of available longterm data, percutaneous access from an antegrade approach with aneurysm exclusion with a stent graft is a reasonable alternative given the medical conditions of this patient. . . . Given the current "state of the art" imaging available at GWUMC, percutaneous placement of such a device is feasible. The team at The George Washington University Medical Center is multidisciplinary and available to treat [the vice president] should he decide to proceed.

On July 23, 2005, we visited the vice president's residence to discuss our recommendations with Mr. and Mrs. Cheney. Lew arranged for a ride, and Tony Venbrux, Dr. Joseph Giordano, GW's chief of surgery, Dr. Ryan Bosch, an internist who replaced Gary Malakoff after Gary's departure from GW the year before, and I piled into an unmarked Secret Service van for the quick trip from our offices in Foggy Bottom to the twelve-acre compound two miles away.

Our meeting was held in the residence's first-floor library amid books about trout and hunting and a Gilbert Stuart painting of John Adams, the first vice president of the United States, above the fireplace. Over coffee, we spoke about the CT findings and the implications of the popliteal aneurysms, the treatment options, and, finally, why we were recommending the novel, less invasive approach. The vice president appeared quite relaxed as he and Mrs. Cheney asked questions; after about an hour, they thanked us for taking the time to come to their home to discuss this with them.

About a week later, I received a request to send a copy of the vice president's scan to Dr. Peter Gloviczki, the chief of vascular surgery at the Mayo Clinic. Dr. Gloviczki was a well-known vascular surgeon who had been asked by the WHMU to review the vice president's case. A few days later, a Mayo cardiologist called and wanted to know the details of the vice president's history and recent cardiac testing.

I spoke by phone with Mr. and Mrs. Cheney to again explain why I thought endovascular repair was the best procedure for the vice president.

"At the risk of being tedious, please allow me, one more time, to explain why I think repairing the aneurysms with stents is a better idea than surgery," I said.

"Dr. Reiner, why do all the other doctors say you're wrong?" Mrs. Cheney asked.

The answer to Mrs. Cheney's question had less to do with specific organ systems or objective data from stress tests, echocardiograms, or heart catheterizations, and more to do with the holistic *cura personalis,* "care for the whole person." The vice president was remarkably well compensated for someone with his level of cardiac impairment, but I thought the stress of open surgery would endanger his stability. I knew that the surgeons at Mayo were focused on how best to repair the legs but couldn't have had a good sense for the nuances of his condition. An old adage in medicine goes, "If you go to a baker, you get a loaf of bread." If you show a vascular surgeon a popliteal aneurysm, he or she will tell you that surgery is the best way to fix it (and it often is). Just not in this patient.

"They don't know the vice president as well as I do," I replied.


The WHMU has a budget item to cover the expense of bringing physicians to Washington for the purpose of consulting in the care of the president or vice president, and Lew Hofmann felt this was the time to do that. At the end of August, Drs. Peter Gloviczki and Barry Katzen graciously took time away from their busy practices in Minnesota and Florida, respectively, and flew to DC to present their recommendations to the vice president.

On Thursday, August 25, Lew, Bosch, and I met Gloviczki and Katzen for dinner at Old Ebbitt Grill near the White House. After dinner, we made the five-minute walk down Pennsylvania Avenue to the Eisenhower Executive Office Building, where Lew had reserved a conference room. I had hoped that by reviewing together Mr. Cheney's clinical data and hashing out the pros and cons of both techniques, we would reach a consensus to present to the vice president the next day. Unfortunately, despite meeting for hours, with Lew acting as facilitator, positions remained unchanged, with Peter Gloviczki advocating surgical repair and Barry Katzen recommending the less invasive endovascular stent graft treatment, which Ryan Bosch and I also strongly supported.

When we called it quits around 11:00 p.m., we were no closer to a unified plan than we were when we started hours before. Walking back to my office along the quiet, late-night streets of downtown DC, I thought about how complicated the treatment of this one patient had become.


Ninety minutes were set aside for our meeting in the West Wing with the vice president and Mrs. Cheney, a huge block of time in their schedules. The consultation had the air of a court proceeding, and I began with an opening statement explaining why the aneurysms needed to be repaired. I then introduced Dr. Gloviczki, who would address the surgical approach to the problem.

Peter had a broad and reassuring smile. His accent was tinged with the Budapest of his youth, but he spoke with precision he'd cultivated in the operating room. Medical illustrators at the Mayo Clinic had produced large, beautiful color drawings that were works of art, and as Peter spoke, he deftly used the exhibits to make his case. One panel showed the vascular anatomy of Cheney's legs and the large clot-filled sacs behind each knee. Another sketch illustrated how the proposed surgery would be accomplished by sewing a segment of vein into the leg to bypass the aneurysm. Gloviczki was an impressive advocate. There was no arrogance about him, just competence and confidence.

Gloviczki concluded his remarks by saying to Vice President Cheney, "If you were my father, I would recommend this surgery."

"If you were my father?" the sixty-four-year-old vice president said, taking mock offense at the fifty-seven-year-old surgeon's remark.

"I mean 'brother,' " Gloviczki quickly corrected, flashing a big, embarrassed smile.

Nothing cuts tension in a room better than laughter.

Next I introduced Dr. Katzen, an interventional radiologist who had helped create the endovascular revolution. Barry's five-day course, the International Symposium on Endovascular Therapy, held annually for the last quarter century in Miami, is the premier conference focusing on cutting-edge vascular therapies. He had brought with him a sample of the kind of stent graft we would use to repair Mr. Cheney's aneurysms. The device, called a VIABAHN Endoprosthesis, manufactured by W. L. Gore & Associates, has the appearance of a large, flexible stent with an integrated fabric liner. The stent itself is constructed of Nitinol, a metal alloy of nickel and titanium that, unlike Julio Palmaz's original stainless-steel stent, has extreme flexibility (superelasticity) and the ability to pop into a preconfigured form (shape memory). The liner is made of Gore-Tex, the ubiquitous fabric that is essentially a porous form of Teflon. Barry described how the stent would be delivered and deployed and said that the procedure would be performed with only sedation and local lidocaine, obviating the need for general anesthesia.

The Cheneys had many questions.

"What is the incidence of infection?"

"What do you use if there isn't enough vein available?"

"Can you do both legs the same day?"

"How long do the stents last?"

"What are the risks?"

"How long is the recovery?"

Before we concluded the meeting, I summarized the two proposals and reiterated the reasons I favored the Venbrux/Katzen approach. Vice President Cheney thanked us for all the time we had spent on this matter and said he would think about it over the weekend and let us know what he wanted to do in a few days.

On Monday morning, Debbie Heiden called and asked if I had a few minutes to talk with the vice president.

"Of course," I said.

When Cheney got on the line, he thanked me again for arranging the meeting and then cut right to the chase.

"I've decided to go with the stent option," he said.

To go all-in in no-limit poker, to bet all your chips, is a sign of either total confidence in your cards or a ballsy bluff. I had gone to great lengths to convince the vice president to undergo the relatively untested endograft procedure. His decision was an enormous demonstration of trust, the weight of which I suddenly felt. I was confident that this was the right thing to do, but there was no denying that I was now definitely all-in.

*The White House*
*Washington*
*September 21, 2005*

*Mr. Vice President*
*Please find enclosed in this envelope a DVD which has a three*

minute video animation of the stent placement procedure. The video does not include animation of the placement of one stent inside another.

With regard to Saturday . . .

Preparation

Please eat a good supper on Friday night. After midnight you should only have water. Take all of your regular medications on Saturday morning.

Remember to bring your "overnight kit" as we discussed by phone on Monday. Attire will be provided for you throughout your stay, however if you desire to have your own pajamas that will be fine. There is a small chance that the groin sites could ooze for the first few hours, so it might not be prudent to put your own clothes on right away.

Procedure

Plan to arrive at George Washington Hospital at 7:00. You will be escorted to a room where you will change into hospital attire. From there you will walk to the procedure lab, arriving around 0715.

In the procedure room, two intravenous lines will be placed, blood will be drawn to prepare for the VERY unlikely possibility of transfusion, and you will be asked to sign the consent form. Your ICD will be disabled.

You will then receive sedation and local anesthesia. We expect the actual procedure to begin by 0800. The procedure may take up to four hours, we expect to be done by noon. Your ICD will be reactivated.

When you have recovered adequately from the sedation, you will be transported to your overnight room on the VIP ward. Although exact times are difficult to predict, we anticipate that you will be fully alert by 1430.

Here is a summary of your operative and medical team:

Dr. Jonathan Reiner

Dr. Ryan Bosch

# HEART

*Dr. Paul Dangerfield, Cardiac Anesthesiologist*
*Dr. Cynthia Tracy, ICD Cardiologist*
*Dr. Anthony Venbrux, Interventional Radiologist*
*Dr. Barry Katzen, Interventional Radiologist*
*Dr. Peter Gloviczki, Vascular Surgeon*
*Dr. Joseph Giordano, Vascular Surgeon*
*I know you are in the best of hands. . . .*
*Very Respectfully*
*Lewis A. Hofmann, MD, FAAFP*
*White House Physician*

When the motorcade bearing Vice President Cheney arrived at George Washington University Hospital early Saturday morning on September 24, 2005, the news media had already assumed their familiar vigil. The aneurysm repair had taken two months to plan and involved dozens of physicians, nurses, technologists, administrators, and security personnel. The VIP wing of the telemetry floor was configured for the vice president's planned overnight stay with freshly painted walls, polished floors, hotel-like furniture, rugs, and new linens. Operating room personnel were placed on standby, just in case, and Secret Service agents were posted throughout the hospital. Dr. Gloviczki and Dr. Katzen were granted temporary DC medical licenses and GW clinical privileges, and they returned to Washington to lend a hand.

The procedure to treat Vice President Cheney's right leg was complex but uncomplicated. After numbing the upper leg with lidocaine, Tony Venbrux placed a large sheath (about the diameter of a soda straw) into the superficial femoral artery. A thin wire was then advanced through the upper leg, into and beyond the aneurysm behind the knee and down to the level of the calf, using X-ray guidance. Two stent grafts were then slid, one at a time, over the wire, positioned within the aneurysm, and deployed by pulling a "rip cord" that released a constraining stitch, allowing the stent with "memory metal" to expand on its own.

Although typically we would opt to treat one leg at a time and separate the procedures by at least a week or two, we had discussed the possibility of repairing both legs during the same session because the logistics for treating the vice president were so intricate. Since Cheney was clinically doing fine, we made the decision to treat the left leg as well, which took another couple of hours to accomplish and again required two stent grafts.

When we were done, I called my wife, Charisse, who asked how it went. Before I could answer, I heard Tony Venbrux, who was speaking nearby into his own phone, respond to the same question.

"It was a triumph," he said.

In early January 2006, only three months after the repair of the popliteal aneurysms, the vice president developed a painful flare of gout in his left foot, a condition he had experienced before. Gout is an inflammatory arthritis, often involving the big toe, caused by the deposition of uric acid crystals in the joint. Nonsteroidal anti-inflammatory drugs (NSAIDs) are usually effective in reducing both the pain and the inflammation of the acute episode, and the vice president had an old supply of indomethacin, which he began.

NSAIDs, a class of drugs that also includes ibuprofen and naproxen, are widely used but not without some risks. The familiar medications can cause gastric irritation or, less commonly, ulcers; they also may increase the risk of a cardiac event, mediated in part by adverse effects on kidney function. In patients with existing heart disease, these agents can result in substantial fluid retention.

Late at night, a few days after beginning the indomethacin, the vice president called the physician's assistant on duty for the WHMU and reported that he was having trouble breathing. He stated that he had gained seven to ten pounds over the prior few days, his legs were swollen, and around midnight he developed shortness of breath. Now, three hours later, his breathing was getting worse.

Five minutes later, Lieutenant Jerald Jarvi, a Coast Guard physician's assistant on call for the WHMU and sleeping in another building on the Observatory grounds, was standing at the vice president's bedside. Jarvi's examination of Mr. Cheney was significant for coarse breath sounds called rales, caused by accumulation of fluid in the lungs, as well as significant edema in both lower legs. Jarvi called me and we agreed that the vice president had congestive heart failure. I said I would meet them at the GW emergency room.

In the ER, Cheney was stable but clearly fluid overloaded. Blood tests showed no evidence of a heart attack, and there were no EKG changes. After a dose of the IV diuretic furosemide (Lasix), the vice president's breathing eased considerably. Although the CHF likely was precipitated by the indomethacin, the episode did vividly illustrate the fragility of Mr. Cheney's clinical balance. It also validated our approach to the aneurysms a few months before. If a few tablets of indomethacin could tip Cheney into heart failure, what might have happened if he had undergone vascular bypass surgery?

## VICE PRESIDENT CHENEY

During my time as vice president, the one instance where the job clearly had a direct impact on my health occurred in February 2007. I was scheduled to make a trip to the western Pacific with stops in Japan, Guam, and Australia. At each stop, I visited with senior government officials and US military personnel. While I was in Australia with Prime Minister John Howard, one of our best allies and friends, President Bush asked me to continue on around the world and add stops in Pakistan and Afghanistan. I was scheduled to see President Musharraf in Islamabad and President Karzai in Kabul. When I arrived in Afghanistan, I first made a stop at our major base at Bagram, north of Kabul, for briefings and meetings with our senior military leaders in the country. Unfortunately, I got snowed in at Bagram and had to spend the night. I planned to continue to Kabul the next day.

As I was preparing to leave the next morning, I heard a loud explosion: a suicide bomber had detonated his bomb at the front gate of the base, killing twenty-three people, including two Americans. When the bomb went off, my security detail took me to a bunker near the room where I had spent the night. A short time later, we resumed my schedule as planned. After the attack, a Taliban spokesman claimed the attack had been aimed at me. That was not credible since I was about a mile away from the site of the explosion, and I was on the base only because of a last-minute schedule change the night before. But it was a demonstration of the kind of violence the Taliban and their allies were visiting on the people of Afghanistan. And it was evidence of the danger our military personnel faced every day.

When I returned to Washington, I had been gone nine days, traveled some twenty-five thousand miles, and spent sixty-five hours in the air. After I had been home a day or two, I noticed a pain in the lower part of my left leg. I reported it to my doctors and arranged for an exam, which included an ultrasound of my left leg. It showed I had developed a blood clot in a vein—a deep vein thrombosis (DVT). It was apparently the result of all those hours on a plane during my recent trip. It was potentially dangerous if it migrated to my lungs or heart and caused a pulmonary embolism. We treated it with regular injections of enoxaparin and oral doses of warfarin, powerful anticoagulants, and over time it dissolved. But managing my medications became more difficult as we had to strike a balance between using the blood thinners to avoid clotting, while at the same time not using so much that we created problems with bleeding.

## DR. REINER

In 2007 Vice President Cheney embarked on a nine-day, twenty-five-thousand-mile trip that included stops in Afghanistan, Pakistan, Oman, Australia, and Japan. A few days after returning, following a speech at the national legislative council of the Veterans of Foreign

Wars, he called to tell me he was experiencing some discomfort in his left calf. There are many potential reasons for discomfort in the leg, but calf pain after extensive air travel is a DVT until proven otherwise, and I recommended that the vice president come to our offices right away for further evaluation.

*Medical Faculty Associates*
*The George Washington University*
*March 5, 2007*

*Dr. Lew Hofmann called late this morning to report that Vice President Richard Cheney had informed him that he had developed discomfort in his left calf. The vice president then presented to the MFA [Medical Faculty Associates] for evaluation at 1:30PM. The vice president was seen with Drs. Lew Hofmann, Ryan Bosch, Joe Giordano, and Michael Hill.*

*Overall, the vice president has felt well. He recently completed a long overseas trip which covered approximately twenty-five thousand miles and sixty-five hours of flight time. Two days ago after arriving back in Washington, DC Mr. Cheney began to note some mild discomfort in his left calf, extending up to the back of the knee. The vice president did not note any swelling in the ankle. There was no chest pain or shortness of breath.*

*On examination the left calf is subtly larger in diameter and mildly more tense than the right calf. The left leg has a mildly positive Homans' sign [pain in the calf when the foot is flexed]. The DP and PT pulses are 2+ bilaterally.*

*Arterial and venous ultrasound of the right leg revealed no evidence of DVT and the popliteal stent graft is widely patent. Venous ultrasound of the left leg shows a prominent thrombus in the left popliteal vein extending into the TP and tibial and peroneal veins. Arterial imaging of the left leg was not performed.*

*In summary, Vice President Richard Cheney has developed a*

*left lower extremity DVT [deep vein thrombosis] most likely caused by his recent extensive plane travel. We have begun enoxaparin 100mg SC q12 hours (first injection given at the time of this examination) and warfarin 5mg qd [blood thinners]. . . . I told Vice President Cheney not to perform his usual exercise regimen. We will plan to repeat the venous imaging study in 1 month's time.*

*Jonathan S. Reiner, MD*

Blood returns to the heart from the long and capacious veins of the legs aided by periodic propulsive compression of surrounding muscles that essentially "milk" the veins of their blood. Clots can form anywhere blood pools, and it has long been recognized that prolonged immobilization, such as that which occurs in a bedridden patient or a long-haul traveler, can lead to the development of thrombi in the legs. In 2003, David Bloom, a thirty-nine-year-old NBC reporter covering the invasion of Iraq, who had spent several days riding in a cramped position inside a tank recovery vehicle, died from a pulmonary embolus that originated in a DVT in his leg.

It has been estimated that 1 in 4,600 people who fly will develop a DVT within two months of travel, a condition erroneously referred to as "economy class syndrome." While there is no evidence that sitting in economy class increases the risk of developing a DVT, the likelihood of developing a clot does increase with flights of more than eight hours and also with assignment to a window seat. Vice President Cheney traveled on Air Force Two, a spacious Boeing C-32 (a modified 757), but even with plenty of room to move around, long flights equal long sedentary stretches. Risk factors for the development of a DVT other than prolonged immobility include a genetic or acquired predisposition to clotting, smoking, cancer, oral contraceptive use, age greater than sixty, and congestive heart failure.

In isolation, the vice president's DVT was a fairly common and very treatable condition, but its occurrence did leave me with some concern about the general trend in his health.

*Medical Faculty Associates*
*The George Washington University*
*June 6, 2007*

*Dr. Lew Hofmann called this afternoon and relayed a message that the vice president needed to talk with me. I called Mr. Cheney and he stated that he has felt more fatigued recently. We saw the vice president 1 week ago for a device check and to discuss plans for routine follow-up. At that time Mr. Cheney stated that he had no chest pain, shortness of breath, palpitations, edema or change in his exercise tolerance. Today Mr. Cheney noted that for the last week to week and a half he has felt more fatigued. He stated that he has been having difficulty keeping the RPM of his exercise bicycle above 60. He notes that he may be a little more short of breath climbing stairs. He has not had any chest pain and . . . has not been short of breath at night. He has not had edema. His weight is down somewhat and is currently around 210.*

*I told Vice President Cheney that we should proceed with our planned echo and nuclear stress test earlier than July and we agreed to have the vice president return on June 8, 2007 for testing. I discussed this plan in detail with Drs. Hofmann and Bosch.*

*Jonathan S. Reiner, MD*

Two days later, the vice president returned to our offices for a comprehensive cardiovascular examination that included an EKG, an exercise stress test with myocardial perfusion imaging (nuclear stress test), and an echocardiogram. Although both the EKG and stress test were unchanged and showed the effects of the earlier heart attacks, the echocardiogram revealed that the vice president's heart function had declined. Prior echos had estimated Cheney's ejection fraction about 30 percent (normal ejection fraction is greater than 50 percent), but now it was closer to 20 percent, a significant drop. In my note summarizing the vice president's evaluation, I wrote:

*Mr. Cheney's increased fatigue is likely the result of a decline in his left ventricular contractility. Although he is remarkably well compensated, he has little reserve. The stress test shows no evidence of active ischemia but he was able to do less exercise compared with his last exam 2 years ago. While the vice president is currently class II, I do believe he would benefit from addition of spironolactone to his regimen. We will also increase the dose of his Cozaar from 50 mg to 100 mg. As he does not get angina I think we can stop the Imdur. This should give us a little more room in terms of systolic blood pressure for maximizing the doses of his heart failure meds. We will start by increasing the Cozaar and then in 1 week add spironolactone 25 mg qd. . . .*

*The vice president's ICD is now near end-of-life and we will plan to have him return in July for elective replacement of the device by Dr. Cindy Tracy.*

Nearly seven years had elapsed since Dick Cheney first told Gary Malakoff and me that he was going to run for vice president, and during those twenty-five hundred days, Cheney's overall health had been stable, although far from uneventful. Now we were beginning to see a not-so-subtle decline in his cardiovascular status. I still had no doubts whatsoever about the capacity of the vice president to perform the duties of his office, but his care was becoming more complex. Congestive heart failure (CHF) is defined as the inability of the heart to maintain an adequate output of blood, and it was becoming abundantly clear that Dick Cheney had CHF.

A few days after the testing at the MFA, Lew Hofmann drafted a summary for the vice president:

*The Naval Observatory*
*June 11, 2007*

*Mr. Vice President*
*I know that we threw quite a bit of information at you in a*

*short period of time on Friday. I thought I would take a moment to review our findings and recommendations. . . .*

Your Heart

*There is no way I can improve on Dr. Reiner's lucid description of the current status of your heart. Both your symptoms and the imaging confirm that there has been some decrease in pumping function. There was no evidence of new blockage.*

The Plan

*Dr. Reiner would like to make medication adjustments which should help preserve your heart's ability to pump effectively.*

*Cozaar is a drug called an "ACE Receptor Blocker" which has been shown to preserve and sometimes improve heart function. You were on a middle-sized dose of 50mg; we will increase it to 100mg. Cozaar is also used to treat high blood pressure, so there is a small risk of lowering your blood pressure to the point where you might feel lightheaded when we make the dose increase.*

*Imdur is a drug in the class of "nitrates" which are used to treat angina. Dr. Reiner started you on this as a precaution when you had a fleeting episode of chest pain some years ago. You have been free of chest pain since. Imdur can lower your blood pressure as well, so we feel that stopping the Imdur may counterbalance the blood-pressure-lowering effect of the higher dose of Cozaar.*

*Inspra and Aldactone [spironolactone] are medications which are also beneficial in preserving heart function. Once you are stable on the new dose of Cozaar, Dr. Reiner may decide to add one of these medications to your regimen.*

*One of the earliest things which will change if your heart is having more trouble is your weight. You will probably gain a few pounds before you begin to develop shortness of breath or changes in exercise tolerance. We want you to <u>record your weight daily</u> from now on, and let us know right away if you experience unexpected weight gain.*

Your ICD

*We are proceeding with plans to change out the ICD in July, most likely on a Saturday morning. This will take place in the main hospital. The new ICD will include the ability to do a very sensitive check on your fluid status. . . .*

*. . . And Some Good News*

*Your cholesterol numbers continue to be excellent:*

*Total cholesterol 171 (normal less than 200)*

*HDL ("good cholesterol") 58 (desirable greater than 40)*

*LDL ("bad cholesterol") 61 (desirable less than 100)*

*Triglycerides 259 (desirable less than 250) . . .*

*Drs. Reiner, Bosch and I are all devoted to not only helping you be the very best vice president you can be, but also to securing for you the healthiest possible future.*

> *Very Respectfully*
> *Lewis A. Hofmann, MD, FAAFP*
> *White House Physician*

The data from the vice president's ICD in June had shown that the battery in the six-year-old device was nearly depleted. Implantable defibrillators have sealed titanium cases, and when the battery is exhausted, the entire "can," electronics and all, must be replaced. The procedure, referred to in cardio slang as a "gen change" (generator change), can usually be accomplished in a thirty-minute outpatient surgical procedure with sedation and local anesthesia, during which the subcutaneous pocket is opened, the old device is unscrewed from its leads, and a new device is inserted. The fact that the old ICD had never been called on to treat a dangerous arrhythmia did not in any way affect our decision to replace it, and one could argue that the decline in the vice president's heart function made a defibrillator even more imperative. Since the original implant, new features had been introduced, and I was particularly interested in its ability to detect the onset of congestive heart failure.

Fluid accumulation, particularly in the lungs, is one of the hallmark features of congestive heart failure, and it often has an insidious onset. Engineers at Medtronic, the Minneapolis-based biomedical device manufacturer, leveraging the fact that an ICD is essentially an implanted electrical circuit, developed a method to detect the early warning signs of CHF by monitoring changes in intrathoracic impedance. Electrical impedance is a measure of the resistance to the passage of current through a circuit and is reduced by the presence of fluid in the chest. One of Medtronic's new ICD models had a feature that they called OptiVol, which had the ability to track daily intrathoracic fluid levels, and I thought this would be useful for monitoring the vice president for incipient heart failure.

ICDs with OptiVol are produced with a usually helpful capability enabling wireless interrogation and programming without the traditional need to rest a mouse-like programming head on the skin above the device. I had learned a lesson from the original implant experience, and since that time had tried to tailor data-driven treatment recommendations to the unusual work and lifestyle of this particular patient. After the vice president received the ICD in 2001, we searched, after the fact, for potential sources of electromagnetic interference in his residence, office, limousine, helicopter, and airplane, and thankfully found none.

This time I wasn't concerned about accidental interference causing the ICD to malfunction; instead I was worried that a sophisticated attacker might wirelessly access the device, reprogram it, and potentially kill the vice president. I broached my concerns with Dr. Cindy Tracy, and she said she would look into it. Medtronic told Cindy that the feature was not customizable, and if she wanted OptiVol, it would also come with wireless. After confidentially disclosing to the company the background for our request, Medtronic agreed to create a one-time change to the new ICD's firmware that disabled its wireless functionality. Medtronic no doubt thought I was paranoid or had seen too many episodes of *24*, but in 2013, a computer hacker disclosed that he had reverse-engineered a device programmer and showed that it was "100 percent possible" to load compromised firmware into an implanted device using a laptop, exactly the way the fictional terrorist Abu Nazir killed the vice president on *Homeland*.

## CHAPTER 12

# Slippery Slope

## VICE PRESIDENT CHENEY

As we approached the end of our second term in office, I was aware that my coronary artery disease was progressing. Some days I had trouble walking up the stairs in the vice president's residence to the second floor. I had had occasional episodes of atrial fibrillation, which caused excessive fluid buildup and sometimes made breathing difficult.

Nevertheless, my health still was not interfering with my ability to do my job. In September 2008, we took our last major international trip to Georgia, Azerbaijan, Ukraine, and Italy. One of the most significant historical events during my years in public office had been the collapse of the Soviet Union, marking the end of the Cold War, the withdrawal of Soviet forces from Eastern Europe, and the liberation of the former Soviet Republics in the "near abroad," the independent republics that lie near to or border Russia. Vladimir Putin once referred to the collapse of the Soviet Union as "the greatest geopolitical catastrophe of the century." In my opinion, he never accepted the notion that former Soviet Republics such as Georgia, Ukraine, and Azerbaijan should be free of Russian domination. In 2008, he used military force to reassert Russian authority in the Near Abroad.

My trip came in the aftermath of the invasion of Georgia by Russian forces. Georgia's president, Mikheil Saakashvili, whom I had known previously, contacted me and told me how deeply concerned he was about what was happening to his country. At one point, the Georgians were convinced the Russian tanks were only a few miles from the capital of Tbilisi. My trip was meant to reinforce the proposition that the United States was committed to the freedom and independence of those states that had gained their freedom when the Soviet Union went out of existence. Ukraine had been threatened by a Russian attempt to install a pro-Russian candidate in the presidency. The people of Ukraine rose up in the Orange Revolution, which led to a second election and the presidency of Viktor Yuschenko. During his campaign he had fallen seriously ill, apparently the result of having been poisoned by pro-Russian elements. Azerbaijan incurred the wrath of the Russians when it tried to build a gas pipeline to southern Europe that would compete with the monopoly the Russians enjoyed as purveyors of natural gas supplies to Western Europe.

The year 2008 was also a presidential election year. I was not actively involved in the campaign, in part because Senator John McCain, the Republican candidate for president, was trying to put as much distance as possible between his campaign and the Bush-Cheney administration. That fall, our administration was also dealing with the global financial crisis. I sat in on many of the meetings and was asked by the president to work to build support for our position among House Republicans. The major responsibility for monitoring developments and developing and implementing the president's policy fell to the secretary of the treasury, Hank Paulson, in close consultation with the chair of the Federal Reserve, Ben Bernanke.

At one point during the fall campaign, McCain asked the president to convene a meeting with the congressional leadership to discuss the economic crisis. McCain suspended his campaign and returned to Washington to attend the meeting organized at his request. When first called on by the president, Senator McCain had nothing to say. When the president called on Harry Reid, majority leader, for his views, he indicated the Democrats had agreed that Senator Barack Obama would speak for all of them. It was clear the Democrats had their act together and the Republicans didn't. After the meeting, it wasn't at all clear why McCain had asked for it in the first place.

As our administration drew to a close, Lynne and I moved from the vice president's residence to a new home in McLean, Virginia, just outside DC. The weekend before the inauguration, I was lifting a box and injured my back. The injury put me in a wheelchair and eventually required surgery to repair a herniated disc.

During the early months of 2009, we adjusted to being private citizens once again as we split our time between our house in McLean, Virginia, and our home in Wyoming. We took the entire family on the vacation of a lifetime: a week cruising the coast of Alaska from Ketchikan to Juneau. Although I had no major problems on the trip, I did have certain limits. When everyone got off the boat to hike to a special area to observe Alaskan brown bears, I had to stay behind because I was concerned the hike would be too strenuous.

For several years in the 1990s, I traveled every year with a group of friends to British Columbia to fish for steelhead, one of the world's great challenges for fly fishermen. I had to give it up when I was vice president because all of the security and logistical arrangements when I traveled involved the use of US governmental resources. I couldn't justify doing so just so I could go out of the country to fish.

October 2009 was the first chance I had to go back, but it required a long, complex trip on commercial flights. When I got to the Babine River in northern British Columbia, I found I had difficulty spending a full day on the river. Steelhead fishing requires wading in fast, often deep water. All I could handle was a couple of hours a day. I spent the rest of my time next to a fire in the lodge. On my annual pheasant-hunting trip to South Dakota, I wasn't strong enough to stay in the field all day with the rest of the party.

A major factor in the transition back to private life from being vice president is the loss of the tremendous support mechanism that surrounded the person who is in that office. Lynne and I lived in the vice-presidential residence that used to be the quarters of the chief of naval operations. For a long time, vice presidents lived in their private homes, but in 1974, Congress decided to provide quarters and moved the chief of naval operations to other facilities. To this day, the Navy provides the personnel who operate the residence, and they are superb.

The enlisted aides take care of all the needs of the vice president and his family, including cooking and cleaning. They take over the daily chores of life so the vice president can focus on the responsibilities of that office. In private life, I used to do most of the grocery shopping and cooking. As Lynne will readily tell you, cooking isn't her greatest strength, although it took both of us a little time to admit it. The first year we were married, we pretended she could cook, and I pretended I liked her cooking, but after that I took over.

Once when I was secretary of defense during Desert Storm, I had my driver stop at the local grocery store on my way home from the Pentagon so I could pick up some needed items. In the checkout line, I was confronted by a woman who made it clear she thought it was totally inappropriate for the secretary of defense to be grocery shopping while there was a war on. When I was vice president, the naval-enlisted aides went to the supermarket.

I am often asked if I miss anything about being vice president. Travel on Air Force Two comes to mind. Counting my time as secretary of defense, the Air Force had taken care of my flight requirements for twelve years. Going back to commercial air travel was a big adjustment. The Secret Service continued to provide protection for me the first year I was out of office. They don't carry luggage, nor should they, since their job is to guard against threats. But there is nothing like having Secret Service agents with you to facilitate passage through airport security.

Another big adjustment was driving myself. Beginning the morning of the day George W. Bush announced I would be his running mate in July 2000, the Secret Service had taken over all responsibility for driving Lynne and me. The only time in eight years that I had gotten my hands on a steering wheel was on one of my trips to Saudi Arabia. Lynne and I were guests of King Abdullah at his farm outside Riyadh. His son took us for a drive in a Cadillac Escalade. Part of the way through the tour, he asked if I would like to drive. I jumped at the chance and got behind the wheel before the Secret Service could stop me. During the year after we left office, I gradually did more and more driving on my own, with the Secret Service following in a separate vehicle.

That is how I came to be backing myself out of my garage in Jackson, Wyoming, on December 9, 2009, when I blacked out. When I regained consciousness a short time later, my car was on top of a large boulder in an aspen grove in front of our house. My Secret Service agents were pounding on the windows with their fists because the doors had locked automatically when I had shifted into gear. I had a large knot on my forehead where I had hit the steering wheel. Aside from that, I felt fine, but in fact I had just been through a very serious incident, a near-death experience.

When I came to, my agents took me to St. John's Medical Center in Jackson. There we were able to download the information from my implanted ICD and transmit it to George Washington University Hospital, where Dr. Reiner confirmed I had indeed experienced ventricular fibrillation. V Fib occurs when the left ventricle, the main pumping chamber of the heart, begins to flutter and is no longer moving blood into the aorta. It is nearly always fatal. The only reason I survived was that eight years earlier, Dr. Reiner had had the judgment and foresight to recommend I get an implantable ICD. That decision saved my life.

## DR. REINER

"Good morning, Jon, it's Lew."

Somehow Lew Hofmann always managed to sound cheerful, even at "o-dark-thirty" when he already had been up for hours.

Lew was no doubt calling about the vice president. Cheney had been under the weather for several days with a lingering cough that initially seemed to improve after antibiotics, only to worsen again. What worried Lew now was that the vice president was short of breath, particularly while climbing stairs, and had noted a several-pound weight gain, which Mr. Cheney attributed to the warm hospitality of hunting lodges he'd visited recently and the Thanksgiving dinner he enjoyed with his family a few days later.

When we replaced Mr. Cheney's defibrillator over the summer, we specifically chose a device with the ability to detect the fluid buildup that accompanies congestive heart failure. I thought the feature would be useful for exactly this type of circumstance: helping to discern whether new symptoms were related to heart failure or something less dire, like a cold. Lew agreed to check the ICD and said he would arrange for us to evaluate the vice president as soon as possible. Later that day I wrote:

> I was called this morning at 5:50 by Dr. Lew Hofmann. Dr. Hofmann stated that he had been called by the vice president who had complained of slightly more shortness of breath than usual. The patient had had a viral syndrome and cough starting about 10 days ago and had used a Z-Pack for 3 days. His symptoms (productive cough, myalgias) improved but recurred a few days ago. . . . I went to see the vice president at the White House. He has not had chest pain. Has not exercised much in past 2 weeks although he has been on several hunting trips. Admits to some dietary indiscretions (including spicy/salty Cajun food). Has gained about 4 pounds over last couple of weeks. Has not noted any edema. Has not noted any palpitations. Does feel a little more SOB [short of breath] going up stairs and feels like he is not getting a full breath. . . .

Overall Mr. Cheney looked okay but he had atrial fibrillation (A Fib), a common arrhythmia affecting more than two million people in the United States, characterized by incessant and chaotic electrical activity that causes the atrial chambers to "fibrillate" (quiver) ineffectively.

For most people, the heart squeezes sub rosa, its cadence unnoticed until it makes itself known through the quick punch of a premature contraction, the gallop of a rapid rate, or the fluttering of a disorderly rhythm. Some patients with atrial fibrillation immediately identify the irregular heartbeat, while others experience a more subtle shortness of breath or a decline in stamina, and some patients have no symptoms at all. Atrial fibrillation can occur in someone with a normal heart or in patients with disorders involving the heart valves, thyroid disease, or congestive heart failure. The major risk of A Fib is a stroke caused by embolization of a clot that can form in the static recesses of the now-immobile left atrium.

In May 1991 President George H. W. Bush experienced unusual fatigue while jogging at Camp David and was found to have atrial fibrillation, later determined to be the result of a hyperactive thyroid gland. Dr. Allan Ross, GW's chief of cardiology and Dick Cheney's doctor at the time, was called in to consult. The president was taken by air to Bethesda Naval Hospital, where he was treated with digoxin to slow his heart rate and procainamide, an antiarrhythmic.

President Bush later made a public service announcement warning about the risks of untreated atrial fibrillation:

> Hi, I'm one of two million Americans who have a type of irregular heartbeat called Atrial Fibrillation, or AF. Left untreated, AF can lead to a stroke, the third leading cause of death in this country. In fact, this year 80,000 Americans will have a stroke because of AF. Luckily, it can be detected and treated. And the first step to seeing if you might have AF could be an easy self-exam. You can learn a simple way to check your pulse to see if you have an irregular heartbeat, and what to do about it. If you're over fifty, it means taking sixty seconds to check your pulse twice a year. Strokes can be prevented. Learn the warning signs and how to reduce your risk. Talk to your doctor.

Blood thinners can greatly reduce the chance of stroke, particularly for patients who have risk factors like congestive heart failure, hypertension, diabetes, or a prior stroke, and we immediately injected the vice president with a quick-acting anticoagulant. Decades of heart disease had left Cheney with a weakened and tenuously compensated heart without much reserve, and when the atrial fibrillation reduced his cardiac function just a little, it was enough to tip him into heart failure. Cindy and I thought that Mr. Cheney would feel better if we could restore his usual rhythm, and we made plans to bring him to GW to electrically reset (defibrillate) his heart. The White House released the following statement:

> The vice president visited with his doctors this morning for evaluation of a lingering cough from a cold. During examination he was incidentally found to have an irregular heartbeat, which on further testing was determined to be atrial fibrillation, an abnormal rhythm involving the upper chambers of the heart. Later this afternoon, the vice president will visit George Washington University Hospital for further evaluation and, if indicated, cardioversion, delivery of an electric impulse to the heart, which is a standard treatment for atrial fibrillation. This will be an outpatient procedure, and the vice president is expected to return home Monday night.

Data retrieved from the memory of the ICD showed that Mr. Cheney had been in atrial fibrillation for ten days, which was exactly as long as he had felt unwell and more than long enough for a clot to form in his heart. Before attempting to convert Mr. Cheney's rhythm back to normal, it was imperative we know whether a potentially devastating thrombus, which can be jarred loose by electrical cardioversion, lurked inside his left atrium, and the best way to do that is with echocardiography.

Cardiac imaging with sound waves (echocardiography) is a technological offshoot of sonar, the naval echo-ranging system developed almost a century ago for tracking submarines. First used in 1953 to examine cardiac structures and refined greatly since then, echocardiography provides detailed cross-sectional cardiac images reconstructed from sound waves that are bounced off the heart. Although often capable of producing vivid pictures, transthoracic echocardiography, obtained with a handheld transducer positioned against the wall of the chest, is not ideal for large patients who have a substantial amount of subcutaneous tissue, or for cardiac structures such as the atria that are located deep and toward the back of the heart. For these applications, and for examining cardiac valves, transesophageal echocardiography (TEE) is a better option.

The esophagus, the muscular conduit for food and drink that connects the pharynx to the stomach, transits the chest directly behind the heart and provides a nearby vantage point from which to examine cardiac structure and function. The transesophageal ultrasound transducer is sealed inside the tip of a long and deflectable endoscope-like probe and is advanced down the throat of a sedated patient to a position adjacent to the heart. The resulting two-dimensional and three-dimensional moving images depict the elegant intracardiac anatomy with a detail previously obtainable only at surgery or necropsy.

We waited several hours for Vice President Cheney to digest his early morning breakfast, and in the late afternoon he came to George Washington University Hospital for a quickly arranged TEE cardioversion. Sara Hennig, an experienced cath lab nurse, placed an IV catheter in Mr. Cheney's right wrist and shaved his chest to provide better electrical conductivity and more humane removal for the saucer-sized adhesive electrode patches that have largely replaced the familiar defibrillator paddles used for decades to deliver the energy. Dr. Paul Dangerfield, a cardiac anesthesiologist familiar with the vice president from prior GW hospitalizations, then administered intravenous sedation. After the vice president was soundly asleep, Dr. Jannet Lewis, GW's director of echocardiography, passed a TEE probe through a hollow plastic bite-block positioned in Cheney's mouth, advancing the long transducer down his esophagus to the level of the heart.

With the lights in the procedure room dimmed, Jannet slowly surveyed the vice president's heart for clots, paying particular attention to the left atrial appendage, a long, tubular outcropping of the left atrium, previously thought to be a relatively unimportant cardiac structure but now known to be the critical location where clots often hide. Satisfied that there was no thrombus in the heart and with the vice president still asleep, we proceeded with the electrical cardioversion.

The use of a defibrillator to restore a normal rhythm has become an iconic medical procedure immortalized in too-numerous-to-count movies and television dramas, two notable examples being the *MacGyver* episode in which the eponymous character resuscitates a friend using two candlesticks and microphone wire and the 2006 remake of *Casino Royale* in which, after being poisoned by a digoxin-laced martini, James Bond attempts to defibrillate himself. In reality, defibrillation (cardioversion) as a treatment for atrial fibrillation is safe and quick and is performed in a highly controlled environment.

Just like in the movies, Cindy called "Clear!" which was Sara's cue to arm the external defibrillator, the device issuing a dramatic high-pitched whine for several seconds as it charged its large capacitor. After double-checking that everyone had heeded Cindy's admonition to move back, Sara depressed the flashing button on the defibrillator control panel.

Secret Service agents watched from the control room as 120 joules of electricity arced through Cheney's chest with a soft, audible "pop," causing a quick spasm of his torso and arms, the patient's response more closely resembling a sudden startle than the violent levitation depicted on television. Our attention then turned from the patient to the EKG monitor, which displayed the newly normalized rhythm.

The successful cardioversion had solved the acute problem, but there remained reason for concern. In general, atrial fibrillation is a very common and treatable disorder, but occurring in the setting of the vice president's long history of ischemic heart disease, impaired ventricular function, deep vein thrombosis, and heart failure, it portended the transition of Mr. Cheney's illness from its long era of stability to the steep slippery slope of end-stage heart disease.

In October 2008 Lew Hofmann was once again called to see the vice president because of a sudden increase in weight.

*The Naval Observatory*

*October 15, 2008*
*06:30*
*The vice president asked me to visit with him this morning at the Naval Observatory when he noticed that his weight had increased by six pounds over the past 5 days. He feels that he has "lost some stamina" over that period, but denies any change in his baseline exertional shortness of breath. No chest pain, palpitations, ankle swelling or orthopnea. He did wake up in the middle of the night two evenings ago with a "coughing fit". He states that he has been carefully compliant with diet restrictions, especially salt, over the past month. No other new symptoms or problems.*

Lew examined the vice president and found that his pulse was irregular, a finding suggestive of atrial fibrillation. Cheney's weight had increased, there were crackles in the lungs, and slight swelling of the ankles, all consistent with congestive heart failure.

Lew arranged for us to come to the White House to see the vice president, and we did confirm that Cheney was back in atrial fibrillation. Data downloaded from the ICD disclosed that the arrhythmia had recurred precisely two days, sixteen hours earlier, and there was a large spike in intrathoracic fluid over the same period of time consistent with congestive heart failure (CHF). It was impossible to know for sure whether the CHF was caused by the atrial fibrillation or the atrial fibrillation was caused by the CHF, but likely it was the former, and although Mr. Cheney didn't look particularly sick, his poor heart function clearly did not tolerate the loss of atrial function that occurs in A Fib. We discussed this at length with the vice president, and he agreed to return to George Washington University Hospital in the afternoon, where we once again successfully cardioverted him.

About a week later, we ran some blood tests and discovered that there had been a decline in the vice president's kidney function, a not entirely unexpected consequence of Mr. Cheney's more pronounced heart failure and the escalating medications we employed to keep the fluid from reaccumulating in his lungs. In a note to Vice President Cheney, Lew Hofmann summarized our assessment:

> We think that your decreased kidney function is due to the combination of your baseline decreased heart strength, your recent brief episode of "atrial fibrillation" (which decreased your heart's efficiency below baseline), and the extra fluid which accumulated. In essence, that "perfect storm" decreased the delivery of blood to your kidney cells, and their ability to function has been slightly compromised.

The first thirty years of Cheney's disease had evolved languorously with widely spaced, important but momentary events that were dealt with and discarded. Now the dominos were dropping quickly, the recovery from each mini-crisis incomplete. I was confident that he would finish out the remainder of his term, but without a doubt Cheney was getting sicker. It was painful to watch. A popular notion maintains that to be an effective physician, you must maintain a protective distance from your patients, an emotional firewall. If that is true, I've never been good at it.

One late summer evening several years ago, Martha, the daughter of a patient, called to share the sad news that her father had died earlier in the day. Her dad's name was Milton, my father's name as well, and I first met the patient when, as a brand-new cardiologist, I repaired a worn-out bypass graft that had been causing him chest pain. He was already eighty years old when I became his doctor, and during his many visits to my office over his last five years, I made some changes to his medications and ordered the occasional test, but mostly we just talked about his long and rich life and politics and the people and things he loved. My care had comprised only a small part of his life, but it had occupied almost the entire span of my young career. Martha graciously thanked me for looking after her father. I told her that I was going to miss him, and when the call ended, I wept for both her loss and mine.

On January 15, 2009, five days before the conclusion of Mr. Cheney's time in office, Lew Hofmann, Ryan Bosch, and I met with the patient in the Eisenhower Executive Office Building to discuss the medical transition plan. Although by law departing vice presidents get an additional six months of Secret Service protection (which President Obama later extended another six months), the coverage of the White House Medical Unit would end at noon on January 20, 2009.

After more than eight years serving the president and vice president of the United States and their families, Lew's time in the White House was coming to an end. At the conclusion of President Obama's inauguration, Lew was going to take one last flight out to Wyoming with Vice President Cheney and then return to Washington to take some well-deserved, and long-overdue, time off before tackling the last assignment of his twenty-six years in the military, flight surgeon for Air Force One.

Our meeting with Vice President Cheney would be our last consultation during his time in office, and as I waited for him, I reflected on how my world, and his, had changed during that time. My beautiful little girls were becoming teenagers, my father and my sister Melanie were now gone, and my career had bloomed and become irrevocably interlaced with the care of this man.

Cheney was a singularly complex patient. First, the sheer duration of his illness was extraordinary. The year 2008 marked the thirtieth anniversary of his first heart attack, the opening act of a drama that no doubt had been in the works for years before the thirty-seven-year-old congressional candidate was admitted to Cheyenne Regional Medical Center. Cheney's remarkable survival was a testament to his dogged determination to live despite his disease and also to key therapeutics like aspirin, beta blockers, coronary care units, bypass surgery, statins, stents, and defibrillators—breakthroughs that were being added to cardiology's armamentarium seemingly just when he needed them.

A single heart attack can kill you, and this patient had outlasted four, but not without paying a steep price. The most recent echocardiogram revealed that the vice president's heart was enormous, the biggest I had ever seen, about twice normal size, the end result of his malignant coronary disease.

Now, three decades into his disease, the intervals between medical crises for Dick Cheney were becoming shorter and shorter and his rebounds not quite back to baseline. The trend, which had been level for so many years, was now clearly on the decline. As the vice president made the transition from public to private life, his illness was also entering a new stage.

We told Vice President Cheney that although Lew Hofmann would be moving on to other duties, the rest of our medical team would ensure that his continued care would be seamless. The vice president seemed very much at ease, but I worried what I would do without Lew. I saw the vice president dozens of times during his two terms in office, but Dr. Hofmann and his colleagues were with Mr. Cheney every day. Whether in the West Wing, the Naval Observatory, Air Force Two, or Jackson Hole, and in war zones, undisclosed locations, and for many thousands of miles around the world, a member of the WHMU was always close by. It's impossible to overstate the impact of their omnipresent, professional vigilance on his longevity. Lew never missed an opportunity to thank me for my help, but it was I who owed him the real debt of gratitude.

I knew that when I next saw Mr. Cheney, he would no longer be the vice president of the United States, and I searched for the right way to acknowledge the moment. The usual platitudes seemed hollow, and instead I simply thanked him for his efforts over the prior eight years, and his long career, to keep my family, and this nation, safe.

Cheney smiled warmly, shook my hand, and said, "Thanks Jon, you made my day."

Our meeting had a bittersweet air. As I watched Mr. Cheney leave the clinic, accompanied by his Secret Service escort for the last time as vice president, I knew this wasn't the end of his story. In some ways, I feared, it was just the beginning.

Well over one million people attended the inauguration of President Obama on Tuesday, January 20, 2009. Because of the enormous assembled crowd and George Washington University Hospital's proximity to the National Mall, the hospital activated an emergency preparedness plan, placing multiple hospital units on standby. I had been a guest at the previous two inaugurations, but I was on call for this event, and as I watched the televised ceremony from the operating room lounge, I was saddened when the cameras showed Vice President Cheney sitting in a wheelchair.

Over the weekend as the Cheneys packed in preparation for their departure from the Naval Observatory, the vice president wrenched his back while reaching for a small box. His left-sided back pain was incapacitating, and on television he looked decidedly uncomfortable as Sarah Creason, a WHMU nurse, pushed his wheelchair onto the podium. It was ironic that for every one of his 2,922 days in office, I had worried about heart attacks, arrhythmias, aneurysms, and heart failure, but what ended up disabling him was something as prosaic as a bad back.

Over the next several months, Mr. Cheney's cardiac status remained relatively stable. He was bothered most by the recurring pain in his lower back and left leg caused by the herniated disc incurred during his last days in office. When physical therapy and epidural injections failed to provide adequate pain control, we considered minimally invasive spine surgery. Although I was loath to expose Mr. Cheney to the stress of an operation, his pain was disabling, and I felt that with careful perioperative care, we could minimize his risks. On the morning of his back surgery, when it was time to go to the operating room, Dr. Paul Dangerfield, the anesthesiologist, asked Mr. Cheney if he wanted to ride down the corridor in a wheelchair.

"No," he said, standing up gingerly. "I want to walk. It will remind me of why I'm having this surgery."

The operation, performed by Dr. Anthony Caputy, GW's chief of neurosurgery, was thankfully uneventful, and it quickly and remarkably resolved Cheney's pain.

A few months later, on December 1, 2009, Mrs. Cheney called and asked if I could see her husband because he was short of breath. After the vice president had left office, Medtronic enhanced our monitoring capabilities by installing devices in the vice president's homes enabling him to upload telemetry and other data from his ICD to a secure website to which we had access. This technology allowed us to keep an eye on Cheney's volume status and heart rhythm even when he was not in Washington, and for the most part, he had been stable. Now something had changed. Later that day the Secret Service, which would continue to provide protection for another month, brought Mr. and Mrs. Cheney to our offices in Foggy Bottom.

A year earlier, a visit to GW would have involved elaborate logistics, including a motorcade with an armored limousine, several Secret Service Suburbans, a Metropolitan Police escort, at least a dozen agents, sometimes a bomb-sniffing dog, and, on one occasion, a black-clad counterassault team, replete with automatic weapons, camped in a stairwell. Now, ten months out of office, the former vice president's protective detail was decidedly lower profile, composed of just a few agents.

Mr. Cheney told us that his leg and back discomfort had completely resolved, but his stamina had worsened to the point that he used a wheelchair to get around airports, he was fairly winded climbing a flight of stairs, and his weight was up about ten pounds.

When I examined the vice president, I found edema in his legs and crackles in his lungs, signs of heart failure. Telemetry data from the ICD revealed that he had been volume overloaded for many weeks, likely since the time of his back surgery.

I told Mr. Cheney that a higher dose of furosemide should help his breathing, and although it might never be necessary, if his symptoms became harder to manage, we might need to consider more aggressive therapeutics, including eventually even heart transplantation. I emphasized that it was way too early to go down those roads, but I thought it was time to tell him that if he got worse we still had options.

Mr. Cheney simply said, "Okay."

One week later Mrs. Cheney called my cell phone.

"Hi, Jon, this is Lynne Cheney," the familiar voice said. "The oddest thing just happened. Dick passed out."

Mrs. Cheney told me that they were in Wyoming, and the vice president had gotten into his car to run an errand. Coming to the end of his Secret Service protection, he often drove his own car, accompanied by agents in another vehicle. As Mr. Cheney put his Jeep into reverse, he suddenly lost consciousness and struck a tree at the end of the driveway. The agents ran to the vehicle and saw that he was unconscious, but they were unable to open the locked doors. As they began to bang on the windows, the vice president regained consciousness. Mrs. Cheney said that her husband appeared to be no worse for wear with the exception of a knot on his forehead.

In phonology, the word *syncope* refers to the loss of sounds from within a word (e.g., *fo'c'sle* instead of *forecastle*), but in the medical lexicon, *syncope* is the term for the loss of consciousness. Syncope has many possible causes, including dehydration, emotional stress, fast heart rates (tachycardias), slow heart rates (bradycardias), medication reactions, seizures, and rapid changes in body position. In 2002, for example, President Bush had briefly passed out after choking on a pretzel. For a patient with severe heart disease like Vice President Cheney, however, the most likely and deadly etiology for syncope is sudden cardiac arrest (SCA), and I told Mrs. Cheney to take him to the nearest hospital.

The human body is composed of trillions of individual cells, each one containing a microscopic metabolic engine fueled by oxygen and glucose supplied continuously via the blood. Some organs can tolerate a temporary interruption in blood flow, but the brain will not. Despite representing only 2 percent of the body's mass, the brain consumes 20 percent of a human's total energy requirement, and a pause in blood flow of as little as five seconds results in a loss of consciousness; after just a few minutes, irreversible brain injury, and subsequently death, can occur. For the nearly one thousand people every day in the United States who suffer a sudden cardiac arrest, the events that occur in the first few minutes of collapse will determine whether they live or die.

Most cases of sudden cardiac arrest are caused by V Fib, the chaotic electrical storm that causes the ventricles to quiver, output of blood from the heart to cease, and blood pressure to drop to zero. Sudden cardiac arrest is a supremely lethal event, afflicting 360,000 Americans each year with a survival rate that varies regionally in the United States but averages only about 11.4 percent. According to the Sudden Cardiac Arrest Foundation, every year SCA kills as many people in the United States as breast cancer, motor vehicle accidents, cervical cancer, Alzheimer's disease, colorectal cancer, HIV, prostate cancer, diabetes, assaults with a firearm, suicides, and house fires combined.

The medical community has long understood the benefits of cardiopulmonary resuscitation (CPR) and prompt electrical defibrillation for patients with SCA, but the time window during which these resuscitative techniques will translate into survival is very narrow, on the order of about five minutes. Unfortunately, there is also often a substantial delay in the arrival of emergency medical services (EMS) personnel, and every minute in delay to defibrillation results in about a 10 percent decline in chance of survival. Nationwide, the average time from a 911 call to EMS arrival is greater than seven minutes, too late for most patients to achieve a meaningful neurological recovery.

Although CPR can attenuate the severe survival penalty that results from a delay in defibrillation, most patients with SCA do not receive bystander CPR prior to EMS arrival, and even when trained responders do provide CPR, its quality is often poor. Ultimately, to improve the survival rate from SCA, the victim must be defibrillated quickly, and to make that more feasible, automated external defibrillators (AEDs) were developed.

Automated external defibrillation (AED), introduced in 1979 and first deployed on offshore drilling platforms, exponentially amplifies the number of potential SCA rescuers by enabling the medically untrained to use a defibrillator. The development of AEDs was made possible by two innovations. The first was the adhesive electrode, invented by R. Lee Heath in the 1980s, which allowed a rescuer to defibrillate a patient without having to hold the potentially perilous paddles, and the second was the development of computer algorithms capable of automatically determining whether a shock is advisable. A modern AED is an intuitive device designed for use by laypersons with no prior medical training. Step-by-step audio prompts walk users through placement of two patches on the victim's chest.

In 1994, the American Heart Association noted that making AEDs more widely available should significantly improve SCA survival and recommended clinical trials to further evaluate AED use by first responders and the lay public. In 1997, American Airlines began to place AEDs on board selected aircraft, later expanding this program to include their entire fleet. Four years later, the Federal Aviation Administration mandated that all commercial aircraft flying with at least one flight attendant carry an AED.

The gaming industry was also an early adopter of this technology, and with its intensely monitored spaces, it turned out to be a unique environment in which to evaluate the impact of AED deployment. Nevada casinos installed AEDs in the late 1990s and found that

SCA victims received a shock on average about four and a half minutes after collapsing, 50 percent faster than the almost ten minutes it took local paramedics to reach the scene. As expected, based on these rapid defibrillation times, survival rates were extraordinarily high, almost 60 percent, and for patients who received their first defibrillation within three minutes of collapse (a virtually unobtainable time without pre-positioned AEDs), the survival rate was a remarkable 74 percent.

Despite the overwhelming data proving the effectiveness and safety of AEDs, many legislative and administrative hurdles have impeded the widespread dissemination of the technology. The Food and Drug Administration (FDA) still classifies AEDs as Class III devices (they require approval from the FDA before they can be marketed), and some models require a physician's prescription. Some states require physician oversight of an AED program or specific training, and some states require registration. Although every state has enacted a Good Samaritan AED law, the details differ from jurisdiction to jurisdiction as to who qualifies for immunity. This national patchwork quilt of AED laws creates an air of liability uncertainty in the minds of potential AED owners and rescuers and is a major reason that many hotels, national retail chains, and big-box stores do not deploy them. A bill before the 113th Congress that I helped to author seeks to solve this problem, but even a topic as apolitical as sudden cardiac arrest is subject to the partisan paralysis endemic in Washington.

You must be lucky to survive a malady that kills nine of the ten people it afflicts. I get to care for the fortunate few who reach the hospital alive, and their stories are always amazing. A fifty-year-old man has a cardiac arrest while jogging on a treadmill at a health club and is resuscitated by the AED that, just months before, he'd urged the club to acquire. A sixty-two-year-old runner drops dead three miles into the Marine Corps Marathon, resuscitated by Dr. Fred Lough, GW's chief of heart surgery, who is running just behind him in the race and does CPR until the AED arrives. An engineer collapses in front of a firehouse in Chinatown and is saved by the firefighters who retrieve their AED. A White House butler develops chest pain, then arrests just as he is being evaluated in the White House Medical Unit. The common thread these survivors share is luck: they all were lucky to have their cardiac arrest in close proximity to both an AED and someone willing to use it.

Over the past two decades, researchers have been able to identify specific patient characteristics that increase the risk of developing sudden cardiac arrest. These include patients with a significant impairment in heart function, survivors of a prior cardiac arrest, and certain inherited predispositions to arrhythmias. For many of these patients, implantable cardioverter defibrillators (ICDs) will dramatically reduce their risk of dying from sudden cardiac arrest.

On December 9, 2009, the European Center for Nuclear Research announced that its new large hadron collider had accelerated protons to a record 1.2 trillion electron volts, Bank of America reported that it had fully repaid its $45 billion TARP loan, and President Obama traveled to Oslo, Norway, to accept the Nobel Peace Prize. December 9, 2009, would also have been the date of Dick Cheney's death had his ICD not terminated the ventricular fibrillation embroiling his heart.

The data downloaded from the vice president's ICD at St. John's Medical Center in Jackson, Wyoming, revealed that at 3:11 p.m., the device detected an abrupt jump in his heart rate to 222 beats per minute, which the implanted computer correctly interpreted as V Fib. The ICD had been programmed to try to disrupt the arrhythmia by rapidly pacing the heart (pace termination), which it attempted five seconds later but without success. The device then charged its capacitor, which took seven seconds to accomplish, rechecked the rhythm, and then discharged 34.5 joules of electricity directly into Dick Cheney's heart, successfully terminating the arrhythmia. The entire event, from recognition to resuscitation, had taken sixteen seconds.

## HEART

When I spoke with Mr. Cheney, he was upbeat, sounding more surprised than upset, and other than a bump on his head, he felt well. In an attempt to reduce the likelihood of a recurrence, I increased the dose of his beta-blocker medication, advised him not to drive until further notice, and told him to rest for a couple of days.

## CHAPTER 13

# Downhill

## VICE PRESIDENT CHENEY

For many years, I had been on various anticoagulants to minimize the possibility of developing blood clots leading to an embolism or a stroke. In January 2010, not long after returning from the holidays in Wyoming, I began to experience serious nosebleeds. The most worrisome was an arterial nosebleed I developed one afternoon when Lynne and I were at our home in McLean. Every time my heart beat, blood shot in a stream from my nose. When I tried to stop the bleeding with pressure, blood ran down the back of my throat. I called Dr. Reiner and told him I was heading for the emergency room at George Washington University Hospital.

Our Secret Service protection had just ended, so Lynne rushed me down the George Washington Parkway to the hospital. Since she hadn't driven herself in almost a decade, the drive there wasn't without its own risks. Once we arrived at GW, the doctors packed my nose and stopped the bleeding. I was released and Lynne and I went home.

Just a few hours later, the bleeding started again, and this time it was even worse. We made the drive again to the emergency room, this time with me holding a trash can in my lap to catch the blood. At the hospital, I was rushed into the operating room, sedated, and the artery cauterized. For a long time afterward, I carried a small packet of materials designed to stop a nosebleed should one occur. It turned out this episode may have been more life threatening than all the coronary episodes that had taken me to emergency rooms over the years.

A month later, in February 2010, Lynne and I were at our house St. Michaels on the Eastern Shore of the Chesapeake Bay, where we had bought a home after the 2004 election. We had a number of friends in the area, enjoyed the beauty of the region, and I loved to hunt duck and geese there in the fall. My health was also a factor in our decision. I knew that as I grew older and my heart disease progressed, I would find it increasingly difficult to spend time in the Tetons in Wyoming because of the high altitude.

After dinner one evening, I developed some chest discomfort that I thought might be related to my heart. I did not have other symptoms, but I was sufficiently concerned that I wanted to check it out. Lynne drove me the twelve miles to the nearest hospital, in Easton, Maryland. On arrival, I was examined, and the preliminary judgment was that it might be another heart attack. After contacting Dr. Reiner at GW, we decided to return and check my condition there. We used a life-flight helicopter service to fly me from Easton back to Washington, DC. I had flown on helicopters thousands of times all over the world, but this was the first time I was flat on my back, strapped to a gurney with an IV and blood pressure cuff on my arm. The crew was experienced and very competent. Since George Washington University Hospital did not have a helicopter landing pad at that time, we had to land in the parking lot at the Washington Nationals baseball stadium and complete the journey to GW by ambulance. At the hospital, doctors determined I had suffered my fifth heart attack. Although it was relatively minor, it was further evidence of my deterioration.

Later that spring, I visited King Abdullah of Saudi Arabia to discuss developments in the Middle East. I also took the opportunity to stop in Abu Dhabi to see my friend the crown prince Mohammed bin Zayed. The meetings in both capitals were good ones, both interesting given the challenging events unfolding across the region. But I recall that between the meetings, all I wanted to do was sleep. I was experiencing a definite decline in energy level that I chalked up to jet lag and time zone changes.

Lynne and I flew to Jackson Hole for Memorial Day as we had

done most years. If any more evidence was needed of my deteriorating situation, it came during that visit to Wyoming. For several years, Memorial Day had marked the beginning of my fishing season. My good friend Dick Scarlett always organizes two days of fly-fishing on the South Fork of the Snake River along the Wyoming-Idaho border. The spring runoff from the mountains is always a problem, but a dam on the border catches the runoff in Palisades Reservoir. The water below the dam is high in May, but it is clear and fishable. The tailwater fishery below the Palisades Dam on the South Fork is one of my favorite stretches of water. I was looking forward to getting back on the river with my fly rod.

The first night home in Jackson, I experienced considerable difficulty breathing. I had trouble climbing stairs. I couldn't sleep. I was going to have trouble spending a week at sixty-two hundred feet. We went to the local hospital and transmitted the data from my ICD to Washington so Dr. Reiner could review it.

The report indicated that I was having an episode of atrial fibrillation. While A Fib is less serious than V Fib, it can lead to the development of blood clots. I needed to go back to Washington, DC. A friend loaned us his plane, and a doctor and nurse from St. John's Medical Center flew with Lynne and me back to Washington. I wasn't sure I would ever see Wyoming again.

By the beginning of June 2010, I was approaching end-stage heart failure. As I went through the month, I found it increasingly difficult to carry out any tasks around the house. Walking to our front gate to get the morning paper was no longer possible. I could no longer climb the stairs to get to the second floor. My world was getting smaller and smaller. The one evening I felt slightly more energized was when we attended the annual reunion of the White House staff and cabinet from the Ford administration. The rest of the time, I just felt exhausted. Every morning when I woke up, all I wanted to do was get to the overstuffed easy chair in my office, put my feet up, and go back to sleep.

I felt no pain or physical discomfort associated with this stage of my disease. But I was conscious I didn't have much more time to live.

Over the years that I had suffered from coronary artery disease, I had believed that sooner or later, I would run out my time and that the end would come as a result of heart failure. What was happening was hardly a surprise.

I was losing my appetite. There wasn't much I wanted to eat, but the things I craved were foods from my childhood—my mother's chocolate chip cookies, for example. Mary baked batches for me using my mom's recipe. My family was trying to keep my strength up, so they also spent a good deal of time making me milk shakes with protein powder sprinkled in. They were deeply worried about me.

I wasn't fearful or anxious about my situation. I had lived a wonderful life, and now it was ending. Contemplating my death was much harder for my family than it was for me. I felt a need to express my wishes with respect to final arrangements, but it was a difficult subject to bring up with my family. They didn't want to face what we all knew was happening.

By this time, we had used nearly all the technology and medical procedures available for dealing with my disease. My doctors had equipped me with a small pump that kept me supplied with a steady dose of milrinone, or "rocket fuel," to assist my weakened heart, but it was a short-term expedient and would soon lose its effectiveness. At this point, there were only two remaining possibilities. One was a transplant. But the demand far outstripped the supply of transplantable organs, and the average waiting period was twelve months. It was clear I would not live long enough to work my way up the transplant list.

There was one other possibility, which Dr. Reiner had mentioned to me earlier in the year: a left ventricular assist device (LVAD). At that time, my condition hadn't deteriorated to the point where I was a candidate. Now I was there. Dr. Reiner arranged for us to visit with the surgical team at Inova Fairfax Hospital in Northern Virginia. The team, headed by Dr. Nelson Burton, briefed us on the LVAD that would be installed in my chest to assist my heart in providing an adequate supply of blood to my vital organs. They showed us a model of the device and explained how it worked. One end would be connected to the bottom of my left ventricle and the other to the aorta. A small pump inside, operating at nine thousand RPM, would push blood from the ventricle through the aorta and the rest of the circulatory system. The pump itself is powered by a driveline that goes from the pump through your chest wall to a control element/computer worn on the outside of your chest, powered by batteries or a base power unit plugged into an electrical outlet.

When I first saw an LVAD, I was intrigued by the technology. Under ordinary circumstances, the idea of putting a device operating at nine thousand RPM into my chest, attached to my heart and to a driveline running through a hole in my chest wall would have seemed a little off-putting. But it was an option, and I was out of other options.

The LVAD was developed as a transition device to sustain a patient long enough to become eligible for a transplant. The original LVADs were not user friendly. They were so large that they were not portable. The patient's bed would be wheeled into the room with the LVAD, and the patient hooked up to the device. Significant progress in recent years, however, had transformed the LVAD to a size that allowed its external elements to be worn on a harness or a vest so the patient could lead a more normal life. Some patients decided to live with the LVAD and not go to a transplant. If the LVAD surgery were successful, I would have the opportunity to decide at some future date if I wanted to go the transplant route.

Surgery was scheduled for July 8, 2010. Because it was expected to be difficult surgery, I checked into the hospital on July 6, two days early, so the doctors could attempt to stabilize my condition and improve my overall health as much as possible before the surgery. I was given additional doses of milrinone on July 6, but it wasn't working. Indeed, it was becoming clear that my heart was failing rapidly and my liver and kidney functions were crashing. I have a vivid memory of that evening with my doctors and my family gathered together around my hospital bed, telling me they believed it was essential to implant the

LVAD on an emergency basis that night. I didn't have two more days. After I heard from the doctors, I asked Lynne, Liz, and Mary, one by one, what they thought. It was unanimous. I looked around the room at everyone and said, "Let's do it."

## DR. REINER

Like a tornado, water entering a drain begins to rotate, forming a cone-shaped whirlpool triggered by the downward suction of the departing fluid. In the idiomatic and indelicate language of medicine, a patient who is "circling the drain" has entered the sinking spiral of accumulating medical issues. In the beginning, the problems gather slowly, but as the patient descends lower, the vortex spins faster and the complications come more quickly, leading inexorably to the patient's demise. It's not always apparent when someone enters the terminal spiral, but once it becomes obvious, it is almost impossible to stop.

The year 2009 was a tough one for Dick Cheney. There had been debilitating back pain requiring spine surgery, an episode of congestive heart failure, and in the final days of the year, a cardiac arrest resuscitated with a shock from his implanted defibrillator. Viewed individually, each of these events had a successful resolution; surgery fixed the back, diuretics resolved the CHF, the defibrillator restored a normal rhythm. In reality, however, these were not isolated incidents but rather a continuum of the same process. The vice president's chronic cardiac disease led to a decrease in his overall physical fitness, which increased the likelihood of a back injury, the surgical repair of which provoked an episode of congestive heart failure, which in turn increased the chance of developing sudden cardiac arrest.

In January 2010, the vice president experienced a nosebleed that required cauterization at George Washington University Hospital. For more than a year, Mr. Cheney had been treated with warfarin (Coumadin), a powerful anticoagulant used to prevent strokes in patients with atrial fibrillation. Warfarin is a synthetic derivative of dicoumerol, a naturally occurring blood thinner that was initially discovered in spoiled sweet clover animal feed and was developed seventy years ago at the University of Wisconsin (part of the name derives from "*Wis*consin *A*lumni *R*esearch *F*oundation") and introduced in 1948 as rat poison. The drug has been used for decades as both a therapy and prophylaxis for clots in a variety of settings, including deep vein thrombosis, pulmonary embolism, the use of mechanical heart valves, and atrial fibrillation. Patients taking the strong anticoagulant must be closely monitored with blood tests and watch their diet, because foods like green leafy vegetables can decrease the effectiveness of the medicine, while other medications taken at the same time, such as antibiotics, can dramatically raise the effectiveness of warfarin. The major side effect of the medication is bleeding, which can be severe or even fatal.

Three weeks later, Cheney's bleeding recurred. A nosebleed is a common ailment, particularly in the dry air of winter. The hemorrhage can be impressive, even in an otherwise healthy person who is not taking any medication. For a patient, such as the vice president, who is being treated with an anticoagulant like warfarin, bleeding, once started, can be hard to stop.

When she called, I told Mrs. Cheney to bring the vice president to the George Washington University Hospital emergency room right away.

"How do I get there?" she asked.

Nine years of Secret Service protection for the Cheneys had concluded just the day before, and Mrs. Cheney was going to have to drive the vice president into Washington by herself, something she hadn't done in almost a decade. I gave Mrs. Cheney directions to the hospital and told her to come to the ER entrance, where we would meet them.

After calling the emergency room to let the attending physician on duty know that the Cheneys were on their way, I tracked down Dr. Nader Sadeghi, a GW ear, nose, and throat surgeon, and Dr. Jehan "Gigi" El-Bayoumi.

Gigi had taken over as Vice President Cheney's internist after Ryan

Bosch left GW several months earlier and had quickly become indispensable to the Cheneys (and to me). She is an extraordinary physician and role model whose exceptional clinical skills are surpassed only by her astonishing compassion and personal care for her patients. Not surprisingly, she cares for many of DC's political elite but somehow manages to deliver her remarkable VIP care to every patient, prominent or not, in her large practice.

Dr. Sadeghi examined Mr. Cheney, identified the problem vessel, which had already mostly stopped bleeding, applied a silver nitrate cautery, and packed the nostril with gauze. We watched the vice president for a while and considered keeping him in the hospital overnight for observation, but a few hours later, when there was no further bleeding, he was allowed to go home.

A little before 10:00 p.m., Mrs. Cheney called again, and now I could hear fear in her voice. Once again, the vice president was bleeding, now much more vigorously than earlier in the day. They were on their way back to the hospital. When Mr. Cheney arrived in the emergency room, blood was pouring from his nose, and a garbage can he had been bleeding into during the ride from Virginia was filled with clots. After manual compression failed to staunch the flow of blood, the vice president was rushed to the operating room, where, under general anesthesia, Dr. Sadeghi located and recauterized the bleeding artery but not before the loss of about one liter of blood (20 percent of his body's total supply).

We had stopped Cheney's Plavix after the first bleed three weeks earlier, and now we needed to stop the warfarin as well. These drugs, both of which impair the ability of blood to clot, had been prescribed in an effort to prevent a host of potentially lethal thrombotic events, such as recurrent DVT, stroke from atrial fibrillation, clotting of his stents, and recurrent heart attack. Unfortunately this last hemorrhagic event was severe: we needed to let the dust settle, and the troublesome vessel heal, before restarting one or both of these drugs.

• • •

## Downhill

During the evening of Sunday, February 21, three weeks after the nearly exsanguinating event, Vice President Cheney experienced about thirty minutes of chest burning. The Cheneys had been spending time on the Eastern Shore of Maryland, and I told them to go to the nearest emergency room, which was Memorial Hospital in Easton, for evaluation. After speaking with the ER doctor there, we decided that in view of the typical cardiac nature of his symptoms, it would be best to bring the vice president back to Washington and arranged to fly him the seventy-five miles by medevac helicopter.

When Cheney arrived at George Washington University Hospital, he was pain free, and his EKG was similar to his prior tracings. Although the first two sets of blood tests used to assess whether the heart muscle had sustained any damage were normal, the third set was mildly elevated, consistent with a small heart attack. The next morning we brought the vice president back to the cath lab to see what had changed.

The last time Cheney had undergone coronary angiography was nine years earlier, in March 2001, when he had developed chest pain caused by restenosis in the coronary stent that had been implanted four months earlier, during the presidential campaign. The procedures in 2000 and 2001 had been performed by accessing the femoral artery through a needle puncture at the top of his right leg. By 2010 we had largely abandoned the groin approach in favor of the radial artery of the wrist because of the increased patient safety and comfort when using this approach. My colleague Dr. Ramesh Mazhari joined me for the procedure, and through a two-millimeter puncture in Cheney's right wrist, we advanced our catheters up through the arteries of his arm, under the clavicle, and down into the chest.

In March 2001, we had been criticized for not performing intracoronary radiation therapy (brachytherapy) when the vice president presented with chest pain and restenosis. The *New York Times* even published an article with the headline "The New Treatment Cheney Did Not Get." In that piece I was quoted as saying, "When you look at a technology in its infancy, I think it is often appropriate to be a little circumspect about applying it, especially using something like gamma radiation." Within a few years, brachytherapy would be shown to mostly only delay the onset of restenosis, not prevent it, and the technology would soon be relegated to the dustbin of abandoned devices by a new generation of "drug-eluting" stents coated with potent inhibitors to the formation of the scar tissue inside stents that causes restenosis.

Now, looking at Cheney's coronaries for the first time in nine years, we noted that the diagonal stent we placed in 2000, and then ballooned again in 2001, was wide open, a very good thing as it supplied blood to a large portion of the vice president's limited amount of remaining viable heart muscle and had likely helped keep him alive. Cheney's coronary anatomy was remarkably similar to what we found almost a decade earlier, with the exception of a grape-sized aneurysm that had since formed in the left anterior descending, the other major artery supplying the still-contractile muscle. We surmised that a clot had probably formed in the aneurysm, eventually tumbling downstream (embolizing) and causing the small heart attack.

It wasn't a coincidence that Vice President Cheney's latest heart attack came less than a month after we stopped his anticoagulants. Blood thinners had precipitated the nosebleeds, but those drugs had also helped to prevent harmful clots like the one that caused this most recent event. If we didn't restart the blood thinners, the vice president would be at risk of another heart attack, but if we did, he would be at risk for another bleed. The medical care of a complex patient like Vice President Cheney is often filled with such conundrums and catch-22s, and after much deliberation we decided to cautiously restart the Plavix.

A little more than one year after leaving office, Cheney had been through worsening heart failure, a sudden cardiac arrest, severe bleeding, and now his fifth heart attack. The vortex was spinning faster.

Although the clinical signs and symptoms of heart failure had been known for hundreds of years, there were only a limited number of options to improve a patient's symptoms and nothing a physician could do to alter its inevitably bad outcome until late in the twentieth century.

For three millennia, the practice of bloodletting, literally the therapeutic draining of blood from a patient, was used to treat a variety of ailments. The Egyptians introduced the technique in about 1000 B.C., and it was continued until about a hundred years ago. When the Council of Tours in A.D. 1163 barred monks and priests from performing bloodletting, barber-surgeons (still identified by the familiar red and white barber pole) became the primary practitioners of the art.

Bloodletting was typically accomplished by incising a vein and was used to release what were thought to be evil spirits or bad humors and treat plethora (an excess of body fluid, that is, congestive heart failure), divert blood away from another actively bleeding site, decrease the body's heat (treat an infection), and treat a variety of other maladies, including gout, "madness," and seizures.

In December 1799, George Washington became ill with "inflammatory quinsy" (probably a peritonsillar abscess). When his pain became so severe that he could no longer swallow, eighty ounces (five pints) of blood was drained from Washington's arm in a single day. That evening, the first president of the United States was dead. More than two centuries later, it is unclear whether General Washington died as a consequence of his likely bacterial throat infection or the well-intended but at best ineffective and probably harmfully exuberant, bloodletting.

Giorgio Baglivi, a seventeenth-century Italian who was physician to Popes Innocent XII and Clement XI, described the use of bloodletting for the pulmonary edema often encountered in heart failure. Although crude, bloodletting did improve the symptoms of congestive heart failure by decreasing the overall volume of blood in the body, and consequently, the amount of blood returning to the heart. This phlebotomy continued into the middle of the twentieth century and was then largely replaced by powerful diuretic medications that harnessed the kidneys' natural ability to remove fluid from the body. When I was a medical resident in New York in the late 1980s, I struggled one night to keep a patient with advanced heart failure alive. Having exhausted all the options I knew, I called the patient's attending to apprise him of the grim situation and to ask if he had any suggestions.

"Take off five hundred cc of blood," he said.

Skeptical of the quaint approach but knowing that there was nothing to lose, I followed the senior physician's recommendation, removing half a liter of blood. I was surprised, and humbled when the patient rallied.

Although both sides of the heart can "fail," impairment of the contractile function of the left ventricle is more common and may occur as a consequence of prior heart attacks, valvular disease, viral infections of the heart, toxins like alcohol, certain types of chemotherapy, or unknown ("idiopathic") causes. When the right ventricle fails, it is most commonly the result of failure of the left ventricle: the blood that backs up into the lungs increases the pressure in the pulmonary vessels, which strains the usually thinner-walled, less muscular right ventricle.

As the left ventricle becomes progressively impaired, it compensates by dilating (getting larger and holding more blood) and beating faster. Over time, its ability to compensate declines, and the patient increasingly develops the symptoms of heart failure, such as fatigue and shortness of breath; toward the end, organs shut down. Right ventricular failure, by contrast, typically presents as swelling in the legs and abdomen, caused by the backup of the blood that would normally be returning to the heart.

As a heart begins to fail, the body responds by activating several compensatory mechanisms resulting in the elaboration of hormones that increase salt and water retention, constrict blood vessels, and increase the heart's contractile force and rate. These responses turn out to be very helpful if the drop in cardiac output is the result of an acute process like bleeding, but they become counterproductive over time if the cardiac output has declined because of an intrinsic problem with the heart. The concept that the physiological response to declining heart function might be "maladaptive" was developed in the 1980s and led to the use of vasodilators and beta blockers for patients with heart failure.

Vasodilators, which include angiotensin II–converting enzyme (ACE) inhibitors like lisinopril or enalapril, are drugs that dilate blood vessels and reduce resistance to cardiac emptying, making it easier for the heart to eject blood, increase cardiac output, and help prevent the heart from dilating. Clinical trials in the late 1980s proved that ACE inhibitors improve the survival of patients with heart failure, and ACE inhibitors and other related vasodilators have become a standard component of therapy for congestive heart failure.

Beta blockers (metoprolol, carvedilol, and others) are drugs that attach to sites on myocardial cells (beta receptors) that normally bind epinephrine and norepinephrine, adrenaline-like hormones that stimulate the heart in the "fight-or-flight" response, and are also elaborated in heart failure. Although it is somewhat counterintuitive, the beta blockers (which are cardioinhibitory) have been shown to decrease mortality and increase the cardiac output in patients with impaired ventricular function.


In April 2010, Liz Cheney called and asked if I had a few minutes to talk. I had been driving home through the mountains of western Maryland, and despite my GPS, I was a little lost, so I pulled over.

"My dad is dying," Liz said plainly.

The vice president had clearly deteriorated over the past few months, and although at the moment he appeared quasi-stable, there was no question where his trajectory was heading. The heart attack in February, although small, had taken muscle Mr. Cheney couldn't spare, and he was requiring higher doses and more frequent adjustments of multiple medications to keep him out of heart failure.

"Is it true that there isn't anything else that can be done for him?" Liz asked, not waiting for me to respond to her first statement. I had gotten to know Liz fairly well over the prior decade and spoke with her occasionally, usually when there was an issue related to her father's care that needed clarification. Although I didn't know it at the time, she was calling because her father had taken her aside to tell her that he thought the end was near and that she needed to accept it.

"No, that's not right," I said. I explained to her that six months earlier, I had told the vice president that should the circumstances warrant, he could be eligible for a mechanical ventricular assist device and even potentially a heart transplant.

"He's not too old for that?" she asked.

I reassured her that he was not. Although the assessment of the severity of her father's illness was correct, I thought he definitely still had options.

Heart failure kills more than fifty-six thousand Americans every year, about the same as breast cancer. Although people with heart failure live longer and better than in the past, 50 percent of people with a new diagnosis of heart failure will be dead within five years. Acknowledging the need for better options for patients with end-stage heart disease, in 1964 the federal government began funding a program intended to spur the development of mechanical cardiac assist devices, eventually investing over $400 million in the technology.

One of the early proponents of this initiative was Dr. Michael DeBakey, the legendary Houston heart surgeon and prolific innovator whose contributions to cardiac and vascular surgery spanned three-quarters of a century. In 1932, at the age of twenty-three, while still a medical student, Dr. DeBakey invented the "roller pump," which was used for decades to transfuse blood and later became a central component of the heart-lung machines created by Dr. John Gibbon and others. Dr. DeBakey developed surgical techniques to repair aortic aneurysms and carotid artery blockages, introduced Dacron as a material for synthetic vascular grafts, invented over fifty surgical instruments, and helped to create the concept for the mobile army surgical hospital (MASH) unit. He was said to have performed over sixty thousand heart operations during his extraordinary life and claimed to have accomplished the world's first coronary bypass graft operation in 1964. At the time of his death in 2008 at age ninety-nine, the *New York Times* fittingly described Dr. DeBakey as a "rebuilder of hearts."

In the early 1960s Dr. DeBakey and his team created several pumps intended to temporarily support or even replace the function of an ailing heart. In David K. C. Cooper's book *Open Heart: The Radical Surgeons Who Revolutionized Medicine*, Dr. DeBakey described his rationale for developing these ventricular assist devices (VADs):

> We became interested in the artificial heart as an extension of the heart-lung machine. As we developed more experience with the heart-lung machine, my feeling was that there were high-risk patients who would only be able to be weaned from the machine if we continued using it for, say, several hours. My reasoning was that if you could support them for a longer period of time, perhaps the heart might recover.

The heart is really composed of two pumps. The pump on the right side (the right ventricle) receives returning venous blood from the body and propels it into the lungs, where oxygen is swapped for carbon dioxide. The oxygenated blood then returns to the left side of the heart, where the thicker and more muscular left ventricle thrusts it back into the body at much higher pressure. Theoretically a mechanical device could replace the function of the left ventricle (left ventricular assist), the right ventricle (right ventricular assist), or the whole heart (total artificial heart).

The earliest designs for these systems were relatively crude and were constantly refined as animal research and clinical experience progressed. In a review article written nearly forty years after the fact, Dr. DeBakey described the first successful implant of a left ventricular assist device (LVAD):

> Our first clinical application of this pump was on August 8, 1966, in a white woman with heart failure caused by severe aortic insuffi-

ciency and mitral stenosis. After replacement of both valves, it was impossible to wean the patient off the heart-lung machine despite prolonged support, and the bypass pump was then attached to the patient. With a pump flow of 1,200 mL/min, it was possible to wean the patient off the heart-lung machine. On the 10th postoperative day, it became possible to discontinue the use of the bypass pump as the heart maintained normal function. The patient recovered completely and returned home to resume normal activities. Unfortunately, she was killed in an automobile accident 6 years after the operation.

On April 4, 1969, Haskell Karp, a forty-seven-year-old man with congestive heart failure awaiting transplant, was taken to the operating room at St. Luke's Hospital in Houston for a procedure scheduled as a surgical excision of a thinned and infarcted segment of his left ventricular wall. The procedure that was ultimately performed would make history and also engender a nearly forty-year feud between two of the world's greatest heart surgeons.

Mr. Karp's surgeon was Dr. Denton Cooley, who years earlier had been recruited to Houston by Dr. DeBakey (and three decades later would be asked by the Bush campaign to vet the health of Dick Cheney). In Cooper's book, Dr. Cooley recounts the events surrounding that operation:

> In 1968, it was evident to me that it was time to try the artificial heart. We were having a number of frustrations in watching people die who could have been saved with a heart transplant. One of my colleagues was a fellow by the name of Dr. Domingo Liotta, who had spent time trying to develop an artificial heart. He came to me rather frustrated, saying DeBakey was apparently not interested in going forward with its clinical application. . . . I knew that if I went to Dr. DeBakey to get permission from our department of surgery, we would get only delay and further negative response. So I decided that the time had come to take a bold step. The opportunity arose

to go ahead and do it, and suffer any repercussions that might follow. We did just that.

We had the ideal candidate who was dying and needed a cardiac transplant, a gentleman named Haskell Karp. We were just interested in seeing if you could sustain a human life with an artificial device. Sure enough, that proved to be the case. The patient did very well with the artificial heart, but unfortunately he died following his transplant because of an infection. I have no regrets for having taken that step.

Dr. DeBakey later countered that since the device could not keep an animal alive for a prolonged period of time, he would not use it in a human. Dr. Cooley's brash implant of the unapproved, and unproven, total artificial heart led to a schism with Dr. DeBakey that continued for nearly four decades. The surgical legends reconciled just months before DeBakey's death.

Over the past two decades, mechanical cardiac assist devices have become the real "time machines," giving patients struggling after cardiac surgery time to recover ("bridge to recovery"), patients on the transplant list the endurance to survive until a donor organ is located ("bridge to transplant"), and an option for patients with advanced heart failure who are ineligible for an organ transplant and have historically had no options ("destination therapy").

The initial VADs created pulsatile flow, mimicking the heart's rhythmic movement of blood, and were driven pneumatically by compressed gas delivered through drivelines mated to a large external console. Later iterations of the technology incorporated electrically powered pumps that could be run from battery packs, offering patients more freedom. Although these systems greatly increased the survival rate of patients waiting for transplants, the pumps were relatively large and prone to mechanical failure.

Newer-generation VADs have moved to a different technology and incorporate a rapidly spinning internal rotor to create a continuous (nonpulsatile) output of blood. Compared to their forerunners, these continuous-flow VADs have far fewer internal moving parts (which increases their reliability and durability), need less anticoagulation therapy, are much smaller, and can run for many hours on easy-to-carry external batteries.

In mid-June 2010, Vice President Cheney redeveloped atrial fibrillation and fluid retention, necessitating the reluctant reinstitution of blood thinners to protect him from a stroke and also a big slug of diuretics to clear the fluid. As is typical for a patient with severe heart failure, it was becoming increasingly difficult to keep him in any semblance of clinical balance.

Dick Cheney had done well for many years, but in less than eighteen months, he had morphed from one of the most powerful men in the world to the sickest patient in my practice, someone requiring nearly constant medical attention. Clearly we were reaching the limits of contemporary medical therapy. If Cheney was going to survive beyond the next few months, he was going to need a VAD. I had broached the topic with the vice president the previous fall, but at that time he was still relatively well and the conversation was brief and maybe a bit premature. Now he was really sick, and it was starting to look as if we may have waited too long.

George Washington University Hospital discontinued its heart transplant program in the 1990s, but over the last several years, our group has collaborated with the advanced heart failure and cardiac transplant program at Inova Fairfax Hospital, about twenty minutes away in Northern Virginia. I asked Dr. Shashank Desai, the director of the program, to join us at GW for a meeting with the vice president to talk about VAD and transplant options.

Desai is an instantly likable, supersmart guy with a big smile and a usually beautiful suit, who several years before had been recruited from the University of Pennsylvania. Shashank brought along Lori Edwards, an experienced nurse practitioner who was the VAD coordinator at Fairfax.

The meeting on Friday, June 18, 2010, with Mr. and Mrs. Cheney lasted about two and a half hours. Earlier in the week, the vice president had been volume overloaded, and although his breathing was better after the diuretic-induced loss of several pounds of fluid, he still had no energy. I took Cheney's blood pressure; it was 86/70, much lower than usual.

The vice president's increased fatigue was likely related to his very low blood pressure, but the more salient matter was that his heart no longer had the capacity to move an amount of blood sufficient to meet his body's needs. Although Mr. Cheney was sick and getting sicker, there were still a few options remaining, and one of them was heart transplantation.

Shashank described in great detail the evaluation process and the general criteria that define a "transplant candidate." And at first glance, Cheney appeared to be eligible, but there was one catch: he had to live long enough to get a heart.

Once a person is accepted for transplant, the wait for a donor heart can be anywhere from six months to three years, depending on the blood type and the patient's level of acuity. At any given time in the United States, about three thousand people are on the wait list for a heart, but annually there are only about two thousand transplants. Shashank told Mr. Cheney that if he chose to be listed for transplant, it might be difficult to sustain him using medical therapy alone until a heart became available, but his odds would improve significantly with a ventricular assist device. Used as a bridge to transplant, a VAD can completely supplant the function of a failing left ventricle and support the patient until a donor heart is found. Recent data from a National Heart Lung and Blood Institute registry show one-year survival rates greater than 80 percent for patients implanted with a continuous-flow VAD used as a bridge to transplantation.

Lori Edwards had brought with her a HeartMate II VAD and all of its necessary accoutrements. Methodically she reviewed the equipment, and what the Cheneys would have to do every day to maintain it.

The HeartMate II LVAD, manufactured by California-based Thoratec, is a ten-ounce titanium cylinder about three inches long, not much bigger than a saltshaker. It has only one moving part, the internal rotor, a modern adaptation of Archimedes' 2,300-year-old pump. The VAD contains an electrically powered motor that magnetically spins the rotor at speeds up to 10,000 RPM, capable of pumping ten liters of blood per minute, enabling the device to replace the function of a dead ventricle. The VAD is surgically implanted in the chest and connected to the heart by an inflow conduit sutured into the left ventricle and by an outflow graft sewn to the aorta. Blood entering the VAD from the heart travels through the inlet conduit, is accelerated by the spinning rotor, and is ejected into the aorta through the outflow graft. The system receives electricity through a driveline that exits the skin at the upper part of the abdomen a few fingerbreadths below the rib cage, and is connected to a controller and two camcorder-sized batteries. The batteries can provide about twelve hours of power; at night, patients usually plug into a tabletop unit. The driveline that exits the skin in the upper abdomen must be kept clean and covered with sterile gauze to prevent an infection from developing in the wire tract, and anticoagulants are prescribed to prevent clots from forming inside the pump.

Shashank and Lori explained to the Cheneys that many patients with a VAD feel well enough to return to work and can resume a variety of recreational activities with the exception of swimming. The Cheneys had a few questions about the durability of the device, and Shashank noted that there were a few patients approaching five years, but since the technology was relatively new, it was difficult to know precisely how long the VAD could last.

I wanted Vice President Cheney to leave the meeting knowing that we had not given up on him, there was still much we could do, and that using a VAD as a bridge to a heart transplant was a realistic possibility and my recommendation. Cheney said he would think about it and let us know.

On Monday morning Mr. Cheney called and said that he was feeling a bit better, and that over the weekend he had spoken with his family and decided that he would be interested in getting a VAD. I told him that I thought that was the right decision and that we would begin the necessary tests. Four days later, Mrs. Cheney called and said that the vice president was much weaker and asked if we could see him right away.

Vice President Cheney arrived in a wheelchair, appearing short of breath and very lethargic. It had been only a week since his last visit, but the deterioration was startling. Shashank, Gigi El-Bayoumi, and Carolyn Rosner, a VAD/transplant nurse practitioner from Fairfax, joined us for the visit. We ran some blood tests in the office suite using a handheld analyzer and found that the vice president's kidney function had worsened over the past week, a marker that his heart could no longer provide an adequate supply of blood to the organs.

I told the vice president that his heart was failing, and I recommended admitting him to the hospital immediately to start intravenous medication that should be able to stabilize him and that we quickly move forward with arrangements for a ventricular assist device. Without much discussion, Mr. Cheney agreed to the plan.

My wife, Charisse, asked me later if the vice president looked sad when I told him he needed a VAD.

"Not sad," I said, "just weary."

*Medical Faculty Associates*
*The George Washington University*
*July 1, 2010*

*Vice President Richard Cheney returned for follow-up today.*
*Mr. Cheney was discharged from GW Hospital 3 days ago after*
*being admitted 3 days before that with deteriorating renal func-*

*tion, severe fatigue and dyspnea and a low flow state. After ad-*
*mission the patient underwent right heart catheterization. . . .*
*IV milrinone was begun and clinical status and cardiac output*
*significantly improved. At discharge serum creatinine had re-*
*turned close to baseline at 1.6. Mr. Cheney was discharged 3 days*
*ago on home IV milrinone at 3.75 mcg/kg/min.*

*On 6/28/10 Dr. Gigi El-Bayoumi and I visited Fairfax Hos-*
*pital where we met with members of the Fairfax LVAD/transplant*
*program including Drs. Desai and Burton. VP Cheney and fam-*
*ily visited Fairfax on 6/29/10 and also met with the medical and*
*surgical team there.*

*Today VP Cheney states that overall he feels a little better*
*than yesterday and much better than last week. He sat outside for*
*2 hours yesterday and was able to walk to Executive Health this*
*afternoon without the aid of a wheelchair. Wt. this AM was 203*
*(down 1lb from yesterday). . . .*

*In summary VP Cheney has made a very nice recovery and is*
*stable on home milrinone.*

*Plan is for LVAD insertion at Fairfax on 7/14/10.*

*Jonathan Samuel Reiner, MD*

Shortly after admitting the vice president to the hospital, we brought him to the cath lab to measure the pressures in his heart. We did this by inserting a catheter in a vein in his leg and passing it through his right atrium and right ventricle into the pulmonary artery, the large vessel that carries blood from the heart to the lungs. The data gained from this procedure, as expected, demonstrated that Cheney's cardiac index was severely reduced and well below the level necessary for adequate perfusion of his organs. The cardiac index is the volume of blood pumped by the heart per minute divided by the patient's body surface area, a measure of the cardiac output adjusted for body size. A normal cardiac index is 2.6 to 4.2 liters per minute per square meter. A cardiac index below 1.8 is considered cardiogenic shock. Cheney's was 1.7. We began to administer intravenous milrinone, a drug that can increase myocardial contractility and at least temporarily increases cardiac output. Soon after the infusion was started, Cheney's hemodynamic parameters and kidney function improved.

Milrinone can improve the performance of a failing heart but not indefinitely. The plan was to continue the drug using home IV infusion, allow Cheney's kidney function, overall clinical status, and nutrition to improve, and then bring him to Fairfax Hospital for a scheduled VAD insertion in about two weeks, at which time he should be better able to withstand the rigors of heart surgery.

Initially the vice president felt quite well and was able to walk modest distances with a small portable intravenous pump nestled in a shoulder bag. After several days, however, his kidney function began to decline again.

*Medical Faculty Associates*
*The George Washington University*
*July 5, 2010*

*9:25 AM*

*I spoke with the patient this am. Mr. Cheney came to the ER yesterday evening for evaluation of right thigh pain. The patient developed this in the morning yesterday. CT scan at GW yesterday revealed hematoma in right thigh. . . . Patient was discharged with morphine for pain control. This am the patient notes discomfort in the right thigh which is improved with the narcotic. He is not SOB [short of breath] but hasn't done much exertion because of the discomfort in his leg. Weight is up 2 lbs compared with yesterday. OptiVol today shows continued rise.*

*I told VP Cheney that it is likely that we will proceed with LVAD sooner than originally scheduled. I think it will be difficult to maintain clinical stability for next 10 days and would prefer to schedule LVAD later this week. The patient is in agreement.*
*9:03 PM*

*I spoke with the VP. Still has significant pain in his right*

*thigh and has been using wheelchair to get around house. Mor-*
*phine helps with the pain. No SOB. Has slept OK. There has been*
*a gradual increase in BUN/creatinine despite recent increase in*
*weight by 2 lbs. I told Mr. and Mrs. Cheney that I do not think*
*it is reasonable to try and temporize until next week for LVAD.*
*I have suggested that we proceed with surgery this week with ad-*
*mission tomorrow AM to Fairfax Hospital for optimization . . .*
*prior to planned LVAD insertion later in the week. The patient is*
*in agreement.*

*Jonathan Samuel Reiner, MD*

On Tuesday morning, July 6, Vice President and Mrs. Cheney drove the short distance from their home in McLean to Inova Fairfax Hospital. Mr. Cheney, unable to walk more than a few steps, was met in the garage by a nurse and brought by wheelchair to the cardiac surgery intensive care unit on the hospital's second floor. The plan was to tune up Cheney for a few days in the ICU using intravenous diuretics and higher doses of milrinone, and toward the end of the week, when he would presumably be in a little better shape, we would take him to the operating room.

I stopped by Fairfax early in the day to make sure that Mr. Cheney was getting settled in. The design of the cardiac surgery ICU contains an ideal corner suite of two adjoining rooms, one of them was set aside for the patient, the other for use as a family lounge. To help ensure his privacy, Mr. Cheney was registered using a pseudonym, and a security guard was posted outside the suite. When I entered the vice president's room, he was in good spirits as nurses tethered him with EKG monitoring leads, IV lines, and nasal oxygen cannula. I stayed just long enough to review the plan with Shashank and the patient, and I told them both that I would see them later in the evening.

After spending the day at GW, I returned to Fairfax in the evening to check on the vice president. Earlier in the day, an echocardiogram was performed, documenting a huge heart, easily twice the normal size, which barely moved. Cheney's ejection fraction (the percentage of the volume of blood in the heart that is ejected with each contraction) was estimated to be 10 percent (normal is 55 to 65 percent).

Shashank repeated a right heart catheterization to measure the pressures in the heart and lungs, and he calculated Cheney's cardiac index at 2.0 liters per minute per square meter—not great, but a little better than before the milrinone was started ten days earlier. In an effort to wring just a little more cardiac performance, we ratcheted up the milrinone another notch.

As I entered the unit through the locked power doors, I could see Shashank standing outside the vice president's room at the end of the corridor. Just as I approached, a nurse exited the room and handed us a printout with Cheney's latest lab values.

Shashank and I reviewed the data in stunned silence. Despite the higher dose of milrinone, Cheney's cardiac index was rapidly dropping.

"These can't be right," I said.

I looked through the window into Cheney's room. He was awake, staring at a TV screen on the opposite wall, a remote control gripped in his right hand. These labs couldn't be correct. They were the numbers of a patient in shock, someone about to die. We asked the nurse to send off a repeat sample of blood to verify the result, an act equal parts prudence and denial. Within a few minutes, the results were back. They were just as bad. In retrospect, I don't know why this final turn for the worse was so surprising. For years, I had known this moment would come, and for the last several months, it looked increasingly imminent, but now that it was here, it still came as a shock. There was no escaping the fact that Dick Cheney had very little time left, probably only hours.

"Where's Nelson?" I asked, referring to Dr. Nelson Burton, a Fairfax cardiac surgeon.

"He's in North Carolina trying to get back," Shashank said.

Most VADs are implanted during elective procedures, and Cheney's had originally been scheduled for the following week. The plan was for Dr. Burton to do the surgery, but he was on the Outer Banks with his family. He was trying to find a flight but might not be able to get back until the morning.

"I don't think we can wait until morning," I said.

Shashank agreed and called Dr. Anthony Rongione, the other designated VAD surgeon at Fairfax, who said he would come right over.

Liz, who had been in her father's room when I arrived, came out to talk with us. I asked Liz where her sister, Mary, was. Liz told me that Mary had a cold and had decided to stay home because she didn't want to risk transmitting it to her father before a big operation.

"Tell her to come," I said.

When Mary arrived, Shashank, Rongione, and I met with the family in the vice president's room to update everyone on where we stood.

I cut right to the chase and told Mr. Cheney that his numbers were worse, and despite the late hour, we thought it was prudent to proceed with the VAD right now.

"Right now?" Cheney asked, his surprise evident.

"Yes, sir," I replied. "Tonight."

We described his drop in cardiac output despite the increase in intravenous medication, and I told the vice president that I was worried he might suddenly get into trouble during the night. We had a window of opportunity to do this, but it was closing fast, and I was afraid that if we waited much longer, it would disappear.

Mrs. Cheney asked if Dr. Burton was back.

"Not yet, but fortunately Dr. Rongione is here."

Anthony Rongione was one of two surgeons at Fairfax who, in addition to the usual portfolio of bypass, valve, and aortic surgery, also had expertise in the placement of VADs.

Vice President Cheney turned to his family and asked what they thought. I would usually leave a family to discuss such matters without hovering, but Mrs. Cheney, Liz, and Mary immediately looked at each other, nodded slightly, and told him he should have the surgery tonight.

"Okay, let's do it," the vice president said, his voice clear.

I've watched tears and fear well in the eyes of patients as I tell them they need surgery. Usually I try to allay their concerns by telling them all the reasons they should do well. In this case, I was the person who was fearful. Cheney was dying. I knew he might not survive the night. Although I had no doubt that he needed the VAD, and right now, the odds were not in his favor. Cheney's kidney and liver function were deteriorating, and as he had gotten sicker, his appetite had dwindled, wrecking his nutritional status. One of the main reasons for trying to buy some time before placing the VAD was to rebuild his overall metabolic state, but we had simply run out of time.

In his eulogy for President Ford in 2006, Vice President Cheney had called his former boss "the still point in the turning wheel." That metaphor aptly described Cheney himself. Despite the tumult attendant to preparations for emergency surgery, Vice President Cheney exhibited an uncommon serenity and personal courage I've rarely witnessed in any patient during my twenty-seven years as a doctor. Come what may, he was ready.

It was past 9:00 p.m., and as the nurses readied the patient, Mrs. Cheney came out into the hallway to talk with us.

"You've already had a long day. Aren't you too tired to operate tonight?" Mrs. Cheney asked Dr. Rongione.

"Are you kidding? I have triplets," a beaming Rongione said. "At this time of the night, I'm just getting started!"


I have a recurring nightmare where I find myself alone late at night in a deserted hospital struggling to keep a supersick patient alive. It's my version of the classic insecurity dream, but it couldn't be further from reality. Even at night, a major medical center like Fairfax or GW is well staffed to take care of a critically ill patient, and when Shashank and I entered the operating room, the place was bristling with people.

When I arrived, Dr. Elmer Choi, a Harvard-trained cardiac anesthesiologist, already had Cheney asleep and was busy adjusting the transesophageal echo probe he had just inserted. On the other side of the anesthesia screen, the surgeons—Dr. Rongione, Dr. Paul Massimiano, and Dr. Alan Speir—were well into the operation.

Surgery to place a VAD requires access to the heart, typically by opening the sternum, but in a patient like the vice president who has had prior cardiac surgery, this can be a bit dicey as important anatomic structures (like the right ventricle) can become adhered to the underside of the bone. Indeed, when Dr. Rongione opened the chest, he found thick adhesions everywhere, requiring a meticulous dissection to free the heart from the surrounding scar tissue.

After the dissection was complete, the VAD's outflow graft was created by sewing a woven Dacron conduit onto the ascending aorta using suture about a tenth of a millimeter in diameter. Next, Tony cored out a piece of the tip of Cheney's heart using a specially designed cylindrical knife, removing a piece of muscle the diameter of a thumb. The VAD's inflow cannula was placed inside the heart and secured with thick sutures. Finally, the VAD itself was placed just below the heart, connected to the inflow and outflow cannulas, and the electric driveline tunneled under the skin, exiting the body over the right side of the upper abdomen. The VAD was then activated, and the revolutions per minute of the device gradually increased until it was more than doubling the output of the depleted left ventricle.

Shortly after the VAD went in, around 2:00 a.m., Dr. Nelson Burton entered the operating room. He'd been unable to get an evening flight from North Carolina, so he got into his car and drove five hours to Virginia. Rongione and Massimiano updated Dr. Burton as he scrubbed into the operation.

Although the VAD had gone in without a hitch, Cheney was not out of the woods. The dissection to free the heart of adhesions and peel off segments of his lungs had taken a very long time, and Cheney had bled a lot. When a person bleeds, intrinsic components of the clotting system are consumed, and the more one bleeds, the harder it becomes to stop. Over the next five hours, Rongione and Burton worked to stop the bleeding. Mr. Cheney would ultimately receive more than twenty units of blood and blood products.

When dawn broke, the bleeding had largely stopped, and the VAD, spinning at more than nine thousand revolutions per minute, was doing its job, providing a cardiac output the vice president hadn't seen since the 1980s. Cheney had been in the operating room all night. Against all odds, the vice president now had a chance of surviving due to the superb skill and dedication of Drs. Anthony Rongione and Nelson Burton and the rest of their team.

Vice President Cheney had gone into surgery sicker than most other patients and his recovery was likely going to take longer than most. Complicating matters was the unhappy surprise of the large amount of scar tissue in the vice president's chest and the bleeding its dissection had precipitated. The net result had been a long operation that would require an even longer recovery.

Cheney returned to the ICU on four intravenous drips to sustain his blood pressure and cardiac function. Although the vice president's left ventricle was fully supported by the VAD, the right ventricle was not, and it was struggling. Dr. Jason Vourlekis, the director of the cardiac surgical ICU, was waiting for Cheney when he returned from the operating room and would oversee the care of the vice president until he was stable for transfer to the step-down unit.

By Friday, only forty-eight hours post-op, Vice President Cheney had improved to the point where he could be taken off the ventilator. Over the next few days, he remained relatively stable, making slow but steady progress, but four days later, on Tuesday, July 13, the vice president became short of breath and a chest X-ray revealed a new abnormality in the right lung consistent with pneumonia. Antibiotics were prescribed, but over the next few days, Cheney's respiratory status declined.

On Sunday, July 18, eleven days following surgery, Shashank Desai, Jason Vourlekis, Gigi El-Bayoumi, Nelson Burton, and I met at Fairfax to discuss Cheney's status. Over the prior few days, the vice president's chest X-ray had worsened. It was becoming increasingly hard for him to breathe. After a long discussion with Mrs. Cheney, Liz, and Mary, we made the decision to place the vice president back on the respirator.

Recovery from a critical illness is often not complication free, and although it was disappointing to lose ground, I remained optimistic.

"This is a setback, not a catastrophe," I explained.

The vice president was kept sedated, his antibiotic regimen was broadened, and he remained on the respirator for the next five days. During these difficult first few weeks, not a moment went by that a member of the vice president's family wasn't with him. Mrs. Cheney, Liz, and Mary took turns sleeping in the room adjacent to his.

On July 23, two and a half weeks after his VAD surgery, Cheney was once again extubated.

Relieved that he was off the respirator, and no doubt anxious to hear how his patient was feeling, Dr. Vourlekis said, "I think you look good, Mr. Vice President. What do you think?"

The room was silent while we awaited Cheney's response. The vice president looked up at Vourlekis and, mist bellowing from the humid-ified oxygen mask on his face, said, "I think you're full of s—t."

# CHAPTER 14

# Transplant

## VICE PRESIDENT CHENEY

Of all the procedures I have undergone since that first heart attack in 1978, the LVAD surgery was by far the toughest. The actual operation was complicated by the fact that I was very weak with a failing heart and rapidly declining liver and kidney functions at the time of the surgery. It was especially difficult because it required going in through the scar tissue left from my bypass surgery in 1988. The network of blood vessels that had developed on the site created serious bleeding problems for the surgical team. I needed twenty units of blood during the surgery, and I was on the operating table for more than nine hours the night of July 6 and the morning of July 7, 2010.

My hospital stay lasted five weeks. Some of that time I spent on a respirator, heavily sedated. At one point, the respirator was removed, but when I contracted pneumonia, I had to go back on it. I was fed intravenously and lost more than forty pounds. When I saw myself in the mirror for the first time some weeks after the surgery, I saw my dad, shortly before he died of heart failure just before his eighty-fourth birthday.

When I came out from under the sedation, I was asked what, if anything, I remembered from that period. I said I had very vivid memories of living in a villa in a small village north of Rome. I recalled the streets of the village and small, attractive cafés where I ate great Italian food and drank good Italian wine. I had walked through the same street every morning to get coffee and a roll for breakfast and to pick up my morning newspaper. There was an American couple there that I talked to on occasion. The man was there for some kind of medical procedure. I had the feeling I was also there for a medical procedure, but it was never clear what kind and I never saw any evidence of any medical facilities or personnel. I also had a vivid recollection of sitting out on a patio overlooking a long dirt road with a car on it climbing up a hill to get to the village, but it never got there. Sometime later, while watching one of my favorite movies, *Saving Private Ryan*, I recognized that scene. In the movie, Private Ryan's mother watches the car from the window of her kitchen. When it arrives in the yard outside her door, two passengers emerge, an army officer and a priest. They are there to notify her that three of her four sons had been killed in action in World War II.

At other times I believed the hospital was located at LAX in Los Angeles or on the Sioux Indian Reservation in South Dakota. I remembered a visit from Dr. El-Bayoumi, our family physician. I had tried to persuade her to help me escape from the hospital because, I told her, "I don't belong here; there has been some kind of mistake." But the overwhelming memory was of my Italian interlude. My family wanted to know if they were with me, and unfortunately I had to tell them they were not—which wasn't the right answer. Their experience had been the direct opposite of mine. They had been extremely worried about my condition and my prospects, especially when I contracted pneumonia and had to go back on the respirator. At the least, they said, I could have taken them to Italy.

When I discussed my long dream with my doctors, they said they had no idea what goes on in the heads of patients when they spend a long time heavily sedated, as I had. My family and I speculated the fact that one of my principal surgeons was named Rongione might have been responsible. I also had been reading a novel by Dan Silva, a friend and one of my favorite authors, set in Italy. Lynne and I and our family have had many occasions over the years to travel to Italy. It is a place we love. It was not at all surprising that if I was going to take a vacation someplace while I underwent everything that was being done to me, I had chosen Italy.


After regaining consciousness and getting off the respirator, I was still very sick and weak. I developed a craving for crushed ice. The doctors didn't want me to drink large quantities of liquids, but they would let me eat ice. I remember lying in bed while Lynne, Liz, and Mary took turns feeding me small spoonfuls. My doctors were most concerned that I had completely lost my appetite. I was wasting away because I didn't want to eat. It wasn't just hospital food. Things had a different taste than they ever had before, and nothing seemed appetizing. Until I resumed eating normally, there was no prospect that I could recover from the surgery or begin the long, demanding process of rehabilitation.

Eventually I regained my appetite when the doctors agreed I could have some of my favorite foods. I developed an immense craving for milk, which I hadn't drunk on a regular basis since I was a youngster. Häagen-Dazs vanilla ice cream was a hit. My daughter Mary brought me homemade chocolate chip cookies baked according to my mother's recipe. I finally convinced my doctors that what I really needed was a Big Mac and a large order of fries. I got them, although they were not part of the normal menu for patients in the ICU.

My biggest problem aside from my loss of appetite was that my weakened state before the surgery, plus the surgery, combined with all those weeks flat on my back, part of it sedated and on a respirator, had destroyed my ability to do anything for myself. For the first time in my life, I was completely and totally disabled. With the exception of breathing, there was no bodily function I could perform without assistance. And to keep breathing, I had to exercise my lungs several times a day with a device designed to expand my lung capacity. The degree of helplessness was extreme. I remember thinking that for the first time, I really understood the enormous challenges facing those who are permanently disabled. I came to understand the courage and determination it takes them to perform functions I had always taken for granted. I was told I could plan on at least one full week of rehab for every day I spent in the hospital. In my case, that meant thirty-five weeks just to recover my normal capabilities.

Once I was off the respirator, the rehabilitation process began. The therapists were dedicated professionals who were very good at their jobs. They saw me every day, often two or three times a day, and never let me duck a session. No excuses were accepted. We started small with simple exercises to begin regaining my strength. At first it took two of them to sit me up in bed or get me to a wheelchair. I was just dead weight because all of my muscles had atrophied. Simple tasks such as taking the cap off a tube of toothpaste were impossible. From my bed, I could see the bathroom, and I longed for the day when I would be able to get out of bed, walk to the facility, and use it on my own.

In the early days of recovery, I had numerous tubes in my chest. The most important was the LVAD driveline, but there were also other tubes draining my chest, which would come out as I healed. I had an IV and a device in an artery in my arm to precisely measure the amount of oxygen in my blood.

One particular memory of Lynne stands out in my mind. The night they wheeled me into the operating room for the emergency surgery, they were concerned that my fingers had swollen so much they might have to cut off my wedding ring. Fortunately they were able to get it off, and Lynne wore it on a gold chain around her neck until she could return it to me some weeks later. It was the first time I had been without my ring in the forty-six years we had been married.

Inova Fairfax Hospital had an innovative program we participated in during my stay. They allowed visits by family dogs, a great morale builder. Of course, there were certain standards that had to be met, but our two labs, Jackson and Nelson, were perfectly well behaved the day they came to see me. They seemed to understand this was a special event and acted accordingly. It was great to see them. My family had also decorated my room with photographs that had been taken by David Bohrer, my official photographer in the White House. As my overall condition improved, I was taken outside to a garden at the hospital for some fresh air.

As I got ready to check out of the hospital, I thought of all the tremendously dedicated and talented people who had performed the surgery and looked after me for the initial five weeks of my recovery. One of the most impressive was Pat Rakers, the nurse in charge of my stay in ICU. She was tough but compassionate and ran her unit with an iron fist. Pat didn't take any lip from anybody, including senior physicians and former vice presidents. She was a veteran of fourteen years' service in the US Army. While I was secretary of defense, Pat had been a member of the crew of a Patriot missile battery. After her time in the army, she went to nursing school and has followed my case in the years since I was her patient.

Being deemed fit to go home didn't mean I could get along without assistance. We made arrangements with a firm to provide health care at home during the early weeks of my recovery, including having someone in the house twenty-four hours a day to help with essential functions. They also made arrangements to transport me home from the hospital. When I was taken to the parking lot on a gurney, I saw a vehicle that didn't look like an ambulance, which is what I had been expecting. It looked exactly like a hearse. It was a long, black limo with room in the back for the gurney and barely enough for the patient. Lying flat on my back, I had only a few inches of space between my nose and the roof of the "hearse." It immediately occurred to me that I was being taken out of the hospital in exactly the kind of vehicle they would have used if my surgery had not been successful. I thought it was pretty funny, but I never shared that with my family. I wasn't certain they would see the humor in it.

When we arrived home, I was moved from the "hearse" to a wheelchair and taken into the master bedroom. Significant changes had been made to accommodate my needs as a patient. Lynne had rented a hospital bed, which could be raised, lowered, or adjusted at the touch of a button. There was also a specially designed chair suitable for use in the shower and the bathroom, but it still required professional help to make use of it. The home health care people were set up in the basement, and I could summon them with a two-way radio from my hospital bed anytime I needed help. Most of them were nurses or EMTs working a second job. They were very good and proved invaluable in the early weeks of my recovery at home.

The LVAD is a tremendous piece of lifesaving equipment, in my case providing the time needed to become eligible for a heart transplant. Initially it takes a lot of getting used to and a good deal of discipline on the part of the patient and the family. Even after you have left the hospital, it is crucial to have someone to help on a continuous basis and, if at all possible, to have a devoted family member who can be your advocate and ask all the tough questions, taking responsibility for your care. In my case, Lynne devoted virtually all her time for many months to focusing on my well-being. She learned everything there was to know about the LVAD and the technology it represents. Liz and Mary, as well as Gus Anies, who works for us, took training on the operation of the equipment so they could help me deal with a crisis should one arise.

My family got deeply involved in other ways with my care while I was still in the hospital. During the most difficult days of my recovery, one of them was present twenty-four hours a day. There was a window in my room that opened out onto the hallway. Each morning I could look out and see doctors making their rounds followed by the usual collection of residents, students, and nurses. One day as I looked out, I saw a familiar face: Liz was in the gaggle following the doctors.

While the up-to-date LVAD I used is a significant improvement over the older machines that required patients to be tethered to a large machine and therefore unable to move about independently, it still requires a lot of effort to adjust to always having to be plugged into a power source. When I came to after the surgery, one of the first things I was aware of was the driveline coming out of my chest into a control element, through the base power unit, and into a wall socket. It was mandatory that I *never* be without power for the LVAD. When we moved out of the vice president's residence in 2009, we had moved into a new home we had built in McLean, where there are a lot of old trees, and much of the power distribution system is aboveground. It is not at all unusual in a thunderstorm or a heavy snowstorm to have major power outages. Without knowing that someday I would be living on an LVAD, we had fortuitously installed at our new house a large generator powered by natural gas that automatically turns on any time there is a power outage.

On one occasion, a TV camera crew came to the house to shoot an interview with me for a documentary. They were determined to set up a lot of lights to supplement the natural light that was available. In doing so, they had knocked out the circuit breaker, shutting off power to that part of the house. I told the producer, tongue in cheek, that I was living on a heart pump that required power twenty-four hours a day. I said I didn't want them to be alarmed, but it made me very nervous every time they shut down the power. (I didn't tell them I was operating on batteries at the time.) They became exceedingly apologetic and cooperative once they believed their zealotry about lighting might be a threat to the continued functioning of my heart.

In my initial period at home, I was in bed most of the time and therefore on the tether connecting my LVAD to the base power unit, which was plugged into an electrical outlet in the wall. As I made progress and became more active, I began to operate off the batteries that came with the LVAD. We had ten or twelve of them that when fully charged were good for up to twelve hours of operation. I wore two at a time. One was supposedly sufficient to run the LVAD, but I never gave one-battery support more than a brief test. Redundancy is a very good thing when your life is at stake. I charged the batteries I wasn't wearing with a machine that fit inside a Rollaboard. When I traveled I carried it that way. The base power unit also fit into a Rollaboard for easy transport. At night in bed, I would switch over to the tether connecting me to the unit, which was much more comfortable for sleeping.

There are numerous alarm systems on the LVAD that signal when the batteries are low or if there is a malfunction in the equipment. I carried a black "go bag," which contained a spare control element as well as extra batteries, so that I could replace all of the external equipment if necessary. On one occasion when Lynne and I were at a cocktail party, there was suddenly a noise that sounded a lot like a cell phone going off. My immediate reaction was to wonder what fool had failed to turn off his phone at the party. Then Lynne came over to me and said, "Dick, I think you are beeping." She was right: an alarm was indicating my batteries were low. We stepped into a nearby room and put in new batteries, trying to draw as little attention as possible.

On more than one occasion, in the middle of press interviews, I deliberately disconnected one of my batteries, which always triggered the alarm. It was disconcerting to those around me, most of whom didn't realize I had a backup and everything was still operating normally. I did it once to Jamie Gangel of NBC, who immediately pleaded, "Please reconnect that!" and forgot the line of questioning she'd been pursuing. Once flying across the country, I had my noise-canceling headphones on, listening to music. I was reading a newspaper when my assistant, riding several rows in back of me, came up and tapped me on the shoulder. When I took my earphones off, she told me I was beeping. Because of my headphones, I hadn't heard it, but everyone else on the plane had.

Once when I left my house in Wilson, Wyoming, to run some errands in downtown Jackson, I forgot the go bag, which presented quite a dilemma when my batteries started beeping. All the instructions say that they are good for only ten minutes after the beeping starts—and replacements were twenty minutes away. I called my daughter Mary, who was visiting, and she grabbed the go bag and headed in her car to the Snake River bridge, the halfway point between our house and Jackson. I set out for there myself and got new batteries from Mary before the old ones ran down.

One of the things LVAD patients have to worry about is the possibility of infection at the site where the driveline passes through the chest wall. It is covered by a dressing that needs daily changing, a task almost impossible to do by yourself because of the measures that have to be taken to keep the wound sterile. The person changing the dressing has to wear sterile gloves and a mask, wash the wound several times with an antiseptic solution, rinse it with sterile water, and cover it with sterile gauze, arranging the dressing so that the driveline emerges from the middle of it. For the twenty months I lived on the LVAD, Lynne was my nurse every time I needed to change the dressing. The few times she wasn't available, Liz or Mary would fill in. The danger of infection was significant because it could be fatal. It was my understanding that if I developed a serious infection, I would go to the head of the transplant list, but there was no guarantee I could get a transplant in time to save my life.

Showering with an LVAD requires putting a waterproof bandage over the driveline site so that it isn't contaminated by unsterile shower water. There is also a shower bag that the external equipment goes in so that it won't get wet and short out.

One of the big concerns was tangling the driveline on a doorknob or dropping the equipment. At all costs, I had to avoid putting the kind of pressure on the driveline that could reopen the wound and allow an infection to develop. As I think about it now, this all seems complicated and technical and important, and it is. But it is also true that over time, with first-class help, you learn to adjust and adapt to the new normal of living with a battery-driven pump keeping you alive.

Thoratec, the company that makes the HeartMate II that I wore, has worked to make the device and its support elements user-friendly. It comes with a belt and mesh vest to hold the batteries and the control element. Lynne found an alternative on the Internet that more closely suited my needs. A woman in Ohio whose husband was a member of the LVAD club had designed and made a cloth vest to hold the gear. Lynne ordered one, and we then adapted it to my requirements. With the help of a local tailor, I soon had vests that I could wear with a suit or sport coat. With some adjustments in my suits to accommodate the vests and holes in my undershirts for the driveline, I had Lynne's approval to be seen in public.

Once I checked out of the hospital, arrangements were made so I could continue my rehabilitation program at home. Two therapists took over the work begun by their colleagues at Inova Fairfax. One focused on basic conditioning and strength and the other on improving my ability to perform the everyday tasks of living. I frankly had been something of a skeptic in the past on the subject of physical therapy. That was before I needed it myself. When I recall how helpless I was after the LVAD surgery, it's impossible not to credit my therapists with working wonders for me. Part of their value lies in their ability to influence your mental attitude, to convince you that you can do anything if you put your mind to it.

When the 2011 fishing season began, I was eager to get back on the river with my fly rod. I had the opportunity that summer to fish with the Rivers of Recovery, a program that assists our wounded warriors, veterans who had served in Afghanistan and Iraq. Fly-fishing is great therapy for those who have been severely wounded or who suffer from post-traumatic stress disorder or traumatic brain injury. Twice now I have had the privilege of fishing with a Marine, Justin Clenard, who lost both of his legs in Afghanistan. Within eight weeks of being wounded, he was up and around on his prostheses. He is now a fully certified guide on the Snake River and a good one. The first time I fished with him, I explained that because I was on the LVAD, I had to be careful not to fall in or my heart pump might short out. He said, "I know what you mean. When I fall in, my legs get rusty."

After I left the White House in 2009, I decided I wanted to explore the possibility of writing my autobiography. I retained the services of attorney Bob Barnett, who had represented Lynne over the years on the many books she had published, as well as numerous other authors. But he has one credential that most people don't know about: in the 2000 presidential campaign, he had played me in Joe Lieberman's practice sessions for the vice-presidential debate. He did the same for John Edwards, the Democratic vice-presidential candidate, in 2004.

I never held it against him since both his candidates lost.

My book, *In My Time,* was published by Simon & Schuster at the end of August 2011. With help from my family, we had been able to get it done even as I dealt with serious health issues. Liz was my co-author, and Lynne and Mary were our in-house readers and editors. When it was released, I had just marked the first anniversary of my LVAD surgery and had recovered sufficiently to undertake an extensive book tour. We traveled from New York to Los Angeles and from Vancouver to Miami, with many stops in between. Travel on the LVAD was a complicated affair. I always had to have someone with me because of all the gear I had to take along. Given the post-9/11 security procedures, we sometimes encountered problems, but in general, the Transportation Security Agency personnel did their best to ease our way while still fulfilling their responsibilities. We occasionally encountered problems of our own making, like the time we left the base power unit in a hotel in Vancouver.

Completing the book and undertaking the book tour were major accomplishments from the standpoint of my health. It proved to me and others that after more than thirty years of coronary artery disease, five heart attacks, a quadruple coronary bypass, one episode of sudden cardiac arrest, end-stage heart failure, and major surgery to implant the LVAD, I still could function and enjoy an active life.

One day in late 2011, I received a phone call from the Cleveland Clinic, one of the foremost heart institutes in our country. The caller indicated the clinic was going to host a conference on innovation in the treatment of heart disease. He said they had a number of suppliers of medical devices and many physicians coming to their conference. Someone had suggested it might be useful to have a patient participate. Someone else said, "Let's get Cheney. He's had everything done to him that you can do to a heart patient!" I agreed and persuaded two of my doctors, Jonathan Reiner and Shashank Desai, to join me for a fascinating afternoon talking about the patient's perspective and answering questions such as, "Which devices or procedures do you believe saved your life?" The list was long.

I had never given much thought to the possibility of a heart transplant. In more than thirty years of living with coronary artery disease, it had never occurred to me that I might someday be a candidate for one. As my disease developed, we always were able to meet the latest challenge with new procedures, devices, or medications. I believed that as I grew older and my disease progressed, we would eventually exhaust all options and my time would be up. I did not look at a heart transplant as one of those options.

I understood from the beginning of the LVAD process, however, that if successful, it could indeed open up the possibility of a new heart. I requested placement on the transplant list at the time of my surgery in case I decided to go that route. Once I started feeling better, I realized that for me the decision whether to live with the LVAD permanently or use it as a transitional device wasn't a close call. A transplant offered the best prospects in terms of longevity and a return to a normal life. I can understand why some people make the decision to stick with the LVAD and not subject themselves to yet another major open heart operation, but the possibility of putting more than thirty years of coronary artery disease behind me with the receipt of a new heart was all the incentive I needed. I also believed that transplant surgery couldn't be any worse than what I had already been through, and I had Dr. Reiner's assurances that transplanting a heart was usually simpler and easier than implanting an LVAD. I started operating on the assumption that the LVAD would buy me the time to work my way up the transplant list. Altogether I spent twenty months on the pump, thankful to be alive. I had learned from experience that my mental attitude was important in getting through any medical crisis, and it was hard not to be positive when I woke up every morning, grateful for another day I never expected to see.

One night during the period we were waiting for the call that a heart was available for me, I was watching the eleven o'clock news. One segment showed two men getting out of a small plane and running across the tarmac carrying a cooler between them. Suddenly they dropped the cooler, it fell open, and a small package, which was, in fact, a heart, rolled out. They quickly scooped it up, put it back in the cooler, jumped in a waiting car, and drove off. I couldn't help thinking, *I hope that's not part of my transplant team!*

As you move up the list, your team can give you some notion that you are getting close to the top. You will get a heart only if one becomes available that meets your requirements in terms of blood type, size, and general suitability, but that can happen even if there are people with the same requirements ahead of you on the list. They might turn down a heart for some reason, giving you a chance at it. During this period, you carefully coordinate your schedule with the transplant team, making certain they can reach you at all times and that you can get to the hospital pretty quickly. If a heart becomes available, two members of the team travel to the site where the donor is located and ascertain the quality and suitability of the donor organ. Usually several organs can be harvested from a single donor, including the heart, kidneys, and liver.

Late in the evening of March 23, 2012, as Lynne and I were getting ready for bed, our phone rang, and Lynne answered. It was Lori Edwards, part of the LVAD transplant team, calling to tell us they had a heart for me. Lynne gave me a thumbs-up signal, and a few minutes later, Dr. Reiner called with the same message—one that's hard to top in terms of good news. We dressed and drove to Inova Fairfax Hospital, about twenty minutes from our house in McLean. When we arrived, we checked into the same room I had been in twenty months before. There was an air of expectation as members of the transplant team drifted in, and we began the process of prepping for the surgery. It was a very different mood from the last time I prepped for open heart surgery. Then I had been dying, my liver and kidneys shutting down because of my failing heart.

Dr. Alan Speir, the surgeon who would perform the operation, came in and introduced himself. He is a tall, slender man with a calm, reassuring air. I had a good feeling about him and what he was going to do for me. Thanks to Dr. Speir, his team, the donor, and the donor's family, I was about to receive the gift of many more years of life.


## DR. REINER

*Choosing an appropriate recipient for a heart transplant is more difficult than you might expect. Even in the patient with advanced coronary artery disease, who is incapacitated to a great degree, the surgeon would hesitate to remove an organ which is, after all, supporting the life of the individual.*

—DR. NORMAN SHUMWAY, 1967

March 23, 2012. Midnight.

There could be only one reason for Shashank Desai to call so late, and I was almost afraid to answer the phone.

"Really?" I asked, not waiting for Shashank to speak.

"Jon, we have a heart, and it is perfect."


Speaking before a joint session of Congress on May 25, 1961, President John F. Kennedy issued a challenge to the nation that would formally begin the race to the moon and usher in a decade of intense scientific advancement:

286

# Transplant

I believe that this nation should commit itself to achieving the goal, before this decade is out, of landing a man on the Moon and returning him safely to Earth. No single space project in this period will be more impressive to mankind, or more important in the long-range exploration of space; and none will be so difficult or expensive to accomplish.

While the general public was riveted by the scientific and symbolic race into space between the Soviet Union and the United States, there was a similarly intense competition during the 1960s among several surgical teams vying to be the first to transplant a human heart.

The competitors were an eclectic group of visionary surgeons who came of age at a time when advances in cardiac surgery, such as the repair of congenital heart defects, valve replacement, and coronary artery bypass grafting were being developed at a dizzying rate, and no obstacle seemed insurmountable. The groups were led by Dr. Norman Shumway at Stanford University in Palo Alto, California; Dr. Adrian Kantrowitz at Maimonides Medical Center in Brooklyn, New York; Dr. James Hardy at the University of Mississippi Medical Center in Jackson, Mississippi; Dr. Richard Lower at the Medical College of Virginia in Richmond; and Dr. Christiaan Barnard at Groote Schuur Hospital in Cape Town, South Africa. There were many problems to solve—technical, biological, and societal—and with relentless perseverance, one by one these barriers would be overcome.

In the late 1950s, Stanford's Dr. Norman Shumway, along with Dr. Richard Lower, had been working on ways to reduce the injury to heart muscle that accompanied surgery in the early years of the heart-lung machine. They found that if the heart was cooled, it would tolerate greater amounts of ischemia than if it was warm. It was during these animal studies that Shumway and Lower began to experiment with techniques to remove and then reimplant an animal's heart. What began as an interesting exercise soon became the focus of their research, and they developed a surgical strategy that would substantially reduce the time required to implant a donor heart.

A human heart connects to eight large-caliber vascular structures in the chest: the inferior vena cava, the superior vena cava, the pulmonary artery, four separate pulmonary veins, and the aorta. Rather than having to reattach eight separate vessels, a time-consuming and technically challenging surgical feat, Lower and Shumway devised a method to suture the back of the donor's heart to a cuff of the recipient's original right and left atria, which were left in place at the time of the excision of the recipient's heart. This technique obviated the need to separately suture the inferior and superior vena cava and the four pulmonary veins, significantly simplifying and shortening the operation, and it became the standard method to transplant a heart.

Before attempting a transplant, it was necessary to understand how long a heart could be preserved outside the body. Shumway showed that a properly cooled canine heart would remain viable for several hours. Although the heart has its own intrinsic pacemaker, it was unclear how a heart would function after all of the nerves supplying it had been severed. Work in the animal lab demonstrated that a donor heart, which has no neural connection to its new host (it is denervated), would begin to beat on its own once the flow of warm blood was restored to the organ. We now know that in some patients, the nerves begin to grow back after many months.

While the various groups working to develop heart transplantation solved many of the technical problems related to the actual surgical procedure, the biological issues generated by implanting an organ from one individual into the body of another were much more challenging and had vexed surgeons for decades.


In 1933, Dr. Yurii Voronoy, a Ukrainian surgeon who was attempting to save the life of a twenty-six-year-old woman with acute mercury poisoning after a suicide attempt, performed the world's first transplant using a cadaveric kidney. Unfortunately, the patient died on post-op day two, likely because her blood type was incompatible with the donor's.

During World War II, Peter Medawar, a British biologist working at the Glasgow Royal Infirmary in Scotland, became interested in understanding why many of the skin grafts used to treat severely burned soldiers failed. Medawar observed that a graft would succeed only if it originated from the same patient, and it would be rejected if it was obtained from a cadaver. Medawar surmised that tissue rejection was an immune-mediated response, a result of the body's recognizing something as "nonself," and his work, for which he received the 1960 Nobel Prize in Physiology or Medicine, ushered in the era of transplant immunobiology.

In 1954, Dr. Joseph Murray, a surgeon at the Peter Bent Brigham Hospital in Boston, performed the world's first successful kidney transplant. Murray overcame the issues related to rejection Voronoy had encountered twenty-one years earlier by transplanting a kidney from one identical twin to the other (one of the techniques Murray used to ensure that the twins were indeed identical was to have their fingerprints analyzed by the local police). Because identical twins share the same immunological identity, the recipient's system saw the new kidney as "self" and did not reject the transplanted organ. The operation was a landmark moment in the history of transplant science, marking the first time a solid organ had been successfully donated from one human being, living or dead, to another.

Relying on the ready availability of an identical twin would obviously not succeed as a durable organ procurement strategy. What was needed was a way to overcome the natural process of tissue rejection. During the 1950s, multiple drugs to attenuate the immune response (immunosuppression) were evaluated, including nitrogen mustard (originally evaluated as a chemical warfare agent) and 6-mercaptopurine (a drug used for cancer chemotherapy). Because of their toxicity, both were deemed unsuitable.

Following the observation that many of the survivors of the atomic bombings of the Japanese cities of Hiroshima and Nagasaki had damaged immune systems, total body irradiation was used in the 1950s. The strategy contributed to the first successful kidney transplant between nonidentical twins, but it was risky and occasionally resulted in the death of the patient.

Shumway and Lower, writing in a 1961 paper, were optimistic that a solution to rejection would be found:

> The precise mechanism by which the host causes the death of the homologous cells is not known. One must assume that, as these mechanisms are clarified, an appropriate means will be found of altering either the elaboration of the homologous antigen or the immunologic response of the host without injury to either graft or host.

The solution soon turned out to be a combination of the drugs azathioprine (a less toxic derivative of 6-mercaptopurine) and prednisone (a steroid). The pair became part of the standard antirejection cocktail for the next twenty years.

At the end of 1963, Dr. James Hardy's team at the University of Mississippi prepared to perform what they hoped would be the world's first heart transplant. Hardy had already made news earlier in the year when he performed the world's first lung transplant. The patient, fifty-eight-year-old John Richard Russell, an inmate sentenced to death for a 1957 killing in Attala County, Mississippi, had been diagnosed with cancer of his left lung. Hardy proposed to remove the diseased lung and transplant a new, cancer-free organ. On June 11, 1963, Russell became the first patient to undergo a lung transplant. Ten days later, the Associated Press reported that Governor Ross Barnett had pardoned Russell because his participation in the surgery would help to "alleviate human misery and suffering [for] years to come." Russell died from renal failure about a week after his pardon.

Six months later, as Hardy and his team readied themselves for what would be historic surgery to transplant a heart, they faced a difficult problem that every other team in the United States encountered: the very definition of death.

Unlike the current era, in which brain death (the irreversible end of all brain activity) defines the end of life, in the 1960s, the cessation of a perceptible heartbeat was the typical criterion used to declare a person dead. This created a difficult technical issue in that a heart could not be harvested from a donor until the donor heart stopped beating. This required a surgical team to stand vigil, awaiting the moment the heart stopped, and then excise the organ immediately in an attempt to retain its viability.

In a 1964 paper in the *Journal of the American Medical Association* describing his first operation, Hardy laid out the technical problem:

> But how soon after "death" of the donor could the heart be removed? If it were not done promptly, irreversible damage might have occurred. To minimize such damage it was planned to insert catheters into the femoral vessels and begin total body perfusion the instant death was announced by a physician not associated with the transplant team. . . . In this way, oxygenation of the body tissues could be affected while thoracotomy was performed to excise the donor heart and begin coronary sinus perfusion.
>
> At the outset, it was expected that months, or even years, might elapse before a suitable donor and recipient died simultaneously in the small University Hospital.

Hardy had been concerned that while there should be no difficulty identifying a suitable recipient for a new heart, it might be hard to find suitable donors. To his surprise, in late December 1963, three patients with fatal brain injuries were admitted to his hospital: one with trauma from a fall, one with a brain tumor, and another with a self-inflicted gunshot wound to the head. All three of the patients died after a period of time on a respirator. Hardy rhetorically asked:

When, if ever, would a physician be justified in switching off the ventilator in a patient whose voluntary respiratory effort had long ceased, to permit the hypoxia that would be followed by cardiac arrest? We were not able to conclude that we would be willing to do this, despite the fact that at some point fruitless resuscitation efforts must cease if a viable kidney, heart, or other organ were to be obtained for transplantation to a recipient.

Lacking today's organized network of hospitals perpetually on the lookout for possible organ donors and the contemporary definition of brain death, Hardy made a bold decision:

> Since we were not willing to stop the ventilator, we had concluded that a situation might arise in which the only heart available for transplant might be that of a lower primate.

On January 21, 1964, Boyd Rush, a sixty-eight-year-old semicomatose, deaf-and-mute male with atrial fibrillation and gangrene of the left leg, was admitted to Dr. Hardy's hospital in critical condition. Although the patient's leg was amputated the next day, his condition continued to deteriorate. It was felt that his gangrene, as well as his declining mental status, was likely the result of embolized blood clots from his heart (probably a consequence of atrial fibrillation). On January 23, as the patient neared death, Dr. Hardy brought him to the operating room and placed him on the heart-lung machine. At the same time, a potential heart donor lay critically ill in the hospital, but his demise was not thought to be imminent. Hardy polled his teammates and by a vote of four to one, they voted to use the heart of a chimpanzee.

In one operating room, the chimpanzee was anesthetized and his heart was removed, preserved with cold oxygenated blood, and brought into the adjacent operating room where Mr. Rush was supported by the heart-lung machine. Using the technique that Hardy had perfected in the animal laboratory, the heart of the patient was carefully excised and the chimpanzee's sutured into its place. In Dr. Hardy's words:

A regular and forceful beat was promptly restored following defibrillation with a single weak shock of the pulse defibrillator.

Unfortunately, the heart of the chimpanzee was too small to support the circulation of the much larger man. The patient died in the operating room. Hardy's bold experiment had failed to save Mr. Rush's life, but it was the first time the surgical techniques to transplant a heart had been tested in a human being, and the experience helped to set the stage for what would come next.

In the fall of 1965, Dr. Richard Lower moved from Stanford University to the Medical College of Virginia to assume the job of chief of cardiac surgery, where he continued his heart transplantation research. In May 1967, Lower was intent on proving that a human heart could be removed from a recently deceased donor, revived, and then used for transplant. Both Lower and Shumway had shown that this could be done with dogs, but it had yet to be proven that it could be accomplished with a human heart.

In a reverse of the procedure performed three years earlier by James Hardy, Lower took the heart from a recently deceased patient, revived it with cold saline, and, using the technique that Shumway and Lower had developed at Stanford, transplanted it into the chest of a baboon. Perfused now with warm and oxygenated blood, the human heart began to beat inside the primate, the first time a human heart had been used as a donor organ. Lower had intended his experiment as proof of the concept that a "fresh" cadaver heart could be successfully resuscitated, and he had done just that. As Donald McRae states in his excellent book *Every Second Counts: The Extraordinary Race to Transplant the First Human Heart*, "It was another measured step toward the first full-scale clinical attempt between a human donor and a human recipient."

• • •

In Brooklyn, Dr. Adrian Kantrowitz was also getting ready to perform a heart transplant. He understood the challenges posed by graft rejection and had focused his attention on cardiac transplantation in infants. Although the surgery "was harder technically and emotionally" than surgery on adults, because infant immune systems are immature, Kantrowitz knew infants were less likely to reject the donor organ. To prepare for his first case, Dr. Kantrowitz and his team worked in the lab for years performing hundreds of procedures on puppies, perfecting a technique to be used for the transplantation of a human heart about the size of a walnut.

Kantrowitz was a remarkable innovator. During his long and distinguished career, first at Maimonides Medical Center in Brooklyn and later at Sinai Hospital in Detroit (now called Sinai-Grace Hospital), he developed more than twenty devices, including an electronic pacemaker, multiple LVADs, and the intra-aortic balloon pump (an easy-to-use temporary heart assist device that I have used hundreds of times to treat critically ill patients).

In June 1966, Kantrowitz and his team had been poised to perform the world's first heart transplant. A baby with anencephaly (a terrible and rapidly fatal congenital malformation marked by absence of the brain) had been born in Portland, Oregon, and in an act of heroic generosity, the parents offered their son's heart to an infant in Brooklyn who was dying from a congenital heart defect. The anencephalic child was flown to New York and prepared for surgery that would make history. As the definition of death in 1966 required the absence of circulation, Kantrowitz was required to wait until the child's heart stopped beating. When that sad moment finally came, the little heart could not be revived, and Kantrowitz was forced to abandon the transplant.

On December 3, 1967, one month after the first test flight of the Saturn V moon rocket, the race to perform the first human heart transplant was won in Cape Town, South Africa.

# Transplant

The surgeon was Dr. Christiaan Barnard, a dynamic forty-five-year-old who early in his career trained in Minnesota with surgical legends Dr. Owen Wangensteen and Dr. Walton Lillehei. After his training, Dr. Barnard returned to Cape Town and joined the staff at Groote Schuur Hospital. In the mid-1960s, Dr. Barnard became interested in heart transplantation and developed an animal lab, but unlike many of his American counterparts, Barnard's team focused mostly on honing their operative technique, relying on the long-term animal results published by some of their counterparts in America. In an interview for David K. C. Cooper's book *Open Heart,* Barnard said, "All we were interested in was perfecting the surgical technique."

Louis Washkansky was a fifty-eighty-year-old man, originally from Lithuania, who had suffered three heart attacks in 1965 and was dying of congestive heart failure at Groote Schuur Hospital. In life, he had never met Denise Darvall, a twenty-five-year-old woman who worked at a bank. On December 2, 1967, Denise's young life ended when a car struck her and her mother, Myrtle, as they crossed a street after leaving a bakery. Myrtle died at the scene, and Denise was brought to Groote Schuur in critical condition with a crushed skull.

When Denise's neurological injury was determined to be nonsurvivable, her father, Edward Darvall, was approached about donating her heart to Mr. Washkansky. Despite having just lost his wife and daughter, Mr. Darvall somehow mustered the strength and selflessness to donate his child's heart.

In 1967, the law in the United States required that the heart stop beating before a patient could be declared dead and an organ harvested. In South Africa, a brain-dead patient with a still-beating heart could be declared dead by the consensus of two neurosurgeons, and theoretically the heart could be removed while it still beat, a far better option from the standpoint of graft and, likely, recipient survival.

On December 3, Louis Washkansky and Denise Darvall were taken to separate operating rooms. Barnard told David Cooper that although South African law would have permitted him to remove the still-contracting heart, he decided to wait for the heartbeat to cease:

> I decided I would not take out Denise's heart while it was beating, not even open the chest. I was scared that I would be criticized. Although we had discussed it with the forensic medicine people, and they said it would be no problem, I decided not to do that. When we had Washkansky's chest open and we were ready to connect him to the heart-lung machine, I went to the donor and I disconnected the respirator myself. We waited. She didn't breathe. After about five or six minutes, her heart went into ventricular fibrillation. I then said to my colleagues to open the chest and remove the heart.

Marius Barnard, Christiaan's brother and a crucial member of the surgical team, told Donald McRae for his book *Every Second Counts* that the process of waiting for the donor's heart to stop beating was more complicated than that. According to Marius, disagreement arose among some team members who were opposed to removing Denise's heart while it was still beating. To shorten the time it would take for the heartbeat to cease after Denise was taken off the ventilator, the donor was given an injection of potassium, which stopped the heart (an at-best ethically ambiguous action), and then harvesting began.

Marius told *Life* magazine:

> Now we've got the heart in a donor, oxygenated and being cooled. We've got the recipient, on the bypass machine, also being cooled and ready. Now things are going. Now the whole thing is on. Now we remove the heart of the recipient and cut out the heart of the donor.

Using the techniques pioneered by Richard Lower and Norman Shumway, Barnard sutured Denise Darvall's twenty-five-year-old heart into Louis Washkansky's chest. After all the suture lines were complete, the heart was defibrillated with an electrical shock. Marius's description in *Life* captured the moment history was made:

> Right away after the shock, the beat started. It was a nice beat, you know. When the heart is beating right, you've got a kind of screwing action. And you can immediately see that it's all right. . . .
>
> Then comes the moment when you stop the bypass. Now the heart is on for the first time, on its own. Now that heart's got to do all the work for the body.

The news of the transplant rocketed around the world, and Christiaan Barnard became a worldwide celebrity.

Three days later, on December 6, 1967, Dr. Adrian Kantrowitz became the first surgeon in the United States to perform a heart transplant and the first surgeon anywhere else in the world to perform the operation on a child when he transplanted the heart of an anencephalic baby into the body of two-and-a-half-week-old Jamie Scudero, an infant dying of a congenital heart defect called tricuspid atresia. The baby initially appeared to do well, with his heart rate and respiration near normal, but seven hours later, the heart suddenly stopped, and the child could not be resuscitated. Kantrowitz told the *New York Times*, "We were trying to make one whole individual out of two individuals who did not have a chance for survival." At his press conference, Kantrowitz credited Dr. Norman Shumway with developing the techniques used for the transplant operation. Kantrowitz also made sure people understood that he considered his first procedure a failure.

Two weeks later in Cape Town, on his eighteenth postoperative day, Louis Washkansky died from pneumonia, probably related to the strong immunosuppressive regimen of radiation, azathioprine, actinomycin C, and prednisone.

Shumway's first transplant would come on January 6, 1968, when he placed the heart of a forty-three-year-old woman, who had died from a cerebral hemorrhage, into the chest of a fifty-four-year-old retired steel worker suffering from congestive heart failure following a large myocardial infarction two years earlier. Shumway's patient lived for fifteen days but died after a steady stream of complications.

A few days before Dr. Shumway's initial transplant, Christiaan Barnard operated again. This patient was Philip Blaiberg, whose surgery was a landmark in its own right. Not only did the fifty-eight-year-old dentist survive to be discharged from the hospital, he lived for another eighteen months, proof of the concept that a patient with a heart transplant could "return to life." The operation pierced another barrier too: Blaiberg, who was white, had received the heart of Clive Haupt, a twenty-four-year-old man described as "colored" in the language of apartheid-era South Africa.

Dr. Blaiberg's longevity helped to fuel explosive enthusiasm for heart transplantation. During the months following Christiaan Barnard's first operation, 102 transplants were performed around the world, unfortunately often with dismal results, some by surgical teams unsuited for the demanding operation. Soon many of the groups would abandon cardiac transplantation.

Shumway persevered and continued to innovate, focusing on strategies to identify patients with rejection and new drugs to prevent it. In the first group of patients transplanted at Stanford University from 1968 to 1971, survival was 49 percent at six months and 30 percent at two years.

In the early years, EKG and echocardiographic changes were used to detect graft rejection, but in 1973, Shumway's program began using endomyocardial biopsy, a safe and easy-to-accomplish procedure whereby a slim biopsy catheter is inserted via a needle stick in the neck and guided to the heart, and a tiny piece of myocardium retrieved for analysis by a pathologist. This technique allowed not only the early identification of rejection, but also the identification of patients in whom the doses of the powerful antirejection drugs might be decreased.

In 1980, Dr. Shumway began using cyclosporin A, a new antirejection drug isolated a decade earlier from a soil fungus, which was very effective in preventing rejection. By 1985, the five-year survival rates for patients undergoing cardiac transplantation had soared to 70 percent.

Norman Shumway died in 2006 at the age of eighty-three, leaving behind a remarkable legacy. According to the United Network for Organ Sharing, in 2011, 21,457 adult heart transplant recipients were alive in the United States.

Mrs. Cheney had a party for the vice president when he finally made it home after getting his VAD. Too weak to walk more than a step or two, Mr. Cheney was assisted to a reclining chair in the master bedroom, and that is where we feted his homecoming. Mrs. Cheney served cake, and she had presents for the doctors and nurses who had cared for her husband. The occasion had the feel of a birthday party.

During the vice president's long hospital stay, Mrs. Cheney had asked me if I was going to take my family on a summer vacation. I told her that I wouldn't be going anywhere until the vice president was out of the hospital and that I would figure it out at that time. Now, in the second week of August, I still hadn't given it much thought. As I stood in the bedroom munching on cake, Mrs. Cheney handed me an envelope, which contained a note and a key to their home in Jackson.

*August 9, 2010*

*Dear Jonathan,*
  *This is a present you have to give back, but only after you & your family have enjoyed Wyoming.*
  *I can't begin to express the enormous gratitude all Cheneys feel for the support & friendship you have been so generous with over the last month—and the last years. You have a special place in our heart and nothing will make us happier than thinking of you in Wyoming with your wonderful family.*

At the end of August, Charisse and I took our daughters, Molly and Jamie, to Wyoming, where we rode horses, rafted the Snake, went to the rodeo, and hiked to a lake where we watched a moose drink from the cold mountain water. Cheney loved this place, its crisp air and jagged Teton skyline. It was easy to understand why. Before the vice president got the VAD, I had promised him he would see Jackson again, and although the summer had been rocky, with a little luck I would keep my word.

The hospitalization to implant the VAD had been an ordeal for the patient and his family. When Cheney was finally taken home by ambulance on August 9, 2010, he had been in the hospital for thirty-five days, the vast majority of that time in the intensive care unit, including a week on a respirator. There had been so much to contend with, including bleeding, a kidney injury, pneumonia, respiratory failure, and a pneumothorax (air leak from the lung), that the ICU director, Dr. Jason Vourlekis, at times looked like a plate spinner at a circus.

Vourlekis, whom I hadn't known prior to the vice president's hospitalization, is a very well trained pulmonary/critical care medicine physician who, prior to coming to Fairfax, had worked at National Jewish Medical and Research Center in Denver and the National Cancer Institute. He distinguished himself during the vice president's complicated ICU stay and somehow managed to retain his dry sense of humor.

The hospitalization had also been hard on Cheney's family. Mrs. Cheney, Liz, or Mary slept in the hospital almost every one of the nights he was hospitalized. When he was in the intensive care unit, a family member was with him 24/7, and on most days Gigi El-Bayoumi would come by to offer her irreplaceable counsel and endlessly compassionate ability to listen.

The vice president left the hospital about forty pounds lighter than when he went in, a consequence of his severe illness and many days without any oral nutrition. Unfortunately, the drop in weight also came at the expense of muscle mass. Cheney was going to require a lot of rehab to regain the strength he had lost, not just during the hospital stay but also in the weeks of declining health leading up to the VAD.

Although the HeartMate II VAD is approved by the FDA for use as either a bridge to transplant or as destination therapy, some patients use it as a bridge to decision, giving them time to decide whether to pursue transplantation or to stick with the VAD. In the immediate aftermath of the vice president's long hospitalization, the question of what to do next was really moot. In the near term, even if a heart were to become available unexpectedly, Cheney was in no condition to undergo another operation or, for that matter, even to decide whether he wanted a transplant. What did make sense was to get in line.

In the United States, organ transplantation is governed by a highly codified system of rules and procedures managed by UNOS (the United Network for Organ Sharing), a nonprofit organization that maintains the Organ Procurement and Transplantation Network, a unified transplant network established by Congress in 1984. UNOS manages the national transplant waiting list, develops the policies and procedures that govern organ allocation, and maintains a database that catalogues every transplant performed in the United States.

Each patient placed on the heart transplant waiting list is assigned a status. Patients who have the highest urgency for transplant (the sickest) are called status 1A; these are patients on high-dose intravenous cardiac medications, those requiring ventilator support, and patients with VADs who are experiencing complications such as clots or infection. Patients in status 1B are those with VADs who are relatively stable, as well as the patients maintained on home intravenous infusions of cardiac medications. Status 2 patients are the least sick and don't meet the criteria for status 1A or 1B.

Two days after the vice president's surgery to implant the VAD, the transplant committee at Fairfax reviewed his case and wrote to him on July 12, 2010, informing him of their decision:

*Dear Mr. Cheney*

*Following completion of your transplant evaluation, your case was recently presented to the Heart Transplant Committee for review. I am happy to report that you have been accepted for listing by the committee. You were listed on July 8, 2010.*

*Insurance authorization has been obtained and you are listed with UNOS (United Network for Organ Sharing) and your referring physician has been notified.*

*Attached is a letter from the United Network for Organ Sharing (UNOS). It describes the services and information offered to patients by UNOS and the Organ Procurement and Transplantation Network.*

*While waiting for your transplant, you will see Dr. Shashank Desai in the transplant clinic at Inova Fairfax Hospital. The frequency of those visits will be determined by your clinical condition.*

*If you get sick or are hospitalized while waiting for your heart transplant, it is your responsibility to ensure that the heart transplant program is notified. Changes in your condition may necessitate a change in your waiting status and therefore your position on the list.*

*Should questions arise prior to your next appointment, please feel free to contact us.*

> *Sincerely*
> *Carolyn Rosner, RN*
> *Heart Transplant and Listing Coordinator*
> *The Heart Transplant Program*
> *Inova Fairfax Hospital*

Entering the transplant queue obviously did not commit Mr. Cheney to receiving a heart, but it started the clock so that if and when he decided to pursue that option, he would have already accrued time.

• • •

I never intended the VAD to be a permanent solution for the vice president. Although Cheney was in his late sixties when his cardiac status began its precipitous slide, his noncardiac-related health was actually quite good. He had no sign of carotid disease and had never had a stroke, he did not have high blood pressure, there was no history of cancer or diabetes, and when his heart was working well, so were his kidneys. Cheney's entire complicated and interlocking puzzle of medical problems was entirely due to his dying heart. The shortness of breath, fatigue, arrhythmias, DVT, renal function, bleeding, and swelling were the consequences of heart failure. If we could fix the heart, everything else would go away.

In spring 2010, as Mr. Cheney required multiple hospitalizations and the interludes of relative stability became shorter and shorter, I spoke with a colleague at GW involved in his care. It quickly became clear that the person he was worrying about was me.

"He's dying, Jon, and there's nothing you can do to stop that," my colleague said.

"No, that's not right," I responded. "He can get a VAD, and then we'll transplant him."

"No, he can't get a heart transplant," he said slowly, as if he were trying to break the bad news to me gently.

"Yes, he can," I said, and I walked away.

I viewed the VAD as a life raft for Cheney, not a destination. The boat was definitely sinking, but we were going to get off that boat, allow him enough time to rehabilitate, and give him time to work his way up the transplant list. That was the plan, and although he had told me early on that he was potentially interested in transplantation, he didn't make his final decision until about six months after the VAD surgery when he was starting to feel well again.

Week by week, Cheney started to improve. The VAD can move a

lot of blood, and it provided the vice president with an essentially normal cardiac output. With reinvigorated blood flow, his kidney function returned to normal, as did his liver. The anorexia that accompanied his end-stage congestive heart failure dissipated, consequently improving his appetite and repleting his nutritional status. As Cheney's metabolic parameters improved, his strength rebounded, and he was able to do more and more exercise.

In a letter to me on September 30, 2010, Shashank Desai wrote:

My impression is that Richard Cheney continues to improve nicely since implantation of his HeartMate II LVAD on July 6, 2010. I am happy to see how well he continues to recondition. I have encouraged him to increase his ambulation, and I am happy to see that he is actually traveling. Logistically, we have helped arrange delivery of oxygen to his high altitude locations, as well as ensuring he has backup batteries and controllers with him at all times. Arrangements have been made for a supply of dressings. Additionally, we have contacted the LVAD programs near to where he will be traveling.

In October 2010, Vice President and Mrs. Cheney finally returned to Jackson, a big step in his recovery. A photo that Mrs. Cheney took exactly three months after his emergency surgery to implant the VAD shows the vice president driving his Jeep (the same vehicle in which he had a sudden cardiac arrest while backing out of his driveway ten months earlier), the beautiful Teton range visible in the distance.

After he came back from Wyoming, the vice president returned for a follow-up visit. Shashank wrote:

An echocardiogram was done in the hospital, which I was able to oversee. He continues with severe LV dysfunction. His aortic valve remains closed throughout the cardiac cycle. He has 1+ aortic insufficiency [mild], which remains stable. . . .

Overall, I am very happy with his continued progress. He will return to VAD clinic in 1 week's time.

The standard protocol for a patient with a VAD includes routine surveillance echocardiograms, and Cheney's echo was startling. For the entire time I knew the vice president, he had always had an abnormal echo, notable for a dilated ventricle that didn't contract well. Now, Mr. Cheney's left ventricle was essentially motionless, and with all the blood flow going through the VAD, the aortic valve no longer opened.

On November 2, Mary Cheney sent me a photo of her dad on a pheasant-hunting trip, resplendent in high-visibility orange, a shotgun in his left hand. What's not visible under all the gear is the VAD spinning at 9,600 RPM, enabling him to do so much more than simply survive.

After the New Year, we met again and the vice president looked even better:

*January 21, 2011*

*Dear Dr. Reiner:*

*I had the pleasure of seeing Mr. Cheney in the VAD clinic today in follow-up. Happily, you were present during this visit. I will reiterate the events of this visit for our records.*

*He has truly turned the corner. His energy level is excellent. He has no shortness of breath with his activities. He is very active and is traveling extensively. He is able to climb up more than one flight of steps energetically and does not have shortness of breath at the top. He has had no difficulties with his VAD driveline or controller. His wound is well healed and he has no further drainage. . . .*

*My impression is that Mr. Cheney is doing well and remains status 1B awaiting orthotopic heart transplantation. His VAD continues to perform well. On interrogation he has had no significant alarms. I am happy to see that he has returned to a near normal quality of life. . . .*

*Thank you for allowing me to participate in the care of Richard Cheney. Contact me directly if questions arise.*

*Sincerely,*
*Shashank Desai, MD*

January 2011 marked two landmark events for Dick Cheney; on the thirtieth of the month, he turned seventy years of age, and after meeting again with the team at Fairfax, he made the final decision to proceed with transplant.

The decision to recommend the VAD had been easy. There was no doubt that Cheney would have died without further support, and a VAD was his only option. Now, seven months later, the decision to push ahead with transplant was a bit harder. Mr. Cheney had just barely survived the last hospitalization, but now that the smoke had cleared, he was well. After all that he had been through, the idea of sending him back for more surgery was almost too much for me to contemplate.

If Cheney was going to opt for transplant, now was the time to do it. Although at seventy, he was still a candidate for the operation, that window would close over the next couple of years, and there would be no going back. If he elected to have surgery, there were no guarantees he wouldn't succumb to the kinds of postoperative complications that nearly killed him in July. It was a difficult choice.

Ultimately it came down to a risk-reward analysis. If the vice president was willing to take the risk, the reward might be great (the first patient to undergo heart transplant surgery at Fairfax, in 1986, was still alive). In the forty-five years since transplant surgery was introduced, refinements in organ preservation, candidate selection, immunosuppression, and rejection surveillance have dramatically increased the life span of patients with a transplanted heart. For patients who underwent heart transplantation in 2009 and survived their first year (the vast majority), the median predicted survival is fourteen years. A successful transplant would give Cheney a legitimate chance of reaching eighty. There were still many rivers to fish and graduations of grandchildren to attend. Cheney wanted the transplant.

The heart transplant waiting list managed by UNOS stratifies patients by level of acuity, time spent on the list, and blood type. To avoid immediate rejection, a donated heart must be the same blood type as or a compatible blood type to the recipient's. Organs from patients with blood types A, B, or O require organs from donors of the same type. Patients with blood type AB (the universal recipient) can receive a heart of any type, and those with blood type O (the universal donor) can donate to a patient of any type. Other factors are important to the allocation of specific organs, including the size of the donor and recipient (you can't put a heart from a hundred-pound donor into a two-hundred-pound recipient), and the presence of certain antibodies in the blood. The vice president's blood type was A, a common group shared by 42 percent of the population. A large percentage of donor hearts are type A, but so are many of the patients on the waiting list.

Despite an increase in the number of people being listed for transplant between the years 2000 and 2011, there was essentially no change in the number of heart transplants performed in the United States during that same period of time (about two thousand per year), a consequence of the lack of growth of organ donation. There are currently about thirty-five hundred patients in the United States waiting for a heart transplant. The mean age for patients on the list is fifty-one, but the number over the age of sixty-five has been rising.

As the months passed, life returned to normal for the vice president, who traveled extensively, adjusting the VAD to his lifestyle rather than his lifestyle to the VAD. The one-year anniversary of the implant surgery came and went, and while there had been movement on the transplant list, there were still several patients with the same blood type ahead of him.

In fall 2011, the vice president started to lose a little ground. Cheney developed some edema, and an echo revealed that his aortic valve was leaking more. For years the vice president had mild aortic insufficiency, a valvular abnormality whereby blood seeps back from the aorta into the left ventricle when the aortic valve is closed. It was starting to get worse and beginning to hamper the effectiveness of the VAD.

The device was still doing its job, pumping blood out of the ventricle, but now some of that blood was immediately leaking back, creating an ineffective loop. Cheney also redeveloped atrial fibrillation, and he had an episode of ventricular tachycardia that his ICD stopped.

*January 20, 2012*

*Dear Jonathan:*

*I had the pleasure of seeing Richard Cheney back in the VAD clinic today in follow-up. He was in Wyoming for the holidays and continues to do well. He had a mild viral illness but does not have any fevers, chills, or sweats currently. He has had one episode of a nosebleed, but this did not progress. . . .*

*On physical examination his mean blood pressure is 92mmHg. His LVAD is set to 9800 rpm with a flow of 5.7 . . . he is well appearing and in no distress. . . . Lungs are clear to auscultation bilaterally. Cardiac exam reveals normal VAD sounds without audible heart sounds. . . . Driveline is clean, dry and intact. . . .*

*My impression is that Richard Cheney has an appropriately functioning LVAD which was implanted on July 6, 2010. He has overall deterioration of his cardiac function under this. He is exercise limited. Additionally he has progressive aortic insufficiency; when last checked, this was moderate in volume. This is very likely the result (cause) of his OptiVol [fluid measurement] being above threshold, as well as the return of his atrial fibrillation. Now he has fast VT requiring therapy. To this end I have asked him to increase his antiarrhythmic therapy of Toprol XL to 100 mg daily. I believe his blood pressure will tolerate this. . . .*

*Overall my general concern about his deteriorating course continues to escalate. . . .*

*Thank you for permitting me to participate in the care of Richard Cheney. Contact me directly if questions arise.*

*Sincerely,*
*Shashank Desai, MD*

## Transplant

A month later the vice president's hematocrit began to drop, prompting a search for a source of his blood loss that included upper and lower endoscopy, both of which were unremarkable. It was unclear whether the VAD was starting to hemolyze (break open) some of Cheney's red blood cells or whether there was another yet-to-be-determined cause of his anemia. What was clear was that once again, the clock was ticking.

March 23, 2012. Midnight.

"Say that again," I whispered, although I heard it clearly the first time.

"We have a heart for Cheney," Shashank said.

Although I had been waiting for this call for more than twenty months, and had known for much longer that one day it would probably come to this, it was still a shock.

Shashank told me what he knew about the donor and that his nurse practitioner, Lori Edwards, had already notified the vice president and arranged for him to be admitted to Fairfax. We discussed logistics for a few minutes and agreed to meet at the hospital in about an hour.

I hung up and dialed the vice president's house in McLean. When he answered the phone, he was unbelievably calm.

"This is going to be a great day," I said, unsure whom I was trying to reassure.

I dressed quickly and gave my wife a quick kiss good-bye. We were already packed and ready to leave in the morning for our annual spring ski trip, but now Charisse and the girls were going to have to fly to Colorado without me. I jumped in my car and sped down the driveway as I had done so many times before in the middle of the night for countless other patients.

Vice President Cheney never asked for, and never received, any special accommodation while he was on the transplant list, as some television pundits later insinuated. Cheney waited twenty months for the call that finally announced his new heart, almost double the usual wait.

When I arrived at Fairfax, the vice president had already changed into a hospital gown and was sitting with Mrs. Cheney and Liz in the same corner ICU suite in which he nearly died following surgery to implant the VAD two summers before. I had an uncomfortable moment of déjà vu when I entered the unit, but I reminded myself that this wasn't the same patient we admitted in July 2010. This patient was well nourished, with great kidney function, excellent physical strength, and no evidence of clinical heart failure. That other patient had been dying.

The nurses were busy with their long preoperative checklist, and it would be several hours before the surgery began. A team would be going out to harvest the heart early in the morning, and Cheney wouldn't be brought to the operating room for several hours. Hopefully he would be able to get a little sleep before then.

Shashank had some lingering questions about the donor and the heart. The only way to answer those questions was to physically evaluate the ultrasound and the donor ourselves. Without telling the Cheneys where we were headed, Shashank and I excused ourselves and left Fairfax.


At 3:00 a.m., we drove through mostly deserted streets to the hospital where the donor was being sustained on a ventilator and IV drips. When we entered the ICU, we found the transplant coordinator busily working the phones. Shashank and I introduced ourselves, and she pulled up the echocardiogram on a computer for us to review.

It's often difficult to get good-quality echo images in a ventilated patient, but what we could see suggested that the heart was normal in size, with normal valves, and good function. It looked like a fine heart.

We asked the coordinator if we could see the donor, and she took us to the room. I entered filled with a mixture of sadness, respect, and gratitude, consciously reminding myself that I wasn't looking at a patient who was dying but someone who had already died. The monitors in the room displayed blood pressure, pulse rate, and blood oxygenation, and they all looked fine, but in this terrible setting, they told me nothing about the patient; they were just individual gauges of organ function. This patient was dead.

I found it impossible to look at this person, a few days ago full of life, and now lifeless, without the humbling reminder of how temporary everything in this world is.

I arrived home as the sun inched over the horizon and caught a couple of hours of sleep before returning again to Fairfax midmorning. The vice president had been brought to the OR early, and his operation began around ten o'clock. Simultaneously, surgery was under way at the other hospital to harvest the donated organs.

Because the success of the transplant is inversely related to how long the donor heart is without blood, surgery to remove the old heart cannot wait for the arrival of the new organ. Conversely, the actual surgery to remove the recipient's damaged heart cannot begin until the team harvesting the donor heart is certain that the donor organ will be suitable, and that happens only when the harvesting surgeon physically examines the heart. Word came that it was a go, and the two surgeons, Dr. Anthony Rongione (who saved Cheney's life twenty months earlier with his brilliant implantation of the VAD) and Dr. Alan Speir, the hospital's director of cardiac surgery, who had trained in cardiothoracic surgery in Texas under Dr. Denton Cooley, got to work.

As was the case during the VAD insertion, the cannulas for the heart-lung machine were placed first, via the large femoral artery and vein at the top of the leg, so that if the surgeons encountered severe bleeding when they opened Cheney's chest, they would be able to support his blood pressure with cardiopulmonary bypass.

Once Cheney was on bypass, Rongione and Speir opened the chest and went about the process of meticulously dissecting scar tissue so that the entire heart and its vascular connections were visible.

Late in the morning, before the new heart arrived, Alan called me over to the table.

"Hey, Jon, take a look."

In Alan's raised right hand, festooned with surgical clamps and now separated from the body that it sustained for seventy-one years, rested the vice president's heart. It was huge, more than twice the size of a normal organ, and it bore the scars of its four-decade battle with the relentless disease that eventually killed it.

I turned from the heart to look down into the chest. Although we had passed the surgical point of no return at least an hour before, the surreal void was a vivid reminder that there was no turning back.

It was surprisingly quiet in the operating room as we awaited the new heart. During the brief interlude, I checked my phone and found a text message from my wife, who was on her way to Colorado with our children. The message read: "Praying for RBC. Thought of him while flying over this vast beautiful country."

Right on cue, the electric doors to the OR slid open and a burly surgeon carrying a small Igloo cooler hustled into the space. The cooler contained the donor heart, which was immersed in a cold electrolyte solution inside a double layer of transparent plastic bags. The surgeon who harvested the heart was Dr. Lucas Collazo, and after handing off the priceless gift to the surgical team, he shook my hand and reminded me that our training had overlapped at North Shore University Hospital twenty-two years earlier.

The new heart was gently handed to Rongione and Speir and placed in the chest of the vice president. First, the back of its left atrium was sewn to a small residual cuff of Cheney's original left atrium. Next to be connected was the inferior vena cava, the large vein that returns venous blood from the lower half of the body. Then one after the other, the superior vena cava, the pulmonary artery, and finally the aorta were joined to the new heart.

When Rongione and Speir were satisfied that all of the anastomoses were secure, the aortic clamp was removed. Now, for the first time in its new home, the heart received warm blood, and after a single shock from defibrillator paddles, it started to beat on its own.

I know that heart transplantation is fundamentally an elegant surgical procedure forged from a century of relentless work by courageous people who refused to believe that it couldn't be done, but for me, like the birth of a child, the awakening of a heart in its new host is a moment filled with divine grace.

As the surgical team started to close the vice president's chest, I stepped out of the operating room to update Mrs. Cheney and Liz, waiting in the same ICU space where they had sat vigil twenty months earlier. I described how different things were this time: how well Cheney had done, the magnificent new heart, and, with a quivering voice, the moment it started to beat. Soon we were joined by Drs. Speir and Rongione, whose beaming smiles telegraphed their news.

# Days of Grace

## VICE PRESIDENT CHENEY

When I awoke after surgery, Dr. Reiner and Dr. Speir were standing by my bed telling me the operation had gone very well. They said that as soon as the new heart had been connected to my blood supply and given a shock, it had started beating, which if you think about it is pretty amazing—an organ from one person happily taking up residence in another—and all because thousands of people have worked in research laboratories and operating rooms over the years perfecting the medicines, the techniques, and the technology that make transplant surgery possible. Getting a new heart is miraculous, but so is the way that researchers and doctors have worked for decades to advance the knowledge and skill that came together for me in a hospital in Northern Virginia.

Of the three open heart surgeries I've had, transplant was by far the easiest. After the operation, I was on a respirator just a few hours, and I experienced only the mildest discomfort, even on the incision. Tylenol 3 was the strongest painkiller I needed. Three days after the surgery, I was out of bed walking the halls of the coronary care unit. I had been told that if everything went perfectly, I might get discharged after two weeks in the hospital. I was out in nine days. Three weeks after the surgery, I was in Wyoming, speaking to the Republican state convention in Cheyenne.

My recovery continues to be trouble free. I take antirejection medications to suppress my immune system so that it does not reject my new heart. With my immune system suppressed, I am more vulnerable to infections, and I have thus become a great consumer of antibacterial hand wipes. I use them on armrests and tray tables when I'm on a plane and keep them handy whenever I'm going to be shaking a lot of hands. Having my immune system suppressed also makes me more vulnerable to skin cancer, so I've learned to apply sunblock first thing every morning and to never go outside without a hat—preferably my Stetson. I also have regular tests—heart biopsies and gene profiling—to look for the signs of rejection, but so far none have appeared.

When I woke up in the hospital, all the paraphernalia connected with the LVAD was gone. I was no longer connected to an electrical source. There was no base power unit. There were no batteries. And other things were gone as well, including my old heart, which after thirty-five years of coronary artery disease, five heart attacks, and episodes of A Fib and V Fib had grown to twice the normal size in an effort to pump blood through my body. Missing was the stent that had been inserted in a coronary artery and the ICD that had saved my life. The only evidence I have been a heart patient—to a layman like me, at least—is the scar on my chest.

Writing this book with Jonathan Reiner has been a great experience. Jon is not only a world-class cardiologist, he is a thoughtful, well-read person who brings a long perspective to his work. He is also a man of unfailing good humor, which is pretty important in someone with whom you spend long hours in the cath lab or going over book revisions. I thought I knew a lot about coronary artery disease when we began this project because I had lived with it for thirty-five years, but now I feel as though I have been through a yearlong advanced seminar on the history of medical cardiology. Studying my medical records has also given me a whole new perspective on what I have been through. As I was living it, I dealt with one crisis at a time, but now I see the long arc of my disease and understand the relationships between what previously had looked like discrete events.

I particularly realize how fortunate I have been that new medications, procedures, and devices in coronary medicine have stayed ahead of my disease. Jon observed one day that it was as though I were traveling down a street, late for work, and all the lights ahead of me were red, but they turned green just before I got there. Most of the innovations that have saved and extended my life weren't available when I had my first heart attack in 1978. The health care system that produced such rapid development and has driven the dramatic reduction in the incidence of death from heart disease over the past forty years is a national treasure and deserves to be preserved and protected.

I find myself thinking a lot about the past these days, about ancestors like Samuel Fletcher Cheney, my great-grandfather, whose Civil War sword hangs on the wall of my office alongside ceremonial swords presented to me by the Corps of Cadets at West Point and by the commandant of the US Marine Corps. I think about my parents and questions I should have asked them while they were here. How I wish they had lived long enough to have been at the inaugural when I was sworn in as vice president on January 20, 2001. What a pleasure it would have been for them to know their great-grandchildren.

I think about the future, too, and how grateful I am to be able to leave a record of my life for my grandchildren and their grandchildren. I spend a lot of time with my four granddaughters and three grandsons, doing things I never thought I would be able to. The other day, before I realized what I had done, I had picked up a forty-pound sack of horse feed and thrown it into my pickup truck with nary a twinge—except maybe in my bad knee. Three years ago, I was in end-stage heart failure and could hardly get out of my chair.

Fifteen months after receiving my new heart, I look on every day as a magnificent gift. I had reconciled myself to dying. I was grateful for having been able to share my life with Lynne and Liz and Mary and the rest of our wonderful family. I considered myself fortunate for all that I had been part of as a result of my career. I had indeed lived in interesting times. I felt I had left nothing undone and was at peace with the idea that I had reached the end of my days.

And now suddenly I have new days ahead—incredible and amazing days that I never expected to see. I owe these days of grace to the donor of my heart and the donor's family, to my medical team, and to family and friends all across America who have sent their prayers my way. They have given me the gift of life, and I thank them. I cannot imagine anything more precious that one human being could bestow on another.

# Acknowledgments

## VICE PRESIDENT CHENEY AND DR. REINER

This story would not have been possible without the tireless, world-class efforts of the physicians, nurses, and staff of the George Washington University Medical Faculty Associates, the George Washington University Hospital, Inova Fairfax Hospital, the White House Medical Unit, and several other institutions. Special recognition goes to Dr. Benjamin Aaron, Dr. Ryan Bosch, Dr. Nelson Burton, Dr. Brian Choi, Dr. Lucas Collazo, Dr. Anthony Caputy, Dr. Paul Dangerfield, Dr. Rick Davis, Dr. Shashank Desai, Lori Edwards, Dr. Gigi El-Bayoumi, Dr. Joseph Giordano, Dr. Peter Gloviczki, Dr. Wes Hiser, Dr. Lew Hofmann, Dr. Andrew Holmes, Dr. Dick Katz, Dr. Barry Katzen, Dr. Sung Lee, Dr. Janet Lewis, Dr. Conor Lundergan, Dr. Gary Malakoff, Julia Mason, Dr. Paul Massimiano, Mary Beth Maydosz, Dr. Ramesh Mazhari, Sarah Murphy, Dr. Wayne Olan, Pat Rakers, Dr. Anthony Rongione, Carolyn Rosner, Dr. Allan Ross, Dr. Nader Sadeghi, Dr. Alan Speir, Dr. Cindy Tracy, Dr. Dick Tubb, Dr. Jacob Varghese, Dr. Anthony Venbrux, Dr. Jason Vourlekis, and Dr. Alan Wasserman.

We would also like to thank those who made the book possible, beginning with attorney Bob Barnett, whose excitement for the project was immediately apparent. Bob's wise counsel and his unique insight every step of the way have been irreplaceable.

We are both grateful to Carolyn Reidy, the CEO of Simon and

# Acknowledgments

Schuster, and Susan Moldow, the publisher of Scribner, for their enthusiasm and support for this project. Our editor Shannon Welch provided seemingly endless encouragement and gently guided us through the amazing and sometimes arduous process of writing this book. We also offer our thanks to the assistance of Simon and Schuster's John Glynn and Brian Belfiglio.

## DR. REINER

Two days after Dick Cheney's heart transplant in March 2012, I sat with Liz and Lynne Cheney in Inova Fairfax Hospital. As it was already quite apparent that the vice president was going to do well, spirits were very high. I told Mrs. Cheney and Liz that the entire history of cardiovascular medicine could be told through the remarkable thirty-five year medical odyssey of Dick Cheney.

Mrs. Cheney said, "That would be a great book!"

"That's my book," I said half jokingly.

"Let me tell Dick," she said as she left the room. In a few minutes Mrs. Cheney returned and said, "Dick loves the idea."

Two weeks later Liz called and asked if I was serious about the book. I said I was. "Good," she said. "Dad's already told Don Rumsfeld he's writing a book with you." Such was the beginning of this project, and it would not have been possible without the warm support of Lynne and Liz Cheney.

Liz was an invaluable collaborator from the very beginning of this project, and I will always be grateful for her assistance, friendship, and constant encouragement.

I had the great good fortune to have an "in-house" medical editor (who also happens to be my wife). Charisse is a pulmonary/critical care–medicine physician, and her input was irreplaceable. The writing of this book consumed the little free time my usual occupation affords me, and without the love, patience, and help of Charisse and my daughters, Molly and Jamie, it simply would not have been possible.

## Acknowledgments

Over the past fifteen years almost every member of the division of cardiology at George Washington University Hospital has had a role in the care of Dick Cheney, and I will forever admire their dedication to the treatment of people with heart disease. The group includes Dick Cheney's former cardiologist, Dr. Allan Ross, who was a mentor to me when I came to GW twenty-three years ago and who gave me my start in academic medicine. Dr. Alan Wasserman, Dr. Dick Katz, and Dr. P. Jacob Varghese were, and continue to be, my teachers, and to them I offer my deepest respect and gratitude. My colleagues Dr. Cindy Tracy and Dr. Sung Lee were important members of the team caring for Vice President Cheney, and their skill and professionalism have always been remarkable. Dr. Gary Malakoff cared for Mr. Cheney for many years, and after his departure his very large shoes were not easy to fill. Dr. Gigi El-Bayoumi, who became the vice president's internist five years ago, is one of the most remarkable physicians I have had the honor of working with, and she continues to teach me much about the art of medicine and the healing power of compassion.

Dr. Lew Hofmann will have my eternal respect and admiration. Lew has the rare combination of competence, professionalism, and humility. Lew spent more than twenty years in service to the Air Force and this country, including eight years caring for Vice President Cheney and his family. If we had a most valuable player award it would go to Lew.

Over the last few years I have had the great pleasure of working with the heart failure team at Inova Fairfax Hospital. Dr. Shashank Desai and his colleagues have built a superb program, and their care for a critically ill Dick Cheney was remarkable. Special thanks go to Dr. Nelson Burton, Dr. Anthony Rongione, Dr. Alan Speir, Dr. Jason Vourelkis, and nurse practitioners Carolyn Rosner, Lori Edwards, and Mary Beth Maydosz.

As the deadline for this manuscript sped closer, my colleague Dr. Ramesh Mazhari very generously assumed some of my clinical duties and shooed me off to the library, enabling me to complete the book. Dr. Miriam Fishman and Gwen Grossman reviewed portions

# Acknowledgments

of the manuscript, and their thoughtful input was helpful and always appreciated.

Finally, I would like to thank Vice President Dick Cheney for his wholehearted commitment to this project. It's not easy to sift through decades of your own medical records, documenting the relentless progression of a lethal illness, but the vice president did just that, always with great curiosity and enthusiasm.

As we were completing the book I asked Vice President Cheney if he was at all apprehensive when he received the call alerting him that a heart had been found and within a few hours he would be undergoing a transplant.

"No," he said.

"The last operation to place the VAD almost killed you. Why weren't you afraid?" I persisted.

"Because you told me the transplant would be easier."

There is no greater honor for a physician than to have a patient place his or her trust in you, and I will forever be humbled by the confidence placed in me by this singular patient and by every patient for whom I am privileged to provide care.

# Notes

## CHAPTER 1: A PRIME CANDIDATE

19 *In 1502, Leonardo da Vinci:* Charles D. O'Malley and J. B. de C. M. Saunders, *Leonardo da Vinci on the Human Body* (New York: Greenwich House, 1982), 22, 300.

19 *The term* atherosclerosis: James L. Young and Peter Libby, "Atherosclerosis," in Leonard S. Lilly, *Pathophysiology of Heart Disease: A Collaborative Project of Medical Students and Faculty* (Philadelphia: Lippincott Williams & Wilkins, 2007), 118.

19 *the Spanish influenza pandemic infected:* US Department of Health and Human Services, *The Great Pandemic: The United States in 1918–1919,* http://www.flu.gov/pandemic/history/1918/the_pandemic/index.html.

20 *Atherosclerotic disease developed in the United States:* J. Michael Gaziano, "Global Burden of Cardiovascular Disease," in Peter Libby et al., *Braunwald's Heart Disease: A Textbook of Cardiovascular Medicine,* 8th ed. (Philadelphia: Saunders, 2008), 1–14.

20 *In 1971, Abdel Omran:* Abdel R. Omran, "The Epidemiologic Transition: A Theory of the Epidemiology of Population Change," *Milbank Memorial Fund Quarterly* 2005, 84:737–741. (Reprinted from *Milbank Memorial Fund Quarterly,* 1971;49:509–538.)

20 *there were steep reductions in deaths:* Gregory L. Armstrong, Laura A. Conn, and Robert W. Pinner, "Trends in Infectious Disease Mortality in the United States during the 20th Century," *Journal of the American Medical Association* 1999;281:63.

21 *On the eve of World War II:* Hardy Green, "How K-Rations Fed Soldiers and Saved American Businesses," Bloomberg.com, February 20, 2013, http://www.bloomberg.com/news/2013-02-20/how-k-rations-fed-soldiers-and-saved-american-businesses.

21 *Following the war, Keys returned:* Patricia Sullivan, "Ancel Keys, K Ration Creator, Dies," *Washington Post,* November 24, 2004.

21 *Beginning in the late 1940s:* Ancel Keys et al., "Coronary Heart Disease among Minnesota Business and Professional Men Followed Fifteen Years," *Circulation* 1963;28:381.

21 *1957 American Heart Association report:* I. H. Page, F. J. Stare, A. C. Corcoran, H. Pollack, and C. F. Wilkinson, "Atherosclerosis and the Fat Content of the Diet," *Journal of the American Medical Association* 1957;164:2051.

22 *Ancel Keys continued to investigate:* Ancel Keys (ed.), "Coronary Heart Disease in Seven Countries," *Circulation* 1970 (suppl. to vol. 41): 1–211.

22 *In 1961, the American Heart Association appeared:* Irving H. Page, Edgar V. Allen, Francis L. Chamberlain, Ancel Keys, et al., "Dietary Fat and Its Relation to Heart Attacks and Strokes," *Circulation,* 1961;23:134–135.

22 *Later that same year:* "The Fat of the Land," *Time,* January 13, 1961.

23 *According to the American Lung Association:* "Trends in Tobacco Use," American Lung Association Research and Program Services, Epidemiology and Statistics Unit, July 2011, http://www.lung.org/finding-cures/our-research/trend-reports/Tobacco -Trend-Report.pdf.

23 *Despite a greater than 50 percent decline:* http://www.lung.org/stop-smoking/ about-smoking/facts-figures/smoking-and-older-adults.html.

24 *There are more than seven thousand chemical substances:* http://www.cdc.gov/tobacco/ data_statistics/sgr/2010/consumer_booklet/chemicals_smoke/.

25 *Framingham investigators had developed:* "History of the Framingham Heart Study," http://www.framinghamheartstudy.org/about/history.html.

26 *In the 1970s, doctors:* J. Judson McNamara, "Coronary Artery Disease in Combat Casualties in Vietnam," *Journal of the American Medical Association,* 1971;216(7):1185–1187.

## CHAPTER 2: ECHOES OF IKE

33 *indigestion while playing golf:* Frank H. Messerli, Adrian W. Messerli, and Thomas Lüscher, "Eisenhower's Billion-Dollar Heart Attack—50 Years Later," *New England Journal of Medicine* 2005; 353;12:1205.

34 *In his exhaustive book:* Clarence G. Lasby, *Eisenhower's Heart Attack: How Ike Beat Heart Disease and Held On to the Presidency* (Lawrence: University Press of Kansas, 1997), 97–98.

35 *In 1880, Karl Weigert, a German pathologist:* Nikhil Sikri and Amit Bardia, "A History of Streptokinase Use in Acute Myocardial Infarction," *Texas Heart Institute Journal* 2007;34:318.

35 *the legendary Sir William Osler:* William Osler, *The Principles and Practice of Medicine* (Birmingham: The Classics of Medicine Library 1978), page 641.

35 *"Obstruction of a coronary artery":* James Herrick, "Clinical Features of Sudden Obstruction of the Coronary Arteries," *Journal of the American Medical Association* 1912;59:2015–2020.

36 *"Which comes first":* William Roberts, "Coronary Thrombosis and Fatal Myocardial Ischemia," *Circulation* 1974;49:1.

36 *"I am happy the doctors":* Dwight D. Eisenhower: "Remarks upon Arrival at the Washington National Airport," November 11, 1955, http://www.presidency.ucsb .edu/ws/?pid=10384.

37 *In 1933, William Kouwenhoven:* Jonas A. Cooper, Joel D. Cooper, and Joshua M. Cooper, "Cardiopulmonary Resuscitation: History, Current Practice, and Future Direction," *Circulation* 2006;114:2841.

37 *The first successful defibrillation:* Ibid.

38 *In 1956, one year after President Eisenhower's:* Paul M. Zoll, Arthur J. Linenthal, William Gibson, Milton H. Paul, et al., *New England Journal of Medicine* 1956;254:727–732.

38 *"Cardiac resuscitation after cardiac arrest":* W. B. Kouwenhoven, Dr. Ing, James R.

Jude, and G. Guy Knickerbocker, "Closed-Chest Cardiac Massage," *Journal of the American Medical Association* 1960;173:1064.

39 *The stage was set:* D. G. Julian, "The History of Coronary Care Units: Ischemia and Infarction," *Lancet* 1961;21:840–844.

39 *Years later, Julian noted:* Ibid., 498.


CHAPTER 3: INTO THE HEART


51 *In ancient Egypt:* James Peto, *The Heart* (New Haven, CT: Yale University Press, 2007), 1012.

51 *Although the Greeks:* C. R. S. Harris, *The Heart and Vascular System in Ancient Greek Medicine, From Alcmaeon to Galen* (Sandpiper Books, Ltd., 2001), 160, 179, 271, 272.

52 *Even Leonardo da Vinci:* Charles D. O'Malley and J. B. de C. M. Saunders, *Leonardo da Vinci on the Human Body* (New York: Greenwich House, 1982), 282.

52 *"That there is one blood stream":* William Harvey, *On the Motion of the Heart and Blood Vessels in Animals,* Alexander Bowie ed. (London: George Bell and Sons, 1889), xviii.

53 *"The heart of animals":* Ibid., 4.

53 *"An organ . . . particularly vulnerable":* Harry M. Sherman, "Suture of Heart Wounds," *Boston Medical and Surgical Journal* 1902;146:653.

53 *In 1929, Werner Forssmann:* David Monagan, *Journey into the Heart* (New York: Gotham Books, 2007), 18–27.

54 *"I checked the catheter position":* Werner Forssmann, "Catheterization of the Right Heart," *Kleinische Wochenschrift* 1929;8:2085–2089.

54 *For the next quarter-century:* "The Nobel Prize in Physiology or Medicine 1956," http://www.nobelprize.org/nobel_prizes/medicine/laureates/1956/.


CHAPTER 5: A TALE OF TWO DRUGS


77 *In the late 1970s:* Marcus A. DeWood, Julie Spores, Robert Notske, et al., "Prevalence of Total Coronary Occlusion during the Early Hours of Transmural Myocardial Infarction," *New England Journal of Medicine* 1980;303:897–902.

78 *Using a laboratory model:* Keith A. Reimer, James E. Lowe, Margaret M. Rasmussen, and Robert B. Jennings, "The Wavefront Phenomenon of Ischemic Cell Death. I. Myocardial Infarct Size vs Duration of Coronary Occlusion in Dogs," *Circulation* 1977;56:786–794.

78 *Progressively longer occlusions:* Keith A. Reimer and Robert B. Jennings, "The Wavefront Phenomenon of Ischemic Cell Death. II. Transmural Progression of Necrosis within the Framework of Ischemic Bed Size (Myocardium at Risk) and Collateral Flow," *Laboratory Investigation* 1979;40:633–644.

78 *In 1933, William Tillett:* William S. Tillett and R. L. Garner, "The Fibrinolytic Activity of Hemolytic Streptococci," *Journal of Experimental Medicine* 1933;58:485–502.

79 *Evgenii Chazov in the Soviet Union:* E. I. Chazov, L. S. Matveeva, A. V. Mazaev, K. E. Sargin, et al., "[Intracoronary Application of Fibrinolysis in Acute Myocardial Infarction]," *Terapevticheskii Arkhiv* 1976;48:8–19.

79   *Peter Rentrop in West Germany:* K. P. Rentrop, H. Blanke, K. R. Karsch, V. Weigand, et al., "Acute Myocardial Infarction: Intracoronary Application of Nitroglycerin and Streptokinase," *Clinical Cardiology* 1979;2:354–363.

79   *In the years that followed:* Nikhil Sikri and Amit Barda, "A History of Streptokinase Use in Acute Myocardial Infarction," *Texas Heart Institute Journal* 2007;34:323–324.

80   *In 1956, researchers:* P. Roy Vagelos, "Are Prescription Drug Prices High?" *Science* 1991252:1082.

80   *In September 1980, Sankyo:* Jonathan A. Tolbert, "Lovastatin and Beyond: The History of the HMG-CoA Reductase Inhibitors," *Nature Reviews* 2003;2:517–526.

81   *Questions concerning the clinical impact:* "Scandinavian Simvastatin Survival Study Group: Randomised Trial of Cholesterol Lowering in 4444 Patients with Coronary Heart Disease: The Scandinavian Simvastatin Survival Study (4S)," *Lancet* 1994;344:1383–1389.

## CHAPTER 6: BYPASS

89   *"Surgery of the Heart":* Stephen Paget, "Wounds of the Heart," in *Surgery of the Chest* (Bristol, CT: John Wright & Co., 1896), 121.

90   *"The sight of the heart beating":* James W. Blatchford III, "Ludwig Rehn: The First Successful Cardiorrhaphy," *Annals of Thoracic Surgery* 1985;39:494.

91   *"The road to the heart":* Harry M. Sherman, "Suture of Heart Wounds," *Boston Medical and Surgical Journal* 1902;146:654.

91   *During that long night:* John H. Gibbon Jr., "Development of the Artificial Heart and Lung Extracorporeal Blood Circuit," *Journal of the American Medical Association* 1968;206;1983.

92   *Determined to solve the problem:* Larry W. Stephenson, "History of Cardiac Surgery," in *Cardiac Surgery in the Adult, Third Edition,* ed. Lawrence H. Cohn (New York: McGraw-Hill Medical, 2008), 8.

92   *The idea for this approach:* William S. Stoney, "Evolution of Cardiopulmonary Bypass," *Circulation* 2009;119:2849.

92   *"a potential mortality of 200 percent":* Ibid., 2849.

92   *In Detroit, Dr. Forest Dodrill:* Manon Caouette, "Research on Cardiopulmonary Bypass in North America," in *Dawn and Evolution of Cardiac Procedures,* ed. Marco Picichè (Milan: Springer-Verlag Italia, 2013), 118.

93   *uncanny resemblance to a Cadillac V-12:* "50th Anniversary of First Open Heart Surgery," Wayne University School of Medicine, October 22, 2002, http://www.med.wayne.edu/news_media/2002/press14.asp

93   *Following his patient's death:* Lawrence H. Cohn, "Fifty Years of Open-Heart Surgery," *Circulation* 2003;107:2168.

93   *monkey lungs:* Stoney, "Evolution of Cardiopulmonary Bypass," 2844.

93   *Gibbon's team finally discovered:* Gibbon, "Development of the Artificial Heart and Lung Extracorporeal Blood Circuit," 1985.

93   *operated on Cecelia Bavolek:* "Medicine: Historic Operation," *Time,* May 18, 1953, http://www.time.com/time/magazine/article/0,9171,818494,00.html.

94   *prestigious Albert Lasker Clinical Medical Research Award:* http://www.laskerfoundation.org/awards/1968_c_description.htm.

# Notes

95   *Vasilii Kolesov, a surgeon from Leningrad:* V. I. Kolessov, "Mammary Artery-Coronary Artery Anastomosis as Method of Treatment for Angina Pectoris," *Journal of Thoracic Cardiovascular Surgery* 1967;54:535–544.

95   *Michael DeBakey, from Baylor in Houston:* H. Edward Garrett, Edward W. Dennis, and Michael DeBakey, "Aortocoronary Bypass with Saphenous Vein Graft," *Journal of the American Medical Association* 1973;223:792–794.

95   *"The opinions concerning":* Igor E. Konstantinov, "Vasilii I. Kolesov: A Surgeon to Remember," *Texas Heart Institute Journal* 2004;31:349–358.

95   *its peak of 190,000:* Chad T. Wilson, Elliott S. Fisher, H. Gilbert Welch, Andrea E. Siewers, et al., "U.S. Trends in CABG Hospital Volume: The Effect of Adding Cardiac Surgery Programs," *Health Affairs* 2007;26:162–168.

## CHAPTER 8: FITNESS TO SERVE

120   *"I felt that was good enough for me":* Lawrence K. Altman, "The Medical Histories: Doctors Say Republican Candidates Are in Good Health," *New York Times,* November 2, 2000.

121   *"normal cardiac function":* Steve Sternberg, "Cheney's Heath Not an Issue, Doctors Say," *USA Today,* July 25, 2000.

121   *"Mr. Cheney's statistical chances":* Altman, " The Medical Histories."

122   *"he's golden":* Sternberg, "Cheney's Heath Not an Issue, Doctors Say."

122   *"it's a disease you control, not cure":* Susan Ferraro, "W.'s Pick May Have Heart for Campaign," *New York Daily News,* July 25, 2000.

122   *Federal aviation regulations:* "Licenses and Certificates: Coronary Artery Disease," August 8, 2011, http://www.faa.gov/licenses_certificates/medical_certification/specialissuance/coronary/.

123   *On March 4, 1841, William Henry Harrison:* http://www.whitehouse.gov/about/presidents/williamhenryharrison.

123   *"The Senator does not now":* Robert A. Caro, *The Passage of Power: The Years of Lyndon Johnson* (New York: Knopf, 2012), 97.

124   *Senator Kennedy told the historian Arthur Schlesinger:* Arthur M. Schlesinger Jr., *Journals, 1952–2000* (New York: Penguin, 2007), 58.

124   *The candidate was, in fact, taking cortisone:* Lee R. Mandel, "Endocrine and Autoimmune Aspects of the Health History of John F. Kennedy," *Annals of Internal Medicine* 2009;151:350–354.

124   *no gross evidence of adrenal tissue:* George D. Lundberg, "Closing the Case in *JAMA* on the John F. Kennedy Autopsy," *Journal of the American Medical Association* 1992;268:1737.

125   *"it expresses its consent and endorsement":* Herbert L. Adams, "Presidential Health and the Public Interest: The Campaign of 1992," *Political Psychology* 1995;16:795–820.

125   *Lawrence Altman, now a senior scholar:* "Lawrence K. Altman," http://www.wilsoncenter.org/staff/lawrence-k-altman.

125   *Dr. Howard Bruenn, a cardiologist:* Howard G. Bruenn, "Clinical Notes on the Illness and Death of President Franklin D. Roosevelt," *Annals of Internal Medicine* 1970;72:580.

126   *"When we got through":* John H. Crider, "President's Health Satisfactory; Unique Report Made by McIntre," *New York Times,* April 5, 1944.

126 *"On Saturday, July 8":* http://www.boston.com/news/local/breaking_news/Lahey%20-%20FDR%20Memorandum.pdf.

## CHAPTER 9: RECOUNT

137 *poor outcomes that sometimes ensue:* Walter Weintraub, " 'The VIP Syndrome': A Clinical Study in Hospital Psychiatry," *Journal of Nervous and Mental Disease* 1964;138:181.

138 *In November 1976:* Spencer B. King III, "Angioplasty from Bench to Bedside," *Circulation* 1996;93:1621–1629, doi: 10.1161/ 01.CIR.93.9.1621.

138 *Gruentzig had to develop all the components:* David Monagan, *Journey into the Heart* (New York: Gotham Books, 2007), 93–94.

139 *"this will never work":* King, "Angioplasty from Bench to Bedside," 1621–1629.

140 *Dr. Elias Hanna, a cardiac surgeon:* Monagan, *Journey into the Heart,* 122.

140 *"Early in the afternoon":* King, "Angioplasty from Bench to Bedside," 1621–1629.

141 *Dr. Andrea Gruentzig and his wife:* Monagan, *Journey into the Heart,* 277–284.

141 *Exactly ten years:* King, "Angioplasty from Bench to Bedside," 1621–1629.

144 *In February 1978:* "An Expert Interview with Dr. Julio Palmaz: Part I—Serendipity and the Stent," http://www.medscape.com/viewarticle/474644.

144 *Dr. Palmaz spent years:* Gernot H. Geisinger, *Materials and Innovative Product Development: Using Common Sense* (Amsterdam: Elsevier, 2009), 213.

145 *"It was total serendipity":* "An Expert Interview with Dr. Julio Palmaz."

145 *Palmaz met Dr. Richard Schatz:* Shawn Tully, "Blood Feud," *Fortune,* May 31, 2004, http://money.cnn.com/magazines/fortune/fortune_archive/2004/05/31/370693/.

145 *"expandable intraluminal vascular graft":* http://www.google.com/patents/US4733665

146 *Cardiologists enthusiastically embraced:* Eric D. Peterson, Alexandra J. Lansky, Kevin J. Anstrom, Lawrence H. Muhlbaier, et al., "Evolving Trends in Interventional Device Use and Outcomes: Results from the National Cardiovascular Network Database," *American Heart Journal* 2000;139:198–207.

146 *In 2009, there were almost:* David I. Auerbach, Jared Lane Maeda, and Claudia Steiner, "Hospital Stays with Cardiac Stents, 2009," Healthcare Cost and Utilization Project, April 2012, http://www.hcup-us.ahrq.gov/reports/statbriefs/sb128.jsp.

151 *"The first value was obtained":* "The American Presidency Project. George Washington U. Doctors Brief Media on Richard B. Cheney's Condition," November 22, 2000, http://www.presidency.ucsb.edu/showflorida2000php?fileid=cheneyheartattack11–22.

152 *"We have biochemical markers":* Ibid.

152 *in an editorial a few days after:* "Mr. Cheney's Heart Attack," *New York Times,* November 25, 2000.

152 *Despite the tumult in the press:* Ron Winslow and Laurie McGinley, "Uncertainty Is Common in Cardiac Cases Like Cheney's," *Wall Street Journal,* December 20, 2000.

# Notes

## CHAPTER 10: WHITE HOUSE CALLS

171    *During the press conference:* http://www.c-spanvideo.org/program/162999–1.

172    *The* Los Angeles Times *published an editorial:* "Cheney's Dilemma," *Los Angeles Times,* March 6, 2001.

172    US News & World Report *speculated:* "A Matter of Heart at the Center of Power," *US News & World Report,* March 19, 2001.

173    *Arianna Huffington wasn't just:* "Dick Cheney's Suicide Mission," March 7, 2001, http://ariannaonline.huffingtonpost.com/columns/printer_friendly.php?id=200.

175    *Mordechai Friedman, a Polish Jew:* John A. Kastor, *You and Your Arrhythmia: A Guide to Heart Rhythm Problems for Patients and Their Families* (Sudbury, MA: Jones and Bartlett, 2006), 109.

175    *Of the 3.3 million Jews:* "The Fate of the Jews across Europe: Murder of the Jews of Poland," http://www.yadvashem.org/yv/en/holocaust/about/09/poland.asp.

176    *After the war:* "Dr. Michel Mirowski Is Dead at Age of 65; Made Heart Implant," *New York Times,* March 28, 1990.

176    *"In 1966, my old boss":* Kastor, *You and Your Arrhythmia,*120.

176    *"I talked to some cardiologists":* Kastor, *You and Your Arrhythmia,*121.

177    *"The initial goal set":* Morton M. Mower, "Building the AICD with Michel Mirowski," *PACE* 1991;14:928.

177    *"More memorable for me":* M. S. Heilman, "Collaboration with Michel Mirowski on the Development of the AICD," *PACE* 1991;14:910.

178    *"Experience teaches":* Bernard Lown and Paul Axelrod, "Implanted Standby Defibrillators," *Circulation* 1972;46:637–639.

178    *"The author's overcautious and negative attitude":* M. Mirowski, Morton M. Mower, and Albert I. Mendeloff, "Letter to the Editor," *Circulation* 1973;47:1135.

178    *"a graphic illustration":* "Heart Machine Sets a New Pace against Disease," *New Scientist,* August 14, 1980, 509.

179    *published in the* New England Journal of Medicine: M. Mirowski, Philip R. Reid, Morton M. Mower, Levi Watkins, et al., "Termination of Malignant Ventricular Arrhythmias with an Implanted Automatic Defibrillator in Human Beings," *New England Journal of Medicine* 1980;303:322–324.

179    *"Although considerable additional work":* James T. Willerson, "Prevention and Control of Ventricular Arrhythmias," *New England Journal of Medicine* 1980;303:332–334.

181    *"The electrophysiology study scheduled":* http://georgewbush-whitehouse.archives.gov/news/releases/2001/06/20010629–2.html.

## CHAPTER 11: TREATING THE VICE PRESIDENT

195    *"an apolitical, professionally focused":* Ludwig M. Deppisch, *The White House Physician: A History from Washington to George W. Bush* (Jefferson: McFarland & Company, 2007), 150.

200    *"Well, no, I've—it's obviously a question":* "Excerpts from Cheney Health Remarks," June 30, 2001, http://www.nytimes.com/2001/06/30/us/excerpts-from-cheney-health-remarks.html?pagewanted=2.

215    *It has been estimated:* Saskia Kulpers, Suzanne C. Cannegeiter, Saskai Middeldorp,

Luc Robyn, et al., "The Absolute Risk of Venous Thrombosis after Air Travel: A Cohort Study of 8,755 Employees of International Organisations," *PLoS Medicine* 2007;4:e290.

220 *a computer hacker disclosed:* Darren Pauli, "Hacked Terminals Capable of Causing Pacemaker Deaths," *SC Magazine,* October 17, 2012, http://www.scmagazine.com .au/News/319508,hacked-terminals-capable-of-causing-pacemaker-mass-murder .aspx.

220 *exactly the way the fictional terrorist:* "The Terrorist Hack That Shocked America—and Why It Matters," *CNBC,* December 12, 2012, http://www.cnbc.com/id/100306578.

## CHAPTER 12: SLIPPERY SLOPE

227 *President Bush later made a public service announcement:* "A Message from George Bush," http://www.strokeheart.org/CYPA/bush.html.

228 *Cardiac imaging with sound waves:* Harvey Feigenbaum, "Evolution of Echocardiography," *Circulation* 1996;93:1321.

228 *First used in 1953 to examine cardiac structures:* Siddarth Singh and Abha Goyal, "The Origin of Echocardiography: A Tribute to Inge Edler," *Texas Heart Institute Journal* 2007;34:431.

238 *afflicting 350,000 Americans each year:* "Sudden Cardiac Arrest: A Healthcare Crisis," http://www.sca-aware.org/about-sca.

238 *The medical community has long understood:* Jonathan S. Reiner, Allen J. Solomon, and Richard J. Katz, "Shock and Law," *Circulation* 2011;124:1391–1394.

239 *the adhesive electrode:* "R. Lee Heath: The Inventor of Hands Free Cardiac Defibrillation and Pacing Pads," http://www.defib.us.com.

239 *In 1994, the American Heart Association:* Myron L. Weisfeldt, Richard E. Kerber, R. Pat McGoldrick, Arthur J. Moss, et al., "Public Access Defibrillation: A Statement for Healthcare Professionals from the American Heart Association Task Force on Automatic External Defibrillation," *Circulation* 1995;92:2763.

239 *The gaming industry:* Terence D. Valenzuela, Denise J. Roe, Graham Nichol, et al., "Outcomes of Rapid Defibrillation by Security Officers after Cardiac Arrest in Casinos," *New England Journal of Medicine* 2000;343:1206–1209.

240 *A bill before the 113th Congress:* H.R. 2135: Cardiac Arrest Survival Act of 2013. To Amend the Public Health Service Act to Clarify Liability Protections regarding Emergency Use of Automated External Defibrillators.

## CHAPTER 13: DOWNHILL

251 *"The New Treatment Cheney Did Not Get":* Lawrence K. Altman, "The New Treatment Cheney Did Not Get," *New York Times,* March 13, 2001.

253 *The Egyptians introduced the technique:* Gilbert R. Seigworth, "Bloodletting over the Centuries," http://www.pbs.org/wnet/redgold/basics/bloodlettinghistory.html.

253 *George Washington became ill:* Herbert Mitgang, "Death of a President: A 200-Year-Old Malpractice Debate," *New York Times,* December 14, 1999, http://www .nytimes.com/1999/12/14/health/death-of-a-president-a-200-year-old-malpractice -debate.html.

# Notes

253 *Giorgio Baglivi, a seventeenth-century:* W. Bruce Fye, "Giogrio Baglivi," *Clinical Cardiology* 2002;25:488.

256 *the federal government began funding a program:* David K. C. Cooper, *Open Heart: The Radical Surgeons Who Revolutionized Medicine* (New York: Kaplan, 2010), 363.

256 *Dr. DeBakey developed surgical techniques:* Lawrence K. Altman, "Michael DeBakey, Rebuilder of Hearts, Dies at 99," *New York Times,* July 13, 2008, http://www.nytimes.com/2008/07/13/health/13debakey.html?pagewanted=all&_r=0.

257 *"We became interested in the artificial heart":* Cooper, *Open Heart,* 362.

257 *"Our first clinical application of this pump":* Michael E. DeBakey, "Development of Mechanical Heart Devices," *Annals of Thoracic Surgery* 2005;79:228–231.

258 *On April 4, 1969:* Lawrence K. Altman, "The Feud," *New York Times,* November 27, 2007, http://www.nytimes.com/2007/11/27/health/27docs.html?pagewanted=all.

258 *"In 1968, it was evident to me":* Cooper, *Open Heart,* 379.

259 *The initial VADs created pulsatile flow:* Douglas J. Hirsch and John R. Cooper, "Cardiac Failure and Left Ventricular Assist Devices," *Anesthesiology Clinics of North America* 2003;21:628.

261 *Recent data from a National Heart Lung:* James K. Kirklin, David C. Naftel, Robert L. Kormos, Lynne W. Stevenson, et al., "Fifth INTERMACS Annual Report: Risk Factor Analysis from More Than 6,000 Mechanical Circulatory Support Patients," *Journal of Heart Lung Transplantation* 2013;32:143.

262 *The HeartMate II LVAD:* Farooq H. Shiekh and Stuart Russell, "HeartMate II Continuous-Flow Left Ventricular Assist System," *Expert Review of Medical Devices* 2011;8:11–21.

## CHAPTER 14: TRANSPLANT

286 *"Choosing an appropriate recipient for a heart transplant":* "Way Is Clear for Heart Transplant," *Journal of the American Medical Association* 1967;202(8):31.

287 *"I believe that this nation":* President John F. Kennedy, excerpt from the Special Message to the Congress on Urgent National Needs, May 25, 1961, http://www.nasa.gov/vision/space/features/jfk_speech_text.html.

288 *It was during these animal studies:* David K. C. Cooper, *Open Heart: The Radical Surgeons Who Revolutionized Medicine* (New York: Kaplan, 2010), 319–320.

288 *Lower and Shumway devised a method to suture:* Donald McRae, *Every Second Counts* (New York: Berkley Books, 2006), 83–86.

289 *Dr. Yurii Voronoy, a Ukrainian:* Edouard Matevossian, Hans Kern, Norbert Hüser, et al.: "Surgeon Yurii Voronoy (1895–1961)—A Pioneer in the History of Clinical Transplantation: In Memoriam at the 75th Anniversary of the First Human Kidney Transplantation," *Transplant International* 2009;22:1132.

289 *Peter Medawar, a British biologist:* "The Nobel Prize in Physiology or Medicine 1960, Peter Medawar—Biographical," http://www.nobelprize.org/nobel_prizes/medicine/laureates/1960/medawar-bio.html.

289 *In 1954, Dr. Joseph Murray:* Thomas E. Starzl, "The Development of Clinical Renal Transplantation," *American Journal of Kidney Diseases* 1990;16:549.

290 *total body irradiation:* Rene J. Duquesnoy, "Early History of Transplant Immunology: Part II," *ASHI Quarterly,* Fourth Quarter 2005, http://www.ashi-hla.org/docs/newsletter/ASHI_Quarterly/29_4_2005/3_ear_hist_trans_part2.pdf.

# Notes

290  *"The precise mechanism"*: Richard R. Lower, Raymond C. Stofer, and Norman E. Shumway, "Homovital Transplantation of the Heart," *Journal of Thoracic and Cardiovascular Surgery* 1961;41:196.10.

290  *On June 11, 1963:* McRae, *Every Second Counts,* 130.

290  *Ten days later:* "Pardon to Reward Convict in Rare Lung Transplant," *Fort Scott Tribune,* June 21, 1963, http://news.google.com/newspapers?nid=1906&dat=19630621& id=8dofAAAAIBAJ&sjid=RNkEAAAAIBAJ&pg=1852,2461432.

291  *"But how soon after":* James D. Hardy, Carlos M. Chavez, Fred D. Kurrus, et al., "Heart Transplantation in Man," *Journal of the American Medical Association* 1964;188:115.

292  *"When, if ever":* Hardy et al., "Heart Transplantation in Man," 115.

292  *"Since we were not willing":* Hardy et al., "Heart Transplantation in Man," 116.

293  *"A regular and forceful beat":* Hardy et al., "Heart Transplantation in Man," 120.

293  *In a reverse of the procedure:* McRae, *Every Second Counts,* 181–182.

294  *"was harder technically and emotionally":* Richard D. Lyons, "Heart Transplant Fails to Save 2-Week-Old Baby in Brooklyn," *New York Times,* December 7, 1967.

294  *immune systems are immature:* Adrian Kantrowitz, "America's First Human Heart Transplantation: The Concept, the Planning and the Furor," *ASAIO Journal* 1998; 44:244.

294  *Kantrowitz was a remarkable innovator:* Jascha Hoffmann, "Dr. Adrian Kantrowitz, Cardiac Pioneer, Dies at 90," *New York Times,* November 19, 2008, http://www.ny times.com/2008/11/19/us/19kantrowiztz.html.

294  *abandon the transplant:* McRae, *Every Second Counts,* 161–162.

295  *"All we were interested in":* Cooper, *Open Heart,* 328–331.

295  *Louis Washkansky was a:* Life, December 15, 1967, 24A.

295  *Denise Darvall, a twenty-five-year-old woman:* McRae, *Every Second Counts,* 200.

296  *"I decided I would not take out Denise's heart":* Cooper, *Open Heart,* 334.

296  *According to Marius:* McRae, *Every Second Counts,* 206–207.

296  *"Now we've got the heart in a donor":* "Gift of a Heart," *Life,* December 15, 1967, 27.

297  *"Right away after the shock":* Ibid.

297  *Adrian Kantrowitz became the first surgeon:* McRae, *Every Second Counts,* 235–236.

297  *"We were trying to make one whole individual out of two individuals":* Lyons, "Heart Transplant Fails to Save 2-Week-Old Baby in Brooklyn."

298  *This patient was Philip Blaiberg:* McRae, *Every Second Counts,* 269–274.

298  *Dr. Shumway began using cyclosporin A:* Daniel J. DiBardino, "The History and Development of Cardiac Transplantation," *Texas Heart Institute Journal* 1999;26:204.

299  *According to the United Network for Organ Sharing:* http://www.unos.org.

301  *heart transplant waiting list:* http://optn.transplant.hrsa.gov/PoliciesandBylaws2/ policies/pdfs/policy_9.pdf

306  *the median predicted survival is fourteen years:* Josef Stehlik, Leah B. Edwards, Anna Y. Kucheryavaya, et al., "The Registry of the International Society for Heart and Lung Transplantation: Twenty-Eighth Adult Heart Transplant Report—2011," *Journal of Heart and Lung Transplantation* 2011;30:1083.

307  *There are currently about thirty-five hundred patients:* http://optn.transplant.hrsa.gov/ latestData/rptData.asp.

# Index

Aaron, Dr. Benjamin, 85, 97, 120, 128
Abdullah, king of Saudi Arabia, 224–25, 244
Abrams, Herbert, 124–25
ABSCAM scandal, 47
ACE inhibitors, 40, 218, 255
Adair, Paul "Red," 141
Addington, David, 106, 153–55
Afghanistan, visit to, 212–13
Agnew, Spiro, 154
Aldactone, 218
Alexander, Keith, 192
Allbaugh, Joe, 111–12, 113, 115
al Qaeda, 191–92
altitude, effects of, 1, 75, 97, 118, 244, 304
altitude sickness, 197–98
Altman, Lawrence, 121, 125
American Heart Association (AHA), 21–22, 36, 138, 139, 141, 178, 239
amyl nitrate, 33
Anies, Gus, 278
angioplasty, balloon, 167–72, 251–52
antiplatelet drugs, 40
anthrax prophylaxis, 194–95
anticoagulants, 2, 4, 33, 34, 213, 227, 243, 248–49, 252, 262
Anturane, 40
Archimedes, 262
Aristotle, 51, 52
arrhythmias
    Cheney's risk for, 175
    early research to detect, 37, 38, 39
    heart failure with, 303
    implantable cardioverter defibrillator to control, 4, 179–83, 219, 231, 241
    sudden cardiac arrest and, 176, 241

*See also* atrial fibrillation; ventricular fibrillation
arteriography. *See* cardiac catheterization
artificial heart, 119, 257–59
aspirin, 40, 197, 234
atherosclerosis, 19–20, 22, 25, 26, 95, 122, 139–40, 142, 167, 202
atorvastatin (Lipitor), 40, 82, 197
atrial fibrillation (A Fib), 221, 226–32, 245, 249, 250, 260, 292, 308
automated external defibrillation (AED), 239–41
Axelrod, Dr. Paul, 178
Azerbaijan, 221, 222

Bachmann, Adolf, 140, 141
Baglivi, Giorgio, 253
Baker, Howard, 69
Baker, Jim, 84, 100, 131
balloon angioplasty, 167–72, 251–52
Barnard, Dr. Christiaan, 287, 295–97, 298
Barnard, Marius, 296, 297
Barnett, Bob, 282–83
Barnett, Ross, 290
Baron, Kenneth, 160
Becker, Dr. Richard, 169
Bennett, Bob, 196–97
Bennett, William, 197
Benson, Merritt, 49
Bernanke, Ben, 222
beta blockers, 40, 234, 241, 255
biological agents, protection against, 194–97
Blaiberg, Philip, 298
bleeding episodes
    anticoagulants and, 249
    bloodletting to prevent, 253

# Index

bleeding episodes (*cont.*)
  end-stage heart failure and, 303
  internal in thigh, 3, 265
  left ventricular assist device and, 271,
    273, 300
  nosebleed incidents and, 243, 248–50
bloodletting, 253
Bloom, David, 215
Bohrer, David, 189, 277
Bosch, Dr. Ryan, 204, 206, 209, 214, 216,
  219, 233, 249
Boswell, Dr. J. T., 124
Bowie, Alexander, 52–53
Bruenn, Dr. Howard, 125–26
Burch, Dean, 28
Burton, Dr. Nelson, 5, 246, 264, 267,
  268, 270–71
Bush, Barbara, 111
Bush, George H. W., 84
  atrial fibrillation of, 227
  cabinet of, 99–100, 101–02, 106
  presidential election and, 83, 85–86, 96
  world situation and, 104, 105
Bush, George W.
  campaigns and, 131, 132, 134, 193
  Cheney as running mate of, 111–15,
    116, 118–19, 121–22, 127–34,
    193, 224
  Cheney's vice presidency under, 115,
    155–56, 161, 189, 190, 193, 212
  Cheney's health and, 133, 150, 173, 193
  9/11 terrorist attack and, 189, 190, 191
  presidency of, 161, 173, 174, 222
Bush, Laura, 113, 132
bypass surgery. *See* coronary bypass surgery
Byrd, Robert, 72

Caputy, Dr. Anthony, 236
cardiac catheterization
  angioplasty with, 145, 146–52, 167–70
  Cheney's monitoring with, 57–58,
    74–75, 76, 77, 120, 122, 127, 133,
    136–38, 142–44, 147–52, 165,
    166, 167–70, 181–82, 251, 264,
    267
  early use of, 53–54, 55, 77, 79, 140–41
  Reiner's administration of, 55–57,
    116, 122, 133, 136–38, 142–44,
    146–52, 167–70, 251
  techniques in, 55–57, 74, 137–38, 251
cardiogenic shock, 120, 264–65

cardiopulmonary resuscitation (CPR), 17,
  238–39, 240
Carrel, Dr. Alexis, 92
Carter, Jimmy, 10–11, 131
Cary, Dr. Freeman, 57
Central Intelligence Agency (CIA), 71,
  103, 159, 192
Channock, Foster, 28
Chazov, Evgenii, 79
chemical agents, protection against, 194–97
Cheney, Bob, 7, 109
Cheney, Dick
  FAMILY AND PERSONAL LIFE
  autobiography authoring, 282–83
  father's death, 109–10
  fishing, 7, 8, 106, 108, 158–60, 223,
    245, 282
  grandchildren, 131, 158, 317
  Halliburton career, 108, 109, 111,
    112, 113, 116
  hunting, 72, 118, 128, 160, 223,
    226, 244, 305
  Jackson Hole, Wyoming, home, 1,
    107–08, 131, 158, 198, 225, 234,
    244–45, 280, 299–300, 304
  McLean, Virginia, home, 1, 132, 223,
    243, 256, 279, 285
  mother's death, 108–09
  skiing, 45, 84, 87, 97, 99, 108, 118,
    158, 309
  vacations, 11, 44, 107, 158, 223, 274
  HEALTH
  altitude sickness, 197–98
  atrial fibrillation (A Fib), 226–32,
    245, 260, 308
  back injury and herniated disk
    surgery, 223, 235–36, 237, 248
  bypass surgery, 84–87, 97–98, 106,
    107, 110, 119–20, 200
  cardiac catheterizations, 57–58,
    74–75, 76, 77, 120, 122, 127, 133,
    136–38, 142–44, 147–52, 165,
    166, 167–70, 181–82, 251, 264,
    267
  "check it out" approach, 15, 48, 69,
    83–84, 114, 133, 135
  chest pain, 4, 34, 40, 57, 76, 134,
    135, 147, 150, 165–66, 174, 197,
    216, 218, 226, 231, 232, 251
  cholesterol levels, 12, 41, 82, 98, 103,
    106, 153, 219

# Index

# Index

# Index

# Index

# Index

# Index

heart failure. *See* congestive heart failure (CHF); end-stage heart failure
heart transplant
    availability of heart for, 285–86, 309, 310–11
    Cheney's consideration of, 261, 284, 285, 306
    Cheney's recovery from, 315–16
    Cheney's reflections on life after, 316–18
    Cheney's surgery in, 285–86, 309–12, 315
    Cheney's waiting period in, 284, 285, 286, 301–02, 307, 309–10
    left ventricular assist device as bridge to, 262–63, 284, 301
    risk-reward analysis and time to proceed with, 306
    waiting list for, 301–02, 306–07
Heath, R. Lee, 239
Heiden, Debbie, 162, 163, 165, 189, 199, 208
Heilman, Dr. Stephen, 177
Heller, Dr. Harry, 176
Hennig, Sara, 229, 230
heparin, 33, 35, 213
Herophilus, 51
Herrick, Dr. James, 35–36
Herschler, Ed, 14
high-altitude pulmonary edema (HAPE), 197
Hill, Michael, 214
Hippocrates, 51
Hiser, Dr. Wes, 29, 32, 40–41, 57–58
Hofmann, Dr. Lewis "Lew"
    concern about biological terrorism and, 195, 196–97
    deep vein thrombosis and, 214–15
    Holter monitoring and, 174, 179
    implantable cardioverter defibrillator and, 187, 217–19, 225, 226
    medical transition plan after vice presidency and, 233–34
    popliteal aneurysm repair and, 206, 208–10
    possible hyperkalemia and, 188–89, 193–94
    Reiner's checkups and, 157, 161, 162, 179, 198, 199, 216, 226, 231
    weight gain and possible atrial fibrillation and, 231–32

White House medical care from, 157, 158, 161–63, 173, 180, 204
Holter monitoring, 164, 165, 174, 175, 179–81
House of Representatives
    campaigns for Wyoming seat in, 12–15, 28–32, 37, 40–41, 43, 50, 69, 71, 85, 87
    Ethics Committee in, 44, 47
    Intelligence Committee in, 48, 71, 155
    Interior Committee in, 43–44, 46
    joint committee on Iran-Contra affair in, 72–73, 75
    Republican Policy Committee in, 47–48, 71–72, 83, 106
Howard, John, 212
Howe, Patty, 73, 106
Huffington, Arianna, 173
hunting, 72, 118, 128, 160, 223, 226, 244, 305
Hussein, Saddam, 103, 104–05
hyperkalemia, 188–89, 193–94

indomethacin, 211–12
Imdur, 217, 218
implantable cardioverter defibrillator (ICD)
    data from, 219–20, 225, 226, 228, 231, 236–37, 245
    decision to use, 181
    electromagnetic interference (EMI) and, 184–85, 220
    Mrs. Cheney's concerns about safety of, 184–85
    periodic evaluation of, 198–99, 209
    procedure to implant, 181–85
    removal after heart transplant, 316
    replacement of, 217, 218–19
    restoring of normal cardiac rhythm by, 4, 241, 248, 308, 316
    risk reduction using, 179, 181, 241
    statement to media about, 180, 181, 200
infarction, 35
*In My Time* (Cheney), 189, 283
Inspra, 218
interviews. *See* media coverage
Iran-Contra affair, 48, 72–73, 75
Iran hostage crisis, 72, 75
Iraq, 103, 104–05

Jarvi, Jerald, 211–12
Jennings, Robert, 78

340

# Index

# Index

# Index

Holter monitoring and, 164, 165, 174, 175, 179–81
implantable cardioverter defibrillator and, 180, 181–85, 198–99
left ventricular assist device and, 246–48, 255, 260, 303–05, 307–09
medical transition plan after vice presidency and, 233–35
nosebleed incidents and, 243, 248–50
popliteal aneurysm repair and, 202–11
possible hyperkalemia and, 188–89, 193–94
ventricular fibrillation and, 225, 241
Reiner, Melanie, 23, 24, 233
Reiner, Molly, 300, 309
Rentrop, Peter, 79
Rhodes, John, 43, 44
Richards, Dr. Dickinson, 54
Ridge, Tom, 116, 173
Rivers of Recovery, 282
Roberts, Dr. William, 36
Rockefeller, Nelson, 112
Romano, Phil, 145, 146
Roncalio, Teno, 13, 14
Rongione, Dr. Anthony "Tony," 268, 269–71, 274, 311, 312, 313
Roosevelt, Franklin Delano, 125–27
Rosner, Carolyn, 263, 302
Ross, Dr. Allan, 6, 70, 71, 74–75, 76, 77, 84, 97, 98, 102–103, 116, 120
rosuvastatin (Crestor), 40, 81–82
Rove, Karl, 114, 131
Rumsfeld, Donald, 9, 173
Rush, Boyd, 292–93
Russell, John Richard, 290
Russert, Tim, 172

Saakashvili, Mikheil, 221
Saddam Hussein, 103, 104–05
Sadeghi, Dr. Nader, 249, 250
Sankyo, 80
Saudi Arabia, visits to, 105, 224–25, 244
Scarlett, Dick, 245
Schatz, Dr. Richard, 145, 146
Schlesinger, Arthur, 124
Scott, Jimmy, 190
Scowcroft, Brent, 100
Scudero, Jamie, 297
Scully, Matthew, 129

secretary of defense
Cheney as, 48, 82, 100–06
Tower's nomination to, 99–100
Senate Armed Services Committee, 28, 96–97, 99–100, 102, 103
Seven Countries Study, 22
Sherman, Dr. Harry, 53, 90–91
shortness of breath
atrial fibrillation with, 227
Cheney's symptoms of, 4, 135, 174, 211, 214, 216, 226, 265, 231, 303
heart failure with, 254, 303
Shumway, Dr. Norman, 287–88, 290, 293, 296, 297–99
Siegel, Dr. Stephen, 122
Silva, Dan, 274
Simpson, Al, 12–13, 48, 71, 102
simvastatin, 81
skiing, 45, 84, 87, 97, 99, 108, 118, 158, 309
sleep apnea, 3
Smith, Dr. Craig, 122
smoking
Cheney and, 8–9, 12, 25, 41, 45, 50, 57
Cheney's family background of, 7, 8
decline in rates of, 23–24
Eisenhower and, 33
quitting after a heart attack, 24, 41, 50
Reiner's sister and, 23
as risk factor, 8–9, 12, 24, 25, 215
Snyder, Howard, 33–34
Sones, Dr. Mason, 54, 95
Sorensen, Theodore, 124
Soviet Union, 10, 48, 67, 75, 102, 103, 104, 200, 221–22, 287
Speir, Dr. Alan M., 269, 286, 311–13, 315
Spiro, Dr. Ronald, 64, 65–66
spironolactone, 218
statin medications, 40, 81–82, 234
Steiger, Bill, 44, 45, 99
Steiger, Janet, 44
Steiner, Dr. Morris, 160
stenting, coronary artery, 147–52, 251, 252
streptokinase, 78–80
stress tests
Cheney's results on, 40, 57, 74, 75, 116, 118, 120, 122, 128, 216, 217
description of mechanism of, 116–18
Reiner's use of, 16, 118, 120, 122, 128, 216, 217

# Index

stroke, 22, 82, 108, 154, 227, 243, 248, 250, 260, 303
Stroock, Tom, 14
sudden cardiac arrest (SCA), 237–38, 239, 240, 241, 248, 252, 283
sulfinpyrazone, 40
Sununu, John, 100–01
Supreme Court, 134

Taliban, 213
Teeter, Bob, 30
terrorist attacks, 189–92, 194–97, 195, 283
Thomas, Bill, 156
Thoratec, 262, 281
Three Mile Island facility, Pennsylvania, 46
Tillett, William, 78–79
tissue plasminogen activator (tPA), 77, 79–80
tobacco use. *See* smoking
Tower, John, 99–100
Tracy, Dr. Cindy, 198–99, 210, 217, 220, 228, 230
triglycerides, 41, 219
Tubb, Dr. Richard "Dick," 163, 173–74, 179, 195
Twelfth Amendment, 114
Twenty-Fifth Amendment, 154, 155
Tyler, John, 123

Ukraine, 221, 222
Union Pacific Railroad, 7
United Network for Organ Sharing (UNOS), 301, 302, 306–07
*U.S. News & World Report,* 45, 172–73

Varghese, Dr. P. Jacob, 76, 77
vasodilators, 33, 255
Venbrux, Dr. P. Anthony "Tony," 203–04, 208, 210, 211
ventricular fibrillation (V Fib), 37, 39, 74, 174–75, 176, 183, 185, 225, 241, 296
ventricular tachycardia, 174, 175, 176, 179–80, 182, 185, 196, 308
Vietnam War, 10, 26

VIP Syndrome, 137
Voronoy, Dr. Yurii, 289
Vourlekis, Dr. Jason, 271, 272, 300

waiting list for heart, 301–02, 306–07
Wallace, Dr. Robert, 87–88
Wallop, Malcolm, 71, 102
*Wall Street Journal,* 152
Walter Reed Army Medical Center, 26
Wangensteen, Dr. Owen, 295
warfarin, 35, 213, 248–49, 250
Washington, George, 253
Washkansky, Louis, 295–97
Wasserman, Dr. Alan, 134, 135, 138, 150–51, 166, 167, 169–71, 182
Waters, Thomas, 198
Weigert, Karl, 35
weight
    Cheney's health and, 5, 41, 164, 174, 197, 216, 218, 225–26, 231, 236, 265, 266, 300
    diet and, 21–22
    fluid retention and, 5
    heart failure and, 231
    as risk factor, 25, 218
    smoking and, 9, 23
Weintraub, Walter, 137
West Nile virus, 196
White House Communications Agency (WHCA), 157, 159, 161
White House Medical Unit (WHMU), 156–58, 159–60, 161–66, 167, 195, 205, 206, 211–12, 214, 235
Whittington, Harry, 160
Whittington, Mercedes, 160
Williams, Dr. John "Skip," 169–70
Williams, Pete, 73–74
Wilson, Woodrow, 154
Witzenburger, Ed, 14, 28
Wright, Jim, 72

Yale University, 102, 114
Yuschenko, Viktor, 222

Zocor, 81
Zoll, Dr. Paul, 38